Protein Power

Succeeds where low-fat diets fail you
- complete, satisfying meal plans, suitable for family dinners or formal entertaining
- a Daily Meal Outline to keep track of your food selections
- ways to modify the foods you love the most to make them fit your diet plan
- tips on making the best selections at fine restaurants or fast-food chains
- a minicookbook filled with nearly 100 easy-to-prepare, inexpensive, and mouthwatering recipes, from Tex-Mex Cheese Flan with Chunky Salsa and Coconut Salmon to Irish Lace Cookies and Chocolate Chip Cheesecake
- supplements that will jump-start your metabolism to burn fat
- ways to include wine in your diet for enjoyment and health
- an invaluable program of strength-building exercises
- tips for maintaining motivation
- and more

Protein Power

Michael R. Eades, M.D.
& Mary Dan Eades, M.D.

BANTAM BOOKS
New York • Toronto • London • Sydney • Auckland

The diet plan presented here is not intended for anyone with kidney problems or for pregnant women or women trying to get pregnant. Readers who are on medication to control cholesterol, blood pressure, fluid retention, or blood sugar or who have an abnormal heart rhythm or have had a heart attack within the last six months must not under any circumstances begin this diet plan without a physician's guidance and close supervision. Even other readers, however, should consult a physician regarding their individual needs before starting any diet or fitness program.

PROTEIN POWER
A Bantam Book

PUBLISHING HISTORY

Bantam hardcover edition published February 1996
Bantam mass market edition published January 1998
Bantam trade paperback edition / June 1999
Figure 12.1 is modified and used with permission of Dr. Barry Sears

Published simultaneously in the United States and Canada

Bantam Books are published by Bantam Books, a division of Random House, Inc. Its trademark, consisting of the words "Bantam Books" and the portrayal of a rooster, is Registered in U.S. Patent and Trademark Office and in other countries. Marca Registrada. Bantam Books, 1540 Broadway, New York, New York 10036.

PRINTED IN THE UNITED STATES OF AMERICA

FFG 10   9   8

To British physician John Yudkin, M.D., Ph.D., who was fighting the good fight before we were born.

And to our sons, Ted, Daniel, and Scott Eades, who will continue to fight it after we're gone.

There was an old man of Tobago,
Who lived on rice, gruel, and sago;
Till, much to his bliss,
His physician said this—
To a leg, sir, of mutton you may go.

Contents

Acknowledgments

We would like to thank the many people who were instrumental in helping us bring this book to you. It's been a long and sometimes difficult process through which we had the unfailing support of our agent and friend Channa Taub, who consoled and cajoled us through some stressful times and was always willing to sharpen her editorial pencil when needed. Channa brought us to Carol Mann, who gets many thanks for bringing our work to the wonderful group at Bantam Books. Thanks to Fran McCullough, our editor, for her interest in and understanding of this project and for all the work she did to streamline and improve the manuscript. And to everyone at Bantam—especially Irwyn Applebaum, Nita Taublib, Allen Goodman, Amanda Mecke, Barb Burg, and Lauren Janis.

To our sons, Ted, Dan, and Scott, who put up with erratic family schedules and cranky parents during the writing of this book, we love you.

Our faithful staff at the clinic, who fielded calls, juggled schedules, and held down the fort while we wrote, deserve special mention—thanks to Rhonda Mallison, Mary Clendaniel, Linda Tullos, Valerie Wilkins, Michelle Denton, and Deya Devorak.

Thanks to Barbara Witt, who contributed most of the recipes.

We are grateful for the support, help, criticism, and advice from our many professional and scientific colleagues who read and commented on this manuscript during its writing. Special thanks to Barry Sears, Ph.D., who has helped us refine our thinking by engaging us in hundreds of hours of how-many-angels-can-dance-on-the-head-of-a-pin-type arguments on the merits of our respective dietary philosophies. And to Allen Hill, M.D., whose suggestions and support have been invaluable, we give heartfelt thanks. Not only has he taken much time from his busy practice to read and help improve our manuscript, he has also graciously taken over the care of our patients innumerable times, often at a moment's notice, during the many absences this project required of us.

And finally, thanks to Cathy Hemming, our erstwhile agent and always our friend, who believed in the merits of this book and this paradigm before anyone else.

Introduction

You may be wondering how a couple of physicians who specialize in weight loss in a relatively small city in Middle America devised a nutritional program that works as well as this one does, while most of the scientists in the major universities are headed off in the opposite direction, puzzling over why their success with low-fat diet plans has been so minimal. In a nutshell, we lucked out. We lucked out because that's how science works. Science progresses because people continue to question why. Researchers propose hypotheses based on their understanding of the natural world and then test them—and most of the time these theories blow up in their faces. The lucky ones stumble onto the hypotheses that turn out to be valid. But of course there's more than luck involved, because as Louis Pasteur said, "Chance favors the prepared mind," and in our case our minds were prepared by many years of clinical practice with patients suffering all the illnesses that are heir to disordered insulin metabolism as well as by our unique combination of medical interests. Mike is a collector of diet books and old medical texts and has a strong interest in paleopathology and biochemistry; Mary Dan is interested in anthropology and has published a book on eating disorders and the deranged metabolic status of eating-disordered patients.

We have a copy of the earliest diet book ever to sweep the nation, *Banting's Letter on Corpulence,* first printed in the middle 1800s. This restricted-carbohydrate diet worked like a charm for Banting and, if sales were any indication, many others. It has always intrigued us because it completely flies in the face of today's low-fat paradigm. At about the same time we ran across Banting we began attending paleopathology conferences and studying anthropology, where we learned what paleopathologists and anthropologists have known for years: the agricultural revolution and the increased consumption of carbohydrates it brought along with it played havoc with the health of early man. Mary Dan's extensive study of eating disorders and metabolic hormonal derangements combined with Mike's interest in biochemistry rounded out the "preparation" of our minds. We looked at Banting's success with carbohydrate restriction along with the paleopathological/anthropological data showing a decline in health accompanying an increase in carbohydrate intake and concluded that maybe the intake of large amounts of carbohydrates wasn't necessarily a good thing. That became our first mini-hypothesis: excess carbohydrate consumption isn't good. But why not?

We knew, as does every doctor, that the immediate effect of carbohydrate consumption is increased blood glucose, then an increased insulin level. We thought that perhaps the increased insulin levels might be to blame for part of the problem. As we studied the medical literature, we found that researchers the world over were finding elevated insulin levels associated with obesity, heart disease, high blood pressure, and diabetes—the common diseases of modern man. We also found that the same researchers were for the most part trying to treat these patients by giving them more of the same thing we were beginning to believe may have caused the problem in the first place: the high-carbohydrate, low-fat diet. It made more sense to us that if excess insulin indeed *causes* these disorders, or at the very least makes them worse, as the increasing mountain of research indicated, perhaps patients would be better off *reducing* their carbohydrate intake, not increasing it.

We took then as our working hypothesis that excess carbohydrate leads to excess insulin, which leads to obesity, high blood pressure, and all the rest. It fit with the anthropological and paleopathological data and, at least as far as obesity was concerned, with Banting's dietary theory. We then began to examine this hypothesis from a basic biochemical perspective and found that it worked beautifully. From all perspectives our hypothesis looked good on paper, so we began to test it carefully, first on ourselves, then on patients in our practice. We found that the results were rapid, dramatic, and pretty much uniform—just what we expected based on the underlying science. As we worked with our patients, we continued to refine our techniques, expand our range of dietary choices, and in general collect those little tips and tricks that make the practice of medicine an art as well as a science. We are still learning and refining every day, and, as with any technique that works, more and more practitioners are beginning to use a restricted-carbohydrate diet for their patients and are adding their own unique refinements to the rapidly growing body of data.

Will this program work for you? In good conscience, we can only say probably. The reason we hedge a little is because of biochemical individuality—we are all as different biochemically as we are in appearance. Every doctor has encountered patients in whom medicines seem to work in an opposite fashion to that intended, patients who are kept awake by sleeping pills and pass out on stimulants. These and similar experiences keep practiced physicians from ever making blanket this-will-work-in-all-circum-stances statements. All we can tell you is that in the almost ten years we have been treating patients with this program we have *never* had a negative outcome. If you're like the vast majority of our patients, you will find the results as striking and life changing as we have and will adopt this program, modified to your own unique lifestyle and tastes, for the rest of your life.

Little Rock
June 1995

Part I

Assessing Your Risk

Chapter I

A New Nutritional Perspective

Every man is the creature of the age in which he lives;
very few are able to raise themselves above the ideas of
the time.

VOLTAIRE

We have a medical book published in 1822 passed down
to Michael from his great-grandfather, a country doctor
from the Ozark Mountains. A long section deals with yellow fever—in the 1800s no one knew what caused it or
how it spread. Now, of course, we understand that the
mosquito is the carrier of the virus that causes yellow
fever, but then the cause eluded the best minds in medical
science. Read what this standard 1822 medical textbook
says about yellow fever:

> . . . it rises from the exposure of putrid animal and veg-
> etable substances on the public wharfs . . . it always begins
> in the lowest part of a populous mercantile town near the
> water, and continues here without much affecting the
> higher parts. It rages most where large quantities of new
> ground have been made by banking out the rivers for the
> purpose of constructing wharfs. . . . the yellow fever is gen-
> erated by the impure air or vapour which issues from the

new-made earth or ground raised on the muddy and filthy bottom of rivers. . . .

From our contemporary vantage point we want to reach back and tell them, "Look, it's a mosquito; why can't you see the big picture?"

The medical problems that confound us today will probably amaze scientists in the twenty-first century as they puzzle over why we medical pioneers of today were unable to reach out and grasp the obvious, why we were so advanced in certain areas of medical treatment yet so abysmally deficient in others. Why, they may ask, could our surgeons perform open-heart surgery so skillfully as to make it a routine operation while at the same time our nutritional experts couldn't determine the optimal diet for preventing most of the problems necessitating that procedure? Why spend so much time and effort developing complex surgical techniques and other wondrous medical procedures that prolong the life of a diseased body for a few months or, at best, a few years instead of focusing on nutritional changes capable of prolonging healthy life for decades? Why can't *we* see the big picture?

The Failure of the Low-Fat, High-Carbohydrate Diet

Yes, doctors today are aware that diet plays a significant role in the development and progression of the major diseases afflicting modern man—heart disease, diabetes, obesity, high blood pressure, and many kinds of cancers. As a consequence dietitians, nutritionists, and physicians constantly exhort us to eat properly to avoid these disorders. By their definition, eating properly means rooting out fat from our diets and replacing it with complex carbohydrate.

Ever since the surgeon general recommended in 1988 that Americans severely reduce their consumption of fat, especially saturated fat, the race to zero-fat products has been on. Eggs, red meat, and other superior protein sources have been virtually drummed out of the American kitchen. Reduce fat intake to almost nothing, we are told by battalions of nutritional experts, and good-bye obesity, heart disease, diabetes, and all the rest. Sounds great in theory, but—and here's why physicians a hundred years from now will be shaking their heads—it doesn't work.

The low-fat, high-complex-carbohydrate approach has proven a failure. It doesn't reduce cholesterol levels to any great degree unless followed to an almost ridiculous extreme, in which case it can actually cause other equally sinister problems, as you will soon discover. It gives diabetes sufferers endless grief in trying to regulate their blood sugar levels. It doesn't reduce high blood pressure unless it brings about significant weight loss. Its success rate for weight loss is almost nonexistent. (You may be surprised to learn that we've treated many people who have *gained* weight on the low-fat diet.) The result of the current no-fat mania has been a fatter and less healthy America, thanks in part to the zeal of food manufacturers who have given us an endless variety of fat-free high-carbohydrate junk to replace the fat-filled junk we were eating before.

In the face of this dismal record, what do we as medical professionals do? Do we write off the low-fat diet as something that sounded good on paper but didn't work in practice, abandon it and begin searching for something better, as we would a new drug that had failed? No. Instead we say, "Bring on more of the same. Let's try harder, let's try longer, let's be more diligent." We tell our patients that it must be *their* fault if their condition doesn't improve on a low-fat diet; they must not be following it correctly. But such thinking flies in the face of metabolic reality because *dietary fat alone is not the problem.* The problem lies in the biochemical structure of the low-fat diet and the mixed signals it gives to the body's essential metabolic processes. Ironically, not only does the low-fat diet fail to solve the health problems it addresses; it actually makes them even worse.

The program we outline in this book triumphs where the low-fat, high-complex-carbohydrate diet fails. It reduces cholesterol rapidly *without* increasing other risk factors; it reverses, or at least significantly improves, adult-onset (type II) diabetes; it drops elevated blood pressure like a rock; it offers a long-term solution for the problem of excess weight—all without asking you to count fat grams or worry about fat percentages. It does all this simply by selecting foods that work *with* your body's metabolic biochemistry instead of against it.

The human body is a remarkably resilient, reactive, regenerative piece of biochemical machinery. Like any piece of complex equipment, it functions best when treated properly. The proponents of low-fat dieting believe the best way to treat the body is by restricting the amount of fat, particularly saturated fat, the body takes in and replacing it with complex carbohydrate. Their flawed thinking goes like this: too much fat accumulation in the arteries causes heart disease and other problems, too much fat accumulation in the fat cells causes obesity, and too much fat intake exacerbates diabetes, so if we reduce fat intake, we'll solve all these problems. Although it seems logical, it doesn't work because it doesn't take into account the body's biochemistry and the ways our metabolic hormones cause us to store fat. When we understand and control these potent body chemicals, we can achieve our health goals by controlling fat from within rather than trying to eliminate it from without. To begin to understand how this works, let's first examine food from a biochemical perspective.

What Is This Thing Called Food?

All food, from pancakes to sushi, is composed of macronutrients, micronutrients, and water. Aside from water, which makes up the lion's share of everything, food is made primarily of the macronutrients protein, fat, and carbohydrate. These three macronutrients are the only food components that provide energy—measured as calories—to maintain life. The micronutrients—vitamins, minerals, and trace elements—provide no caloric energy but are nevertheless essential for life. They perform a multitude of cellular functions, many of which involve the efficient use and disposal of the macronutrients. Without macronutrients we would suffer malnutrition, starvation, and death; without the micronutrients we would suffer deficiency diseases, a precipitous health decline, and death. The nutrients from both groups are necessary for life.

BALANCING THE BIG THREE

Since the entire caloric content of food comes from the three macronutrients, it is obvious that decreasing any one macronutrient—fat, for instance—requires increasing another (carbohydrate or protein or both) to maintain any given caloric level. If your metabolic needs for a day require 2,000 calories, and, in accordance with the recommendations of the nutritional establishment, you reduce your fat intake, what happens? You increase your intake of carbohydrate and protein to make up for the calories lost by removing the fat, right? Actually, it's a little more complicated than that. You don't go to the grocery store and buy three scoops of protein, five scoops of carbohydrate, and two scoops of fat; you buy meat, eggs, vegetables, fruits, dairy products. Some foods, meat and eggs, for instance, contain only protein and fat, while others such as apples and grapes are practically all carbohydrate with only a trace of protein. You can trim the visible fat from cuts of meat to reduce fat content, but otherwise it's difficult to extract just one macronutrient from a particular food item. So the only way to change the ratios of fat, protein, and carbohydrate is to change the types of foods eaten. If you want to decrease your fat intake, you simply eat less meat, eggs, and dairy products and replace them with fruits and vegetables. Sounds reasonable, but is it?

Not really, and here's why. Humans don't require equal amounts of the three macronutrients for optimal health. The average person requires at least 70 to 100 grams of protein per day, or about 300 calories' worth, and at least 6 to 10 grams of linoleic acid (a type of fat that is essential to health), about 75 calories' worth. What about carbohydrate? The actual amount of carbohydrate *required* by humans for health is *zero*.[1] We haven't made these fig-

---

[1] As you will discover in a later chapter, your body has all the biochemical machinery necessary to make all the blood sugar you need to nourish the tissues that require it—red blood cells, some parts of the eye, brain, and kidney.

ures up; they represent the consensus of scientific wisdom today. Now, this doesn't mean that as long as you get 75 grams of protein and 6 grams of fat you'll do fine. You need more calories to provide energy for your bodily functions. It does mean that if you got enough energy from either protein or fat and maintained your minimum intake of each, you would do fine. Eskimos eat very little carbohydrate, in fact no carbohydrate during the winter, and survive nicely to a ripe old age. Although their traditional diet is composed of a large quantity of protein and an enormous amount of fat, Eskimos suffer very little heart disease, diabetes, obesity (despite the cartoons), high blood pressure, and all the other diseases we associate with a more civilized lifestyle. Furthermore, Eskimos don't have metabolic systems from an alien planet; they have the exact same biochemistry and physiology that we do. Yes, *you* could eat the same diet and tolerate it nicely.[2]

Bearing in mind that protein and fat are essential to health and carbohydrate isn't, what happens when we cut back our fat as the nutritional establishment recommends? Since we can't for the most part remove the fat from the food, we end up replacing foods that contain fat with

---

[2] We know this because of the famous study done in 1929 and 1930 using the explorers Vilhjalmur Stefansson and Karsten Anderson. These men returned from the Arctic reporting that Eskimos were able to live on nothing but caribou meat all winter while performing arduous work, expending great amounts of energy without consequence. To prove that not only Eskimos had this capability, both explorers volunteered to be studied while hospitalized in Bellevue Hospital in New York City for one year. During this time they ate a meat diet composed of more than 2,500 calories a day, which was 75 percent fat. At the end of the year both had lost about 6 pounds of weight, their cholesterol levels and other blood chemistry values were normal, and neither experienced any adverse effects.

those that don't. Since most sources of good-quality protein—meat, eggs, and dairy products—contain a fair amount of fat, to cut back on fat we end up cutting back on protein as well and replacing them both with carbohydrate. Most vegetable sources of protein—beans and grains—are incomplete unless combined carefully and contain far more carbohydrate than protein. In the end if we strictly follow the low-fat prescription we can end up deficient in protein (it's difficult to be deficient in fat because the only essential fat is linoleic acid, which is found in vegetable oils).

But possibly the worst news of all is that eating more carbohydrates stimulates your body's fat storage. In attempting to reduce fat intake, you wind up actually getting fatter, because some macronutrients stimulate profound metabolic hormonal changes. Surprisingly, fat doesn't do much. If you were to swill down a dish of lard while hooked up to a laboratory device to measure the levels of your metabolic hormones—chiefly insulin and glucagon—you wouldn't see much activity, because fat is essentially metabolically inert. Carbohydrate, however, would set off a Mad Hatter's tea party of metabolic activity. Eating a handful of grapes while hooked to the same device would initiate a wild swinging of gauge needles indicating a rapid increase in insulin and a decrease in its opposing hormone glucagon, all perfectly normal metabolic responses kindled by the consumption of carbohydrate. It follows logically that the constant consumption of large quantities of carbohydrate would then produce large quantities of insulin, which indeed it does.

Even complex carbohydrates stimulate the response because *all* carbohydrates are basically sugar. Various sugar molecules—primarily glucose—hooked together chemically compose the entire family of carbohydrates. Your body has digestive enzymes that break these chemical bonds and release the sugar molecules into the blood, where they stimulate insulin and the other metabolic hormones. This means that if you follow a 2,200-calorie diet that is 60 percent carbohydrate—the very one most nutritionists recommend—your body will end up having to contend metabolically with *almost 2 cups of pure sugar per day.*

What's Insulin Got to Do with It?

So, what does insulin have to do with anything other than diabetes? And if you don't have diabetes, why should you care about insulin at all? Because it's important to your health.

Insulin, a hormone produced and released into the blood by the pancreas, affects virtually every cell in the body. Insulin occupies a chapter or two in every medical biochemistry and physiology textbook, entire sections in endocrinology texts, and even two pages of tiny print in our fifteen-year-old *Encyclopaedia Britannica.* Whole textbooks are devoted to its myriad activities. Insulin regulates blood sugar, yes, but it does much more. It controls the storage of fat, it directs the flow of amino acids, fatty acids, and carbohydrate to the tissues, it regulates the liver's synthesis of cholesterol, it functions as a growth hormone, it is involved in appetite control, it drives the kidneys to retain fluid, and much, much more. This master hormone of metabolism is a substance absolutely essential to life; without it, you would perish—quickly.

But insulin is also a monster hormone; it has a dark side. In the proper amount it is life sustaining; too much of it causes enormous health problems. Reams of scientific studies, with more added to the stack daily, implicate excess insulin as a *primary* cause of or significant risk factor for high blood pressure, heart disease, obesity, elevated cholesterol and other blood fats, and diabetes (yes, insulin itself can *cause* diabetes, a concept we will explore at length later in this book).

If you don't have diabetes now, that doesn't mean you won't develop it in the future, especially if it runs in your family. The same goes for heart disease, high blood pressure, and all the rest. Insulin problems have a strong genetic basis, so a good way to determine if you are at risk for any of the insulin-related disorders is to examine your family tree closely. If your parents or grandparents had or have any of the following, you are at risk:

- heart disease,
- high blood pressure,
- accumulation of fat around the waistline,
- elevated cholesterol,
- elevated triglycerides and other blood fats,
- type II diabetes,
- excess fluid retention (swelling of ankles).

As you consider the health profiles of your family members, be aware that the more of these disorders you identify, the more at risk you are for developing them. If you are at risk, you have a pressing reason to care about insulin, because controlling it can literally save your life; if you have already been afflicted with one (or more) of these disorders, controlling your insulin can restore your health.

Taming the Monster: Controlling Insulin Through Diet

How do you go about controlling it? With our nutritional regimen—a carbohydrate-restricted, moderate-fat, adequate-protein diet that modulates the body's metabolic hormones, including insulin. Diet is what makes insulin levels go haywire in the first place, so it stands to reason that dietary changes should be able to reverse the problem. Diet is, in fact, the *only* way to solve this problem.

The foods we eat exert a profound influence on what happens within our bodies hormonally—both for good and for bad. By eating the correct balance of foods we can almost medicinally alter what goes on inside us in a healthful way; by eating the wrong foods we can precipitate health disasters. We can more easily dig our graves with a fork and spoon than with a shovel.

Our plan uses food as a tool to reverse, or at the very least markedly improve, disorders engendered by a metabolic system out of whack. Our easy-to-follow dietary regimen is tasty, filling, nutritionally complete, and even allows for the consumption of alcoholic beverages—in moderation. It works. And best of all it works quickly.

How quickly? In terms of feeling better and more energetic, within a week or less; for cholesterol reduction, substantial reductions in blood levels by three weeks, maybe sooner (we say maybe sooner because we've never checked anyone before three weeks). Victims of high blood pressure—a condition that is usually insulin related—typically achieve a greatly lowered, or normal, blood pressure within a week or two. Those with diabetes and related problems generally find their blood sugar levels normalized or at least greatly improved within just a few weeks—

sometimes only days. High blood pressure, elevated cholesterol, type II diabetes—this program corrects or greatly improves them all in short order by normalizing the body's disrupted metabolic hormonal status, which causes all these problems in the first place.

Obesity, the other major health problem rooted in a disturbed insulin metabolism, doesn't disappear as quickly, of course. Although our nutritional program opens all the metabolic pathways to allow an efficient burning of body fat for energy, the body fat still has to be burned—and depending on how much there is to burn, that can take some time. The good news is, however, that long before our patients lose much weight on the program the medical problems afflicting most of them—high blood pressure, elevated cholesterol, diabetes, gout, and a host of others—improve dramatically or even vanish. Now, granted, on the typical low-calorie, low-fat, high-complex-carbohydrate weight-reduction diet these medical disorders will sometimes *gradually* improve as body weight falls, but on our diet these improvements are almost immediate due to the rapid metabolic changes effected.

Of course we don't have all the answers; but we do have a nutritional program that we've tested on ourselves, our three sons, thousands of our patients, and countless people nationwide, without a single adverse reaction.[3]

Our approach is scientifically valid, historically valid, and can be explained using not a few obscure scientific articles but standard medical textbooks. This is important

---

[3] In 1989 Michael wrote a book, *Thin So Fast,* published by Warner Books that described our nutritional regimen as applied solely to weight loss. Since then we've received countless letters from readers all over the world, recounting their successes after years of failure on more conventional diets.

because it means that we've based our conclusions on scientific fact, not theory. Medical scientists doing cutting-edge research publish their findings in medical/scientific journals, initiating a firestorm of debate and a flurry of activity in other laboratories the world over. Many scientists then repeat the experiments, sometimes obtaining the same results, sometimes not. Before any particular piece of scientific knowledge is generally considered valid, it must be confirmed by multiple long-term tests, performed in many different labs, all with the same result. Only then does it enter the medical literature as fact, and only then is it published in medical textbooks. Not only can *all* the concepts underlying our program be found in every basic medical textbook, but studies confirming our approach are beginning to appear throughout the medical journals (again, write to us in care of our publisher for a bibliography).

Could anyone have seen this big picture earlier?

Interestingly enough, the answer is a qualified yes. The history of dieting begins in 1825, when the Frenchman Jean-Anthelme Brillat-Savarin published an essay entitled "Preventative or Curative Treatment of Obesity" in his gastronomic classic *The Physiology of Taste* in which he stated: "Now, an antifat diet is based on the commonest and most active cause of obesity, since, as it has already been clearly shown, it is only because of grains and starches that fatty congestion can occur, as much in a man as in the animals; this effect . . . plays a large part in the commerce of fattened beasts for our markets, and it can be deduced, as an exact consequence, that a more or less rigid abstinence from everything that is starchy or floury will lead to the lessening of weight." Brillat-Savarin had obviously empirically stumbled onto the virtues of a restricted-carbohydrate diet and published his findings. In 1862 William Banting, an upscale London undertaker, found himself so obese that he could not tie his shoes and had to walk downstairs backward. He tried all the fashionable cures of the day without success until his physician put him on a diet free of starchy and sugary foods. Banting followed this diet to the letter and lost a pound a week until he reached a normal weight and restored his health and his ability to walk down the stairs face first. He was so overjoyed with his success that, at his own expense, he published and distributed 2,500 copies of his *Letter on Corpulence,* describing his treatment and his own modifications of the plan. Demand was so great for this pamphlet that it rapidly went through many editions on both sides of the Atlantic before his death in 1878 at eighty-one years of age. His diet was so well known that his name became synonymous with dieting; people weren't dieting; they were banting. In America, Banting's lean-meat diet led to the development of the American Salisbury steak, a staple of life in the late 1800s.

The next popular weight loss and health book was *Eat and Grow Thin* by Vance Thompson, husband of actress Lillian Spencer and founder of *M'lle New York* magazine. This slim book touting the virtues of a restricted-carbohydrate diet (allegedly written by the Asian sage Mahdah) was an enormous best-seller that went through its 112th printing in 1931.

These early diet books all have in common the fact that their authors were untrained as physicians or scientists (Brillat-Savarin was a lawyer) and basically promoted and adhered to these diets simply because they worked, as testified to by the hundreds of thousands of "patients" who followed them. In the late 1920s mainstream medical scientists observed and reported on the efficacy of the restricted-carbohydrate diet when the Arctic explorer Vilhjalmur Stefansson and a colleague submitted themselves to a meat-only diet for a year (see footnote 2).

In England in more recent times T. L. Cleave, the surgeon-captain of the Royal Navy, and John Yudkin, M.D., Ph.D., professor of nutrition at Queen Elizabeth College, London University, have studied and written extensively on the merits of the restricted-carbohydrate diet. Dr. Yudkin has published papers on restricted-carbohydrate dieting from both a scientific and a natural history perspective in most of the prestigious medical journals during a career spanning six decades. At eighty-five, he continues to write and publish. His books, *This Slimming Business* and *A-Z of Slimming,* are classics on the subject.

The three most popular diet books in America in recent years were all written by physicians detailing their own versions of the restricted-carbohydrate diet. Dr. Irwin Stillman published his *Quick Weight Loss Diet* in 1967, describing how he overcame middle-aged obesity and a heart attack by cutting carbohydrates and drinking large quantities of water. Dr. Robert Atkins wrote *Dr. Atkins' Diet Revolution,* another multimillion-copy best-seller, in 1972, detailing his own experiences as well as those of his many patients with low-carbohydrate dieting. In 1979 Dr. Herman Tarnower explained his approach to low-carbohydrate dieting with his cardiology and internal medicine patients in *The Complete Scarsdale Medical Diet.* These books in hardcover and paperback have sold over 20 million copies (amazingly, the last two are still in print twenty years later), and there is probably not a dieter alive who hasn't at least heard of one of these books, if not all. Why are they so popular? Because they work.

None of the authors of any of these popular diet books wrote about the underlying science involved; they just found carbohydrate restriction to be an effective means to bring about weight loss and health improvement in an easy-to-follow diet. In essence these authors "discovered" by trial and error the same thing that Brillat-Savarin, Banting, and the others found the same way. There has been no doubt that these diets work. The only question has been: why? In the chapters to come, you will learn the biochemistry and physiology of the why. And in learning how carbohydrate restriction works through insulin reduction, you will be able to use our techniques to expand on the restricted programs of those who came before us.

First let's look at the most extensive study of the low-fat, high-complex-carbohydrate nutritional approach ever undertaken—the civilization of ancient Egypt. You can draw your own conclusions from the pages of history.

The Bottom Line

At the end of each chapter you'll find a succinct summary of everything you need to remember.

Chapter 2

The Symptom Treatment Trap

All great truths begin as blasphemies.

GEORGE BERNARD SHAW

"You want me to eat *what?*"

The middle-aged lady sitting across the desk from us was incredulous and becoming more so by the second as we explained to her the changes she needed to make in her diet—changes necessary to reduce the dangerously elevated level of fat in her blood. She didn't have a serious weight problem; she had come to us seeking advice on the treatment of her cholesterol problem, but she was having difficulty accepting that advice.

"But if I eat all these foods you're telling me to eat, won't my cholesterol just go higher? I can't see how I can eat an egg or red meat in my condition. Are you sure this is going to work?"

We explained how her physiology worked and why her cholesterol was high. Her metabolism would change as she followed our nutritional plan, and these changes would result in a dramatic reduction in her cholesterol levels. We told her that once she got started on the proper diet she would see major results within just a few weeks instead of the months it usually takes for diets to work—if they do at all. Then she could judge for herself whether or not she was on the right track. She may not have been convinced by the scientific explanations of her problem and its solution, but she brightened at the thought of seeing results so quickly.

"Six weeks!? Do you really think I will have improved much by then?" she asked.

"You will be pleasantly surprised."

"I hope so. I don't know if I can go through another experience like the last time. I worked so hard with my previous doctor. I faithfully followed the diet he prescribed, and for what? Practically nothing. I don't mean to be such a whiner, but you've got to understand that I'm at my wit's end with this. If I don't get this cholesterol under control and start feeling better, I'm going to be a basket case."

We certainly understood. Although her problem is more serious than most, Jayne Bledsoe[1] is fairly typical of the patients we treat in our metabolic practice. We have heard variations of her history from countless other patients who have gotten stuck on the cholesterol treadmill.

Treating the Symptom, Missing the Problem

Jayne had been unaware that she even had a problem until she went for a routine physical examination. Her doc-

---

[1] Most of the case histories in this book are, like this one, actual patients whose names have been changed. Occasionally a composite patient history is used to illustrate a particular point.

tor checked her over, told her she appeared to be in good health, drew some blood, and told her he would call her when the results came back from the lab. He called the next day and dropped the bombshell: her blood fats were dangerously elevated. Her serum cholesterol was 750 mg/dl (milligrams/deciliter)—normal is anything below 200 and her triglycerides (another blood fat usually measured in the 100-to-250-mg/dl range) were a whopping 3,000 mg/dl! Most physicians get excited over a cholesterol of 300 mg/dl, let alone 750, and become outright alarmed at such a triglyceride level. So it's no surprise that her doctor—following standard medical protocol—completely bypassed Step One and immediately started her on the National Cholesterol Awareness Program Step-Two Diet *and* two potent cholesterol-lowering medications.[2]

Jayne faithfully followed her doctor's orders for six months, although not without difficulty. The medications nauseated her, and the diet kept her constantly hungry. Her condition was the talk of her friends and relatives, one of whom actually remarked to her, "I didn't know a person could still be alive with a cholesterol of 750!" By the

---

[2] From the "Report of the National Cholesterol Education Program Expert Panel on Detection, Evaluation, and Treatment of High Blood Cholesterol in Adults," *Archives of Internal Medicine* 148:36–69, January 1988. Under these guidelines physicians treat patients with elevated cholesterol in a stepwise fashion starting with dietary modification that limits fat to 30 percent and protein to 10 to 20 percent of calories and encourages the consumption of large amounts of carbohydrate. This is called the Step-One Diet. If the blood cholesterol level refuses to fall or doesn't fall far enough on the Step-One Diet, a more stringent one that further reduces fat intake—the Step-Two Diet—follows. In those cases in which diet alone fails, most physicians turn to one or more of the many cholesterol-lowering drugs.

time Jayne returned for her recheck, she was desperate for improvement. And she had improved some, but not nearly enough. Her cholesterol had dropped from 750 mg/dl to 475 mg/dl and her triglycerides from 3,000 mg/dl to 2,000 mg/dl—an improvement to be sure, but still cause for great concern to both Jayne and her physician. They discussed her treatment options. Her doctor suggested either increasing the dosage of her cholesterol-lowering medications or adding yet another medicine to her regimen. Jayne wanted to think about it before she decided which option to take. She decided to do neither until she got a second opinion from another physician, so she came to our clinic.

After listening to her history, we drew another blood sample and found that indeed she did have extraordinarily elevated levels of cholesterol and triglycerides in her blood—495 mg/dl and 1,900 mg/dl, respectively. In addition, her blood sugar was elevated to 155 mg/dl (normal is below 115 mg/dl), an ominous sign of impending diabetes.

We instructed Jayne to stop taking both of her cholesterol-lowering medications and to change her diet drastically. Her new nutritional regimen allowed meat (even red meat), eggs, cheese, and many other foods that most people view as *causing* cholesterol problems, not solving them. We told her to call in three weeks to check in and to come back to have her blood checked in six weeks.

She called at her appointed time and reported that she "felt grand" and that her nausea and hunger had vanished. The results of her blood work astounded her. Jayne's cholesterol level had fallen to 186 mg/dl and her triglycerides to 86 mg/dl. Her blood sugar had dropped to 90 mg/dl;

everything was back in the normal range. As you might imagine, she was ecstatic.

How could this happen? How can a diet virtually everyone believes should raise cholesterol actually lower it—and in a person who doesn't have just a slight cholesterol elevation but a major one? We know Jayne Bledsoe's case is not a freak happenstance or an aberration because we've tried variations of the same regimen on countless other patients—all with the same results. The results make perfect sense, because Jayne's problem, her illness, is not the elevated cholesterol level—that's merely a sign of the underlying problem. Her problem is *hyperinsulinemia,* a chronic elevation of serum insulin.

When Jayne first came to our office, her insulin level was almost 20 mU/ml (milliUnits/milliliter), about double what we consider normal, which is anything below 10 mU/ml. After six weeks on a diet designed to lower her insulin level, Jayne's lab work showed that she had dropped hers to 12 mU/ml, almost normal. By treating her real problem—excess insulin—we were able to solve her secondary problems of elevated cholesterol, triglycerides, and blood sugar. Standard medical therapies treat the symptoms of excess insulin—elevated cholesterol, triglycerides, blood sugar, blood pressure, and obesity—instead of treating the excess insulin itself. Unfortunately, the standard treatment of the symptoms may even *raise* the insulin levels and worsen the underlying problem.

Excess Insulin: The Real Culprit

A substance that fundamentally influences every cell in the body, insulin is the master controller of the metabolic system without which all metabolic processes would be rudderless. Insulin is a hormone produced and secreted into the bloodstream by the pancreas, a glandular organ located behind the stomach, deep in the abdominal cavity. As it travels through the circulatory system insulin regulates the level of sugar in the blood—its most important function—and performs a thousand other tasks. Insulin, by activating or inhibiting various metabolic pathways, can make us sleepy, hungry, satisfied, dizzy, stuporous, or bloated. It can raise blood pressure, elevate cholesterol levels (as it did in Jayne Bledsoe's case), cram fat into fat cells, cause the body to retain excess fluid, damage arteries, and even change protein and sugar into fat. In the appropriate amount insulin keeps the metabolic system humming along smoothly with everything in balance; in great excess it becomes a rogue hormone ranging throughout the body, wreaking metabolic havoc and leaving a trail of chaos and disease in its wake.

Although medical researchers have known of the beneficial effects of insulin since the 1920s, when it was discovered, they have also generated an enormous amount of data over the past three decades showing that some of the effects are not so beneficial.

Because there are no drugs available that can significantly reduce insulin levels, dietary manipulation is the *only* effective treatment of insulin excess and the diseases it promotes (although exercise helps). That's not to say that high blood pressure, for example, can't be treated by medications; as everyone knows, it can be. But treating high blood pressure treats only the symptom and not the underlying cause.

Hypertension and Heart Disease: The Insulin Connection

Epidemiologists had long known that people with high blood pressure die from strokes and heart attacks at a much greater rate than those with normal blood pressure. By treating hypertension on a grand scale, medical scientists reasoned that they could significantly reduce the incidence of death caused by stroke and heart disease. Based on this reasoning and very little hard evidence, since no long-term hypertensive control studies had ever been done, the push was on to get Americans with high blood pressure diagnosed and medicated. At this point the first long-term studies of the benefits of treatment were just being started. Researchers at medical centers across the country were gathering groups of subjects with hypertension so that they could treat and carefully monitor them for the many years necessary for such studies to be valid. Statisticians performed their analytical alchemy and estimated that hypertension controlled with drugs decreased the incidence of deaths from heart disease and stroke—by 40 percent and 25 percent, respectively.

How accurate were the statisticians? Not very, as it turns out. When the results were in, the researchers were astonished. The incidence of deaths due to stroke had fallen by approximately 25 percent—precisely what the statisticians had predicted; the figures for heart disease, however, weren't even close. Rather than the predicted 40 percent decrease, the experts found *no statistically significant decrease* in deaths from heart disease compared to people who were not treated at all. People who ignored their hypertension and went on about their business didn't develop heart disease at any greater rate than those who went to the expense and trouble of taking daily medications and assiduously monitoring their blood pressure. As you might imagine, this discrepancy prompted a lot of head scratching among the scientific establishment—especially in view of the fact that, based on their predictions, 19 million Americans were now spending upward of $4 billion annually on medicines to lower their blood pressure. What happened? How did the calculations go so far afield?

As the researchers examined the data more closely, they found hypertension and heart disease are related through the common denominator of too much insulin—a discovery that spurred a tidal wave of new research. Since the excess insulin caused both the high blood pressure *and* the heart disease (through mechanisms we will explore in coming chapters), it becomes immediately obvious why reducing the blood pressure without reducing insulin levels would have little effect on the progression of heart disease.

A dismal postscript is that many of the medicines—diuretics and beta-blockers—actually *increased* insulin levels as they reduced blood pressure. So, ironically, many hypertensive patients taking medicine in the hope of preventing heart disease were encouraging the real culprit—excess insulin. In a great majority of these cases dietary control of elevated insulin levels could have eliminated *both* the high blood pressure *and* the threat of heart disease.

Elevated insulin is Jayne Bledsoe's problem. The diseases that insulin affects directly—high blood pressure, elevated levels of cholesterol and other fats in the blood, diabetes, heart disease, and obesity—are the cause of the vast majority of death and disability in America today. They are the grim reapers of Western civilization. They kill more than twice the number of Americans *each year* than died in World War I, World War II, the Korean War, and Vietnam combined.

How do we know that these disorders are actually caused by diet and not by some other factor or combination of factors? Just as with most aspects of medicine, some degree of uncertainty persists, but we've got a pretty good idea from data from three different research approaches—historical, current epidemiological, and direct experimental. And nothing in this book is theoretical—it's all proven biochemistry found in any standard medical text—it's simply never been put together in this way before.

The scientific evidence will speak eloquently for itself, so let's begin to examine these biochemical connections of diet and disease.

The Bottom Line

Virtually everyone is familiar with insulin as a regulator of blood sugar, and indeed that's its main job in your body. But far beyond that, insulin can be called the *master hormone of human metabolism*, involved in the regulation of blood pressure, the production of cholesterol and triglycerides, and the storage of fat. When insulin levels become too high—a topic we'll devote considerable discussion to throughout this book—metabolic havoc ensues with elevated blood pressure, elevated cholesterol and triglycerides, diabetes, and obesity all trailing along in its wake. These disorders are merely *symptoms* of a single more basic disturbance in metabolism—excess insulin and insulin resistance.

There are no medications that treat excess insulin; a properly structured diet is the *only* means to bring it in line. (The usual low-fat, high-complex-carbohydrate approach won't do it; it has just the opposite effect.) Some medications—especially the beta-blockers and some diuretic medications, the very ones used to treat blood pressure and heart problems—actually make matters worse by causing the body to produce even more insulin, and doctor and patient get caught in the "symptom treatment trap."

Here's what usually happens: a patient gains weight and subsequently develops high blood pressure, for which the doctor prescribes a mild diuretic and low salt. The patient returns with better blood pressure but now a slight elevation in cholesterol and is put on a low-fat diet. He returns no lighter, with little change in cholesterol, but now his triglycerides or blood sugar have risen, too. The progression occurs because *all* these disorders are related through a single disturbance (excess insulin) that is actually being aggravated by the treatment.

These disorders occur so commonly in our society that we've become numb to the staggering toll they take: heart disease, high blood pressure, and diabetes kill twice as many people every year as were killed in both world wars, Korea, and Vietnam *combined.*

How do we know that these disorders are actually caused by diet and not by some other factor or combination of factors? Just as with most aspects of medicine, some degree of uncertainty persists, but we've got a pretty good idea from data from three different research approaches—historical, current epidemiological, and direct experimental.

Chapter 3

Excess Insulin and the Insulin Resistance Syndrome

*One is unable to notice something—because it is
always before one's eyes.*

LUDWIG WITTGENSTEIN
Philosophical Investigations

Consider how different life would be if we didn't have the
ability to store excess energy from the food we eat. Like
the electric mixer that works only when it's plugged in, we
would have to be constantly hooked up to our energy
source—food. At first glance, this might not seem like
such a bad idea. Many people nibble, snack, and munch
their way through the day anyway, so wouldn't it be grand
if they could continue without the consequences of obesity, elevated cholesterol, and the other diseases of over-
consumption?

One obvious disadvantage would be that we would
have to eat more food faster as we increased our intensity
of activity. Let's say we're involved in a strenuous activity—swimming, for example. We could stuff ourselves just

before we jumped into the water, but that wouldn't help. It would be like keeping the mixer plugged in for two hours before we used it, then unplugging it and turning it on. Nothing would happen because the mixer can't store electricity. So we would have to eat while swimming. It would be cumbersome and inconvenient to have to figure out a way to consume food at all times—even during sleep.

If we ate too much, it might be like plugging a mixer designed for 120 volts of electricity into a 240-volt circuit. What if we got stuck in an elevator and ate our way through all the food we had with us? As soon as the food was gone, we would sputter and choke out our last few moments like a car out of gas. Our survival would depend on always having adequate foodstuffs immediately at hand, and any activity that had the potential to separate us from our food would be fraught with mortal danger.

Our Built-In Battery

Did you know that, theoretically, most people could go for a couple of months without eating a single bite—some even up to a year or longer, depending on their degree of obesity? We can all eat ten meals a day or one or none; we can expend prodigious amounts of energy while eating little or no food, or we can eat prodigious amounts of food and expend almost no energy. In short, we have the capacity to use the energy from food we eat to meet our immediate needs and store the rest for later use. We have a built-in battery—the fat we carry on our bodies, which is replenished every time we eat and used for energy when we don't. In fact the amount of fat on the body of an average person weighing 150 pounds contains enough energy to allow that person to walk from Miami to New York City without eating.

Insulin and a few other hormones coordinate the activities of metabolism and ensure that our fat batteries work, making it possible for us to live unfettered by a constant power supply. Our metabolic systems precisely regulate the storage of excess food energy as fat and the release and breakdown of this body fat for the energy necessary for life. The metabolic system performs these tasks silently and without conscious effort on our part, but it is not foolproof.

The Yin-Yang of Metabolism

Insulin and glucagon are the primary hormones involved in the storage and release of energy within the body. When we eat, insulin drives our metabolism to store the excess food energy for use later. When later comes, glucagon drives the metabolism the other way, letting us burn our stored fat for the energy we need to swim or walk or sleep in the hours long after we've eaten. If we think of insulin as the hormone of feeding and storing and glucagon as the hormone of fasting and burning, it's easy to see how people living in today's America—with its abundance of food and never-stop-eating lifestyle—could be in the insulin-dominant mode most of the time.

Although it performs countless other tasks throughout the body, insulin's chief priority is to keep the blood sugar level from rising too high. Glucagon's main function is to prevent the blood sugar level from falling too low. The importance of this minute-by-minute regulation of the level of sugar in the blood is underscored by the fact that without either one of these hormones we would be dead in a matter of days or perhaps even hours. Without insulin the blood sugar would skyrocket, causing profound metabolic disturbances, dehydration, coma, and death. An absence of glucagon would allow the blood sugar to fall rapidly, bringing on brain dysfunction, somnolence, coma, and then death, because the brain requires blood sugar to operate properly. Because of this critical need to maintain the blood sugar in a narrow physiological band, the body doesn't really much care about the secondary activities of these hormones as long as they keep the blood sugar where it's supposed to be. And that's what gets us in trouble.

Can blood sugar regulate insulin and glucagon? Obviously it does. If blood sugar goes up, insulin goes up; conversely, if blood sugar falls, so does the insulin level, and the glucagon level rises. It's this mechanism that gives us indirect control over our insulin and glucagon by manipulating our blood sugar level. No matter how hard we try, we can't change our insulin and glucagon directly: we can't use meditation or biofeedback, and we can't take insulin or glucagon pills because these hormones are destroyed in the digestive process. Short of injecting ourselves with these hormones, the only way we can change our insulin and glucagon levels is to change our blood sugar level—which we can do in a hurry.

If you want your insulin level to increase, just drink a sugary soft drink. Your blood sugar will climb, and so will your insulin level—within minutes. It's a little more difficult, however, to increase glucagon levels. You'd somehow have to get your blood sugar level low enough to stimulate the pancreas to release glucagon. The only way to do this quickly is to give yourself an insulin injection. This extra insulin will drive the blood sugar low enough to stimulate the pancreas to release glucagon. Alternatively, you can wait around several hours without eating until your blood sugar falls enough on its own to bring about a surge of glucagon.

Our blood sugar level governs the functioning of our entire metabolic system. It's at the top of the chain of command. When our blood sugar rises, it orders the metabolism to proceed along a certain course; when it falls, it gives the opposite orders. If our blood sugar, through the efforts of glucagon and insulin, controls our metabolism, and we can control our blood sugar level by eating or not eating certain foods, doesn't it stand to reason that we can control our metabolism? Indeed we can. In fact this ability to control our metabolism is the foundation of our dietary program.

INSULIN VS. GLUCAGON: TIPPING THE BALANCE

Insulin—as part of its energy-storing behavior—activates a number of metabolic systems that we would just as soon not have activated, at least not on a perpetual basis. They were designed to operate on an intermittent, as-needed basis, but thanks to the aging process and the typical American diet, they tend to operate overtime. What systems are we talking about? The cholesterol synthesis system, for one. Insulin activates the enzymes that run the cholesterol-making apparatus, resulting in overproduction of cholesterol. Our own cells make cholesterol and lots of it. In fact, 70 to 80 percent of the cholesterol burbling along in your blood vessels was made by your own body.

Only 20 to 30 percent came from your diet. Every cell in the body has the capacity to make cholesterol, but most is made in the liver, the intestines, and the skin, with the vast majority coming from the liver cells. Elevated levels of insulin spur these cells to churn out vast amounts of cholesterol, leading to elevated blood levels. You might wonder why nature designed it this way. Storing excess food energy as fat seems reasonable, but why make cholesterol?

Excess food energy increases blood sugar, which increases insulin, which triggers the storage cycle leading to fat accumulation. To store fat and build muscle, the body must make new cells, and insulin acts as a growth hormone for this process. Cholesterol plays a vital role in this building and storing process; cholesterol provides the structural framework for all cells. In fact, if all of the cholesterol in your body were suddenly to vanish, you would dissolve into a puddle just like the Wicked Witch in *The Wizard of Oz* when Dorothy threw the water on her. Unfortunately, *excess* insulin stimulates *excess* cholesterol, and therein lies the problem.

Excess insulin also encourages the proliferation and growth of smooth muscle cells in the linings of our arteries, an activity that causes a couple of problems. The larger muscle cells thicken the arterial walls, making them less elastic and reducing the volume inside the arteries. Less elastic, smaller coronary arteries are more prone to develop plaque and arterial spasm, the underlying causes of heart disease. Because the heart has to develop greater pressure to force the blood through the narrow, thickened arteries throughout the rest of the body, elevated blood pressure results. To compound this problem, insulin also causes the kidneys to retain salt and fluid, which adds to the blood volume, increasing the pressure even more.

Let's not, however, neglect glucagon, its opposite. Because glucagon is the hormone of fat burning and fatty tissue breakdown, it reverses the building and storage processes set in motion by insulin. Under glucagon stimulation, the body gets rid of fat by burning it for energy. Since the body requires no extra cholesterol to help rid itself of cells, glucagon shuts down the production of cholesterol and helps send it on its way out of the circulation. The body doesn't need extra fluid to burn fat, so glucagon prompts the kidneys to get rid of it. Glucagon stimulates the breakdown and disappearance of the smooth muscle overgrowth in the arteries and lessens the incidence of arterial spasm. It's easier to see the whole scenario for these two master hormones in chart form so that you can compare them more easily.

THE ROLES OF INSULIN AND GLUCAGON

INSULIN	GLUCAGON
lowers elevated blood sugar	raises low blood sugar
shifts metabolism into storage mode	shifts metabolism into burning mode
converts glucose and protein to fat	converts protein and fat to glucose
converts dietary fat to storage	converts dietary fats to ketones and sends them to the tissues for energy
removes fat from blood and transports it into fat cells	releases fat from fat cells into the blood for use by tissues as energy
increases the body's production of cholesterol	decreases the body's production of cholesterol
makes the kidneys retain excess fluid	makes the kidneys release excess fluid
stimulates the growth of arterial smooth muscle cells	stimulates the regression of arterial smooth muscle cells
stimulates the use of glucose for energy	stimulates the use of fat for energy

Scanning this chart, it doesn't take a rocket scientist to see that the more time we spend on the glucagon side, the better off we are. Remember, however, that metabolism control is *not* a one-or-the-other phenomenon: all insulin *or* all glucagon. Both hormones are present in the blood all the time. What drives the metabolism to store or to burn is a *dominance* of one or the other.

How Food Affects Insulin and Glucagon

Scientists have fed research subjects all kinds of food in all kinds of combinations, drawn their blood, and measured its insulin and glucagon to discover how foods affect these hormones. The results of these experiments are in the following chart.

INFLUENCE OF FOOD ON INSULIN AND GLUCAGON

TYPE OF FOOD	INSULIN	GLUCAGON
Carbohydrate	+++++	no change
Protein	++	++
Fat	no change	no change
Carbohydrate and Fat	++++	no change
Protein and Fat	++	++
High Protein and Low Carbo	++	+
High Carbo and Low Protein	+++++++++	+

As you can see from the chart, of the three basic constituents of food—fat, protein, and carbohydrate—carbohydrate makes the most profound change in insulin, because it makes the most profound change in blood sugar level. Fat doesn't do anything; as far as insulin is concerned, fat doesn't exist. The combination of carbohydrate and protein, especially large amounts of carbohydrate with small amounts of protein, causes the greatest increase in insulin, a most enlightening fact, considering the typical American diet.

What We Eat

What does the typical American eat? How about the old standard: meat and potatoes—protein and carbohydrate. A hamburger and fries—protein and carbohydrate. A pizza, which is basically cheese, meat, and a crust—carbohydrate and protein. Macaroni and cheese—carbohydrate and protein. Think of anything we commonly eat: eggs and hash browns, milk and cereal, pork and beans, chicken and dumplings, peanut butter and jelly, ice cream, chili con carne, lasagne—the list could go on forever; every one of these popular foods is a combination of lots of carbohydrate and some protein. And lots of fat, of course, which we will consider shortly.

Let's forget about the protein for a minute and concentrate on just the carbohydrates that we eat, which do an outstanding job of raising insulin all by themselves. The second National Health and Nutrition Examination Survey (NHANES II) conducted by the National Center for Health Statistics published data in 1983 on the food consumption patterns of Americans.[1] What would you guess

---

[1] The newest NHANES information (NHANES III) has not yet been completely tabulated, but partial results show a reduction in fat intake, an increase in carbohydrate intake, and an almost 25 percent increase in the incidence of obesity.

as the number-one food consumed by the most Americans? White bread, rolls, and crackers—almost pure carbohydrate. How about number two? Doughnuts, cookies, and cake—more carbohydrate and fat. Number three, alcoholic beverages. All in all, of the top twenty foods Americans eat, eleven are virtually pure carbohydrate, four are a combination of carbohydrate and protein, and only five are pure protein or a combination of protein and fat. These last five represent only 12 percent of the calories we eat.

What *about* the fat and cholesterol we've shrugged off in our discussion so far? Do we not have to worry about them at all? Don't they cause some problems? Sure they do, but not nearly the problems that carbohydrates do. And when dietary fat and cholesterol do cause problems, it's usually *because* of the carbohydrate eaten along with them. It is true that fat is the raw material from which the body makes cholesterol, and it is also true that if you add more fat to your diet your cholesterol will increase, *but only if you continue to eat a lot of carbohydrate at the same time that you add the fat*. Although fat is the raw material the body uses to make cholesterol, insulin runs the cellular machinery that actually makes it. If you reduce the level of insulin, the cells can't convert the fat to cholesterol, almost no matter how much fat is available. Eating fat in the absence of carbohydrate and expecting it to be converted to cholesterol is like trying to make your car go faster by putting a larger gas tank in it. If you reduce the amount of carbohydrate when you add the fat, not only will you probably not see any increase; you could even see a *reduction* in cholesterol levels.

Sadly, the typical American diet is almost all fat and carbohydrate. According to the National Research Council's

Committee on Diet and Health in 1985, 46 percent of calories in the average American's diet came from carbohydrate, 43 percent from fat, and a paltry 11 percent from protein: *89 percent of the American diet is fat and carbohydrate.*

THE SKINNY JUNK-FOOD JUNKIE AND OTHER PARADOXES

Knowing how insulin works can help us analyze and make sense of seemingly contradictory data. The Harris poll completed in 1990 for *Prevention* magazine presents what appears on the surface to be inconsistent data. Americans scored 66.2 out of 100 in this survey on a variety of health-promoting practices, up from 61.5 percent in 1983, the first year the survey was taken. What health-promoting practices? Eating less fat, eating less cholesterol, as we'd expect. The survey reported that although fewer Americans were making an effort to avoid or restrict sugar, sweets, and other refined carbohydrates, all in all our healthful behavior "has improved significantly since 1983, with greater numbers of individuals actively watching key elements of their diet such as their cholesterol level." You would think that with this "significant" improvement in dietary behavior over the past seven years and the reported reduction of fat and cholesterol intake the population would have less high blood pressure and obesity, and fewer cholesterol problems. The survey didn't look into the first two, but it did address obesity. It reported that 64 percent of adult Americans, or about 100 million people, were overweight, up from 58 percent in 1983. If the nutritional establishment is right, and fat and cholesterol are the problems, with more people following such a "healthful" diet you would expect to see a reduction in obesity. The survey found just the opposite.

You may find specific examples that seem to run contrary to the idea that elevated insulin causes the host of problems we've been discussing. We have a friend, for example, who has a son who might as well be connected by hose to a tank of sugar water. This kid always has a can of some kind of soft drink in his hand. He eats candy bars, cookies, cupcakes, and ice cream nonstop. His favorite foods are "spaghetti, pizza, Cap'n Crunch cereal, and toast." He eats at least 500 grams of carbohydrate per day, a figure that converts to over *2 cups* of pure sugar. (*Any* carbohydrate is metabolized exactly like sugar.)

But the kid is rail thin, and his cholesterol is only 135 mg/dl. What's going on? Is he a statistical aberration, like the one relative in every family who smokes and drinks unremittingly, and lives to be ninety-five?

Although he does eat more sugar than many teenagers, this young man is not very different from most youngsters in America today. They all eat way too much sugar and other refined carbohydrates but seem to suffer no ill effects from it. Studies done both in the United States and in England indicate that many children from the ages of about five up to adolescence consume approximately 200 grams, or about 1 cup, of sugar per day. That's 1 cup of pure sugar, not total carbohydrate; total carbohydrate intake is much greater, about twice as much. So the data show that children eat excessive amounts of sugar and other carbohydrate, but anyone who looks can see that the vast majority of children are not fat. And if you checked their cholesterol levels and blood pressure—as we have done—you'd find that almost all would be within the normal range or even low.

Although today's kids are twice as fat as they were a generation ago,[2] you still see relatively few fat kids because most children don't have an insulin problem—yet. But age and their diet and their genes finally catch up with them. After thirty or forty years of growing older on a high-carbohydrate diet, their intricately meshed metabolic gears start to slip, and they begin to develop obesity, high blood pressure, and all the rest. By then they *will* have an insulin problem.

In childhood the insulin–blood sugar regulation mechanism works perfectly. When you're a kid and you eat ice cream or drink a soda loaded with sugar, your blood sugar starts to rise and your pancreas releases a little insulin, which drives your blood sugar back down pronto. The pancreas releases just a small amount of insulin to force the blood sugar back down to normal because in childhood the cells are extremely sensitive to insulin. Small amounts of insulin translate into low insulin levels. And due to this delicate sensitivity, small amounts of insulin easily handle even the outrageous amounts of sugar and other carbohydrates that kids stuff themselves with—but not without a price. That price is a developing loss of sensitivity of the sensors to insulin—a condition known as *insulin resistance*—and chronically elevated insulin levels.

---

[2] *Archives of Pediatrics and Adolescent Medicine,* 1995.

Insulin Resistance: When Only Too Much Is Enough

When cells become resistant to insulin, the receptors on their surfaces designed to respond to insulin have begun to malfunction. No clear cause for this malfunctioning has yet emerged from ongoing research, but the odds are it will be a combination of inherited tendency and lifestyle abuse. It simply means that the receptors require more insulin to make them work properly in removing sugar from the blood. Whereas before they needed just a touch to lower it, now they need a continuous supply of excess insulin to keep blood sugar within the normal range.

As time goes by, blood sugar rises higher and stays up longer after the carbohydrate meal despite the enormous amount of insulin mustered to lower it. Bear in mind that were your doctor to check blood sugar during this stage of developing insulin resistance, your blood sugar would be perfectly normal. The major silent change taking place is the ever-growing quantity of insulin needed to keep it that way. Only by checking your blood insulin level—a lab test most doctors don't even consider yet—can you determine whether you have an elevated insulin level (the condition called *hyperinsulinemia*) or *insulin resistance.* *Hyperinsulinemia* means simply having too much insulin in the blood, whereas *insulin resistance* means that the receptors no longer respond properly to insulin. This is the classic story of the chicken and the egg: which came first? Researchers are not yet certain, but the preponderance of evidence points to excess insulin as the culprit.

It's not the little spurts of insulin that we see in children and adolescents after they eat carbohydrates that cause problems; these are perfectly normal. It is the sustained elevated insulin levels—hyperinsulinemia—of the insulin-resistant adult that lead to the high blood pressure, cholesterol elevation, diabetes, and excess weight of midlife. Hyperinsulinemia is the real problem; all the other "problems" are merely the symptoms. If you look back at the chart showing the roles of insulin and glucagon, you can easily see what kinds of mischief hyperinsulinemia causes and how all these symptoms develop. Picture all the processes listed on the left side operating full blast—as they do under full insulin stimulation—and you can imagine the degree of harm being done silently.

Unfortunately, most doctors treat only the symptoms and often in a way that makes the real problem worse. If you go on a low-fat diet, what happens? By decreasing your fat intake you usually decrease your protein intake, because virtually all foods that are protein-rich contain substantial amounts of fat. Meat, eggs, cheese, most dairy products—the best sources of complete dietary protein—are all either taboo or severely restricted on a low-fat diet. With this protein and fat restriction, the only food component left in the diet is carbohydrate, which by default results in your eating a high-carbohydrate, low-protein diet—the very diet that maximizes insulin production. If you had hyperinsulinemia to begin with—and if you have elevated triglycerides and cholesterol and high blood pressure, you can bet that you do—increasing your body's production of insulin isn't going to help. Instead of attacking the root cause of the problem, you'll leave the doctor's office with a prescription for a high blood pressure medicine, a more stringent diet, and perhaps a prescription for a cholesterol-lowering medicine as well.

You are relieved, your doctor is happy, and the drug

companies are ecstatic: they have just signed you on as a new customer to the tune of between $50 and $200 per month for life.

If these methods bring about only cosmetic solutions to blood pressure, cholesterol, and other problems, how can we actually treat these disorders and make them go away? All you need to do is treat the hyperinsulinemia, and the other disorders improve or disappear.

The only method available to treat hyperinsulinemia is diet. Fortunately the dietary approach works spectacularly well. You can treat elevated cholesterol with the standard low-fat cholesterol-lowering diet with limited success until the cows come home, but you can reduce your insulin level with our program in a matter of days and see an almost immediate reduction of blood pressure, a significant reduction in your cholesterol or triglyceride levels in a few weeks, and a steady loss of excess stored body fat in the weeks and months ahead.

It's important to remember, however, that even though the regimen works rapidly to return insulin sensitivity to normal in most people, *it works only as long as you follow it.* It doesn't return you to your childhood levels of imperviousness to carbohydrate assault. You must continue to follow the guidelines to maintain the changes; a return to your former eating habits will return you to your former problems. This nutritional structure is successful because it works *with* your metabolic system instead of counter to it; it's been proven again and again around the world.

Better in the Bush: Aborigines and Insulin Resistance

The concept of undertaking nutritional therapy for disease by constructing a diet of reduced carbohydrate is beautifully illustrated in the work of Dr. Kerin O'Dea, an Australian physician, and her colleagues, who have extensively studied the Australian aborigines over the past decade or so. The aborigines are an interesting group in that they develop a high incidence of hyperinsulinemia and type II diabetes when exposed to an urbanized, Western diet. Like a huge number of Americans, they are genetically predisposed to the development of these disorders, but they develop them much more quickly. This situation, although unfortunate for the aborigines, makes them ideal candidates for the study of the relationship between diet and hyperinsulinemia.

Dr. O'Dea began her studies by looking at the baseline insulin and glucose levels of urbanized aborigine subjects who were consuming a Western diet. She found that both the insulin and the glucose levels were significantly elevated, which should come as no surprise when we consider the diet they were eating: "white flour, white sugar, white rice, carbonated drinks, alcoholic beverages (beer, port), powdered milk and cheap fatty meat." This sounds a lot like the diet of the majority of teenagers in America today. When we look at the composition of this diet in terms of the three nutrient types, we find that it is "high in refined carbohydrate (40–50%) and fat (40–50%) and relatively low in protein (< or = 10%)" or almost precisely the same composition as the typical American diet.

Dr. O'Dea then started these people on her experimental diet, which she designed to approximate the original native diet they would consume were they back in the bush: considerable protein, not a lot of fat, and very little carbohydrate. The nutrient composition was "protein 70–75%, fat 20–25%, [and] carbohydrate <5%." She kept the aborigines on this "very low carbohydrate–high protein diet" for two weeks and then rechecked their blood values. She found that her subjects had developed "a small but significant improvement in glucose tolerance which was accompanied by a similar small reduction in insulin response." She concluded that "these findings suggest an improvement in glucose utilization and insulin sensitivity after the high protein–low carbohydrate diet."

This success inspired Dr. O'Dea to undertake what turned out to be a prolonged and exceptionally enlightening study. She gathered a group of middle-aged, hyperinsulinemic, diabetic, mildly overweight aborigine subjects who had been living on a Western diet much like the one just detailed. These subjects agreed to return to "their traditional country in an isolated location" in western Australia for seven weeks, during which they would live the lives of hunter-gatherers.

During the seven weeks that the aborigines lived off the land in the bush Dr. O'Dea and her group kept careful records of the various foods the subjects ate as they wandered from area to area and tabulated them for later analysis. Depending on whether the group was on the coast or traveled inland, the diet varied, with protein ranging from 54 to 80 percent, fat from 13 to 40 percent, and carbohydrate from less than 5 percent to a high of 33 percent. How did these subjects fare on this high-protein, restricted-carbohydrate diet? Their blood glucose levels fell from an average of about 210 mg/dl to 118 mg/dl. Insulin levels dropped almost by half, from 23 mU/ml to 12 mU/ml, near the normal range. Triglycerides, which are storage fat molecules synthesized in the liver under the stimulus of insulin, fell by a factor of three, from 354 mg/dl all the way down to 106 mg/dl. All this improvement came in just seven weeks from a diet that was predominantly (64 percent) animal in origin. (Exercise wasn't a factor in their improvement. Dr. O'Dea determined that the aborigines were surprisingly *less* active in the bush than in the city.)

Dr. O'Dea summed it up succinctly: ". . . all of the metabolic abnormalities of type II diabetes were either greatly improved (glucose tolerance, insulin response to glucose) or completely normalized (plasma lipids) in a group of diabetic aborigines by a relatively short (7 week) reversion to traditional hunter-gatherer lifestyle." Dr. O'Dea discovered by actual experimentation with a group of people afflicted with one of the diseases of civilization the same thing that anthropologists learned by examining the mummy and skeletal data: the carbohydrate-restricted, high-protein diet confers optimal health on its followers.

Where does this leave us? You are probably wondering if you need to start subsisting on snails, turtles, kangaroo, crocodiles, crickets, and other diverse beasts to get your cholesterol down. That would work, but you don't have to go to those lengths. Our regimen provides all the benefits of the hunter-gatherer diet but uses foods that you capture at the grocery store and even in the wilds of the nearest fast-food outlet. All we need do to gain the benefits of the hunter-gatherer diet is to consume a diet that approximates it in nutritional composition, which we can do easily.

The Bottom Line

Insulin and its counterbalancing partner, glucagon, are the master hormones controlling human metabolism. The word *insulin* may immediately call up a mental association with diabetes, and the connection is a valid one. Controlling blood sugar is definitely insulin's most important job in the human body.

Many people—especially those with heart disease, diabetes, high blood pressure, elevated cholesterol, or obesity in their families—have inherited a tendency for the insulin sensors on the cells to malfunction with age, illness, stress, or assault by years of high sugar and starch consumption. As these sensors become sluggish, the condition of *insulin resistance* develops. Because it's crucial to get the sugar out of the blood and into the cells, the pancreas will compensate by making more and more insulin to force the sluggish sensors to respond. Thus begins a vicious cycle of requiring ever more insulin to keep the system going. Finally, some people become so resistant to insulin that the amount necessary to make the sensors respond and clear the sugar from the blood is more than their pancreas can make; that person becomes an adult diabetic.

Excess insulin stimulates a wide variety of other metabolic systems: it encourages the kidneys to retain salt and fluid; it stimulates the production of cholesterol by the liver; it fuels an increase in triglyceride production; it thickens the muscular portion of the artery walls, increasing the risk for high blood pressure; and it sends a strong message to the fat cells to store incoming sugar and fat.

Insulin's actions are countered by the second metabolic hormone, glucagon. Glucagon sends signals to the kidneys to release excess salt and fluid, to the liver to slow down the production of cholesterol and triglycerides, to the artery wall to relax and drop blood pressure, and to the fat cells to release stored fat to be burned for energy. When insulin levels in the blood are high, however, they so overwhelm the system that they suppress glucagon's actions.

Since food is what mainly controls the production of these two hormones, we have been able to create a nutritional structure that maximizes the release of glucagon and minimizes the release of insulin, creating a closer balance between these two hormones. Under these conditions the actions of the glucagon predominate, allowing the metabolism to heal and the malfunctioning sensors to regain their sensitivity. Once this healing occurs, the metabolic disturbances that insulin resistance caused improve or disappear. If elevated, your cholesterol and triglycerides return to normal, your blood pressure returns to normal, blood sugar stabilizes, and you can effectively lose excess stored body fat. All these benefits accrue not by treating the symptoms—the blood pressure, cholesterol problem, overweight, or diabetes—but the root cause, chronically elevated insulin and insulin resistance. There are no medications yet to treat this disorder—the right diet is the only remedy, but it works extremely well.

52 PROTEIN POWER
• Score 20 points if
have ad

Chapter 4

Assessing Your Risk

Middle age is when your age starts to sho   nd the middle.

BOB HOPE

Now that you understand the role that diet plays in regulating metabolism (especially the production of the hormones insulin and glucagon) and you know that a diet high in complex carbohydrates and low in protein will actually *increase* your risk for obesity and other insulin-related health problems, you're probably asking, "How does this information apply to me?" Good question. How do you determine your risk for these disorders? You can begin in just the way we begin when a patient comes to us for help in losing weight, controlling cholesterol or triglycerides, or treating diabetic problems: by looking into your own and your family's medical history. Simply knowing the kinds of problems you or members of your family have suffered will shed light on your risk for insulin-related disorders.

Take this medical history quiz to find out more:

you:

...ult-onset diabetes or developed diabetes dur-
...ng pregnancy

Score 10 points for each *yes* response if you:

- have elevated triglycerides
- have a *low* level of HDL ("good") cholesterol
- are overweight mainly around your middle

Score 5 points for each *yes* response if you:

- have high blood pressure
- are overweight mostly in your legs and hips
- have elevated cholesterol
- retain fluid
- crave sugar and starchy foods

Score 3 points for each parent with a *yes* response:

- has/had high blood pressure
- has/had heart disease
- has/had adult-onset diabetes

Check your scores against the following totals to assess your risk:

- Less than 10: low risk for developing insulin problems
- 10 to 15: moderate risk for insulin problems
- 15 to 20: high risk for insulin problems
- 20 or more: you very likely *have* an insulin disorder

While your history points up your risk, laboratory tests confirm these suspicions and assess the extent of your metabolic disturbance and your overall state of health. Blood tests and other such measurements also give you a benchmark against which to track your progress as you heal yourself nutritionally. What kind of testing do we recommend?

The Laboratory Evaluation of Ri

With the help of your physician you shou
of fasting laboratory tests performed. In pr
your blood tests, you should eat no solid food an
liquids other than water for a minimum of eight
hours beforehand. If you take medications, please cho
with your physician for instructions on which medicines to
take prior to your tests. The easiest time to have your
blood work done is first thing in the morning after an
overnight fast, rather than trying to fast throughout the
day. Ask your doctor to perform the following tests:

SERUM INSULIN

The handling of this test is very important. The specimen
should be kept frozen and the test completed within 24
hours of the blood draw. Be sure that the test is performed
by a national reference laboratory, such as Smith-Kline,
Roche Biomedical, or Nichols, or by a research laboratory
accustomed to doing this test. Results can vary widely—
even from the same specimen—if it's not handled properly. Remember that even though most laboratories will
set values of over 25 to 30 as abnormally high, the "normal" samples include many people with insulin resistance
who have not yet developed diabetes. General clinical
evaluation of insulin levels as a marker for disease is still in
its infancy. In our clinic, as in many research settings, we
use the fasting insulin normal values of healthy young
people as the standard against which we should measure
ourselves. If your insulin reading is over 10 mU/ml you
can consider yourself to have developed some degree of
insulin resistance. The more over 10 your reading, the

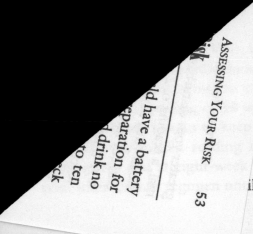

as the upper end of nor-
that it's taking 2½ times
control blood sugar at its
uld mean it's taking over
blood sugar at its current
s high, repeat the test at
intervals thereafter during
il normal.

d have a battery
eparation for
d drink no
o ten
ck

SMA-24 OR C   PROFILE

This battery of tests goes by a variety of names but usually includes blood glucose, the electrolytes (sodium, potassium, chloride, bicarbonate), measures of heart, liver, and kidney function, uric acid, cholesterol, and sometimes triglycerides. Important points to note:

1. Your blood sugar level: If your fasting level is greater than 115 mg/dl, you are already starting to lose blood sugar control. It's also important to note how much insulin it's taking to keep your blood sugar at its current level. The ratio of blood sugar (measured in mg/dl) divided by insulin should be greater than 7. If your ratio is less than 7, you are developing or have developed insulin resistance. (A level of over 7 doesn't clear you, however.) To assess your progress, repeat this test at eight weeks and every eight weeks thereafter until normal.

2. Your potassium level: If it's at or below the bottom of the normal range, you must be very aware of the need to supplement your diet with extra potassium unless you take blood pressure medications that could interact with it. (Ask your doctor or pharmacist.) If your level was low initially, repeat after one week of extra supplementation to see if your level has returned to normal. If still low, double your supplementation and repeat weekly until your level is normal again.

3. *Your kidney function tests:* If normal, you should have no problem handling any protein intake level. If your tests show kidney damage, you probably already know that you suffer from kidney problems. In that case you should not eat more protein than your minimum daily protein requirement. If your values were abnormal, repeat this test in six to eight weeks. You should see improvement in these values, or at least they should be no worse. If they are worse, discontinue the program.

4. *Your liver function tests:* Often people with an unrecognized insulin-related disorder will show mild to moderate elevations in some of their liver enzymes. This elevation usually occurs because of fat deposits' being laid down within the liver itself. If this is the case for you, you should see these test numbers return to normal as you proceed through your nutritional program. If your liver tests were abnormal, your physician should repeat them after you've been on the program for about eight weeks and at eight-week intervals until they are normal again. If your alkaline phosphatase (one of the liver tests) was abnormal, it could be a sign of gallbladder disease, which often occurs in people with insulin-related problems. If you still have your gallbladder and this test result is elevated, you should have a gallbladder ultrasound to be certain you don't have gallstones.

5. *Cholesterol and triglycerides:* See "Lipid Profile," on page 56.

6. *Uric acid:* This test helps to assess your risk for gout, which frequently afflicts people with insulin-related problems. If this value is high and you do not currently suffer

from gout, count yourself lucky. The reading should improve as you progress through the diet. Repeat the test at eight weeks for high readings.

LIPID PROFILE

This test subdivides the blood fats into their various components of total cholesterol, triglycerides, VLDL cholesterol, LDL cholesterol, and HDL cholesterol. The most telling indicators of insulin-related problems are elevation of triglycerides and a low HDL cholesterol, but you may also discover elevated VLDL and LDL cholesterol as well. Whatever the actual cholesterol numbers, as stated in Chapter 13, what's most important in assessment of heart disease risk is the ratio of your total cholesterol to the HDL "good" cholesterol. If you divide your total cholesterol number (in mg/dl) by the HDL number, your ratio should be 4 or less. If your ratio is above 4, you should consider yourself at increased risk for heart disease. As you progress through our nutritional program, these readings should improve. You should see a sharp, rapid drop in triglycerides, accompanied by a decrease in your total cholesterol-to-HDL ratio. Reevaluate these readings at eight weeks if they were elevated. If you are on medication to lower cholesterol or triglycerides, your doctor will need to evaluate them sooner (at about three or four weeks) and will probably need to reduce the doses of your medication. Following the readings at three- to four-week intervals, your doctor will most likely be able to wean you slowly off your medication as you regain metabolic control. Repeat the lipid tests after you've been off your medication for eight weeks and stable on your diet during that time and then every six months to one year thereafter.

HEMOGLOBIN A₁C

This test measures the amount of the red blood cell pigment hemoglobin that has been bound to blood sugar. The reaction that binds these two together is irreversible and depends on how much sugar is in the blood. Because red blood cells remain in circulation for about 90 to 120 days before they are removed and recycled, this test gives us a way to measure what your blood sugar has been *on average* for the last 30 to 60 days. In this test the lower your number, the better. Even if your reading falls within what the laboratory deems as "normal," you must remember that these normals include many people with insulin resistance, which shifts the levels upward. If your reading is outside the laboratory's normal, consider yourself already very insulin resistant. If you fall within the normal range, assess yourself according to the scale that follows.

Take note of the top and bottom of the normal range for Hgb A₁c for the laboratory your physician used. Determine the average value for that lab by adding the high value and the low value and dividing by 2. The middle of the range (this average number) represents an average blood sugar reading of 100. Each tenth of a point above that average correlates with 4 additional blood sugar points in mg/dl. In our lab, a reading of 5 is the average Hgb A₁c reading. Based on that average, the following scale would apply:

4.0 = 60	4.5 = 80	5.0 = 100	5.5 = 120
4.1 = 64	4.6 = 84	5.1 = 104	5.6 = 124
4.2 = 68	4.7 = 88	5.2 = 108	5.7 = 128
4.3 = 72	4.8 = 92	5.3 = 112	5.8 = 132
4.4 = 76	4.9 = 96	5.4 = 116	5.9 = 136

6.0 = 140	6.5 = 160	7.0 = 180	7.5 = 200
6.1 = 144	6.6 = 164	7.1 = 184	7.6 = 204
6.2 = 148	6.7 = 168	7.2 = 188	7.7 = 208
6.3 = 152	6.8 = 172	7.3 = 192	7.8 = 212
6.4 = 156	6.9 = 176	7.4 = 196	7.9 = 216

12-LEAD ELECTROCARDIOGRAM

Any dietary change, but especially this regimen, will result in a sometimes dramatic loss of water and electrolytes such as sodium and potassium. In people who have certain abnormal heart rhythm patterns such an abrupt change could be dangerous.[1] Although most people don't have these problems, it's wise to check first. Your physician can determine if your heart rhythm and the heart's electrical function are normal by checking the heart tracings of a standard electrocardiogram (EKG). A normal electrocardiogram within the last year or two, unless you've had any heart problems in the meantime, should be sufficient to assure you're not at risk for this kind of rhythm problem.

---

[1] If your heart rhythm is abnormal, you will need to approach this program with great care, slowly reducing your carbohydrate intake in 20-gram/day drops from your current level to the level recommended in the phases described in Chapter 5 over a period of several weeks instead of making the dramatic drop we normally suggest. This method, while more difficult, will allow you to slowly waste your excess body fluid. You must stay in close contact with your physician during this time.

URINALYSIS

This test checks for sugar in yo[...]
tor of diabetes—but also to make[...]
have any blood or protein (signs of [...]
age) or signs of urinary infection that [...]
der the stress of a dietary change.

COMPLETE BLOOD COUNT (CBC)

This test evaluates your red blood cells for number,[...]
and shape to uncover anemias and your white blood c[...]
for number and type to assess your immune function[...]
Some nutritional clues from the CBC include (1) large,
pale red blood cells indicate a need for more B vitamins,
especially B_{12}; and (2) small, pale red blood cells may indicate iron deficiency. If you are anemic or your white blood
count is abnormal, your physician needs to evaluate these
problems fully before you make any nutritional changes.

THYROID PANEL

Evaluation of your thyroid gland activity is important if
you're overweight, have high cholesterol, retain fluid, or
have no energy. Trying to correct these problems in the
face of low thyroid function is quite difficult. Your evaluation should include levels for thyroid hormone (at least
T_3, free T_4) and a high-sensitivity TSH, the brain stimulator that signals to the thyroid gland that it needs to make
more hormone. Even in the face of normal thyroid hormone levels, if your TSH is elevated, your brain is saying
you need more thyroid activity. If this is the case, your

tal thyroid hor- r readings. Re- ill help your ou and to ad-

f the insulin- llowing note

r urine—a strong indica- certain that you don't ossible kidney dam- ight blossom un-

size, ells

ntion after control in- have used treat these conditions in our clinical practice for nearly a decade.

Hypertension: Using these dietary guidelines, your hypertensive patients will rapidly reduce blood pressure, so quickly in fact that if they currently take diuretic medications you will need to taper and discontinue these medications quickly when the patients begin the intervention protocol. You can taper and withdraw other classes of antihypertensives, such as ACE inhibitors, calcium channel blockers, or beta blockers more slowly, monitoring their blood pressure response weekly over a three- to four-week period. In rare cases diet alone will not control their blood pressure, and in these cases your best choice is a small dose of ACE inhibitor, calcium channel blocker, or alpha agonist. None of these medications elevate insulin, whereas the beta blockers and thiazide diuretics do.

If blood pressure fails to normalize, or if it normalizes and then returns to an elevated level (this is more common in very overweight people), the cause may be an excess of arachidonic acid coming into circulation from fat breakdown. If the patient can take aspirin, place him or her on low-dose aspirin therapy to block the production of series two prostaglandins from arachidonic acid. One-half aspirin per day is enough.

Fluid Retention: Usually fluid retention disappears quickly. If it remains, however, and you need to diurese the patient, choose a loop diuretic, such as Bumex or Lasix in tiny doses, taken along with an extra potassium supplement (such as Micro-K 10). Again, because the thiazides cause elevation of insulin, their use in fluid retention would be counterproductive.

Hyperlipidemias: Because of insulin's stimulation in cholesterol synthesis (stimulation of HMG CoA Reductase in the rate-limiting step), correction of insulin resistance through dietary reduction of carbohydrates will quickly bring elevated LDL, VLDL, and total cholesterol back to normal. With the regimen and exercise, HDL remains unchanged or often rises. Triglycerides fall sharply and quickly. If your patients are on lipid-lowering agents, you will likely be able to taper them over the next several weeks and in all probability discontinue them in compliant patients. Reduce the doses incrementally (we usually halve them) and after three to four weeks check lipid levels and drop again if indicated. We've seen this regimen return cholesterol readings of over 600 and triglyceride readings of over 3,000 to normal in three weeks. The metabolic power of the right nutritional regimen for this condition is startling.

Adult-Onset Diabetes Mellitus: In patients on no medications, the regimen will return their blood sugar readings to normal in a few weeks. In patients taking oral hypoglycemic agents, you will need to keep in close contact to help taper their medication doses during the first week or two. In most cases by three weeks they will be off all oral agents for sugar control if they carefully follow the intervention protocol. We usually halve their dose the first full day on the plan, then halve it again the next. The patient should be well versed in the use of a glucometer and should take his or her blood sugar readings frequently during this period. Some patients respond so rapidly that we can totally eliminate their medication in a few days if they comply with the regimen.

You will need to watch your adult-onset patients who take insulin very closely. Before these patients can begin the protocol, we always check a C peptide level (not a fasting insulin since that would measure what they inject as well as any beta cell production) to see just how much native insulin they're making. If they've got a good solid amount of C peptide, then the problem is truly one of insulin resistance; they will respond quite well, and you will very likely be able to work their insulin dose down to zero in time as long as they adhere to the regimen.

In patients who make little C peptide, the regimen will definitely improve their health, help to restore balance to their metabolic hormones, and you will be able to reduce their doses of insulin significantly. But you won't be able to eliminate insulin entirely, since their beta cells have "burned out" or been otherwise damaged. This regimen works so dramatically to improve sugar control that you must be close at hand to interpret blood sugar changes and help your diabetic patients adjust their insulin doses accordingly.

If you have questions about managing your patients with insulin-related disorders on this regimen, please feel free to contact us at our office: 11025 Anderson Road, Suite 130, Little Rock, AR 72212.

Michael R. Eades, M.D., and
Mary Dan Eades, M.D.

The Other Half of the Risk Factor: Are You an Apple or a Pear?

We don't care what you weigh! That may seem like a strange statement for two doctors who devote their clinical time to health, nutrition, weight loss, and fitness. But in fact what you weigh is not as important as what your weight is made of—how much is lean and how much fat. So we'll give you an easy method to determine your body composition. You'll be able to calculate how many of your pounds are active lean tissue (muscle, organs, hair, skin, nails, skeleton, and water) and how many pounds are fat so that you can assess your nutritional requirements and have a realistic estimate of where you're beginning as well as a good tool to track your progress. We'll also give you some guidelines to help you set a healthy goal for recomposing your body to new lean, healthy fat-to-muscle percentages.

Although being overfat is an important health risk, *where* you carry your fat is even more important. If you likened your shape to that of a fruit, would you call yourself an apple, with most of your weight around your middle? Or are you more like a pear, with the weight aggregated mostly in your hips and thighs?

When your body stores fat in the abdominal region—the apple distribution—it doesn't lay the fat down just under the skin around the abdomen and waist but also inside the abdominal cavity, around the heart, liver, kidneys, and intestine and even within these organs. This apple-shaped fat pattern occurs most frequently in men, and for that reason you may have heard it referred to as an android or male fat distribution. But since this pattern is not exclusive to men, we prefer to use the more accurately descriptive term *abdominal fat*. Although many women also develop this apple shape, more often women store their excess body fat in the pear-shaped pattern: slimmer in the chest and upper body, with the main accumulation of fat around their hips and thighs—what's been called the female or gynoid pattern. And again, since some men take on this pear shape, too, we'll simply call it *hip and leg fat* for the sake of clarity.

Insulin has a much greater influence on the fat cells in the abdominal area, and for this reason people who suffer from faulty insulin metabolism and who develop insulin resistance are more likely to store abdominal fat and take on the apple shape. Because excess insulin strongly drives the storage here, excess abdominal fat carries with it a greater risk for all the insulin-related metabolic problems: high blood pressure, elevated cholesterol, heart disease, and diabetes. Recognize that storing the fat in the abdominal region doesn't *cause* these problems; it's simply another symptom of the underlying metabolic disorder, insulin resistance.

Hip and leg fat, on the other hand, is less a consequence of underlying metabolic disorder. That is not to say there is no connection; fat cells throughout the body respond to insulin's signal to store fat. But the storage here is deposited primarily underneath the skin (subcutaneous fat) and marbles the muscles of the hips and legs. In these areas, which are outside the major body cavities, there are no vital organs for fat deposits to surround and infiltrate. For these reasons excess fat accumulation that stays confined to the hip and leg region doesn't carry with it the increased risk to health that comes with excess abdominal fat. Usually, however, if the fat accumulation continues long enough, the pear-shaped body will finally begin to store abdominal fat, too, and then the same host of insulin-related metabolic problems begins to arise. Often blood pressure goes up a little, then cholesterol, triglycerides, and finally blood sugar. For many women who have carried hip and leg fat for much of their lives and seemed perfectly healthy otherwise, these additional health problems may not occur until after the childbearing years but then come on with a vengeance as menopause approaches.

The Waist-to-Hip Ratio

Sometimes just looking at your shape in silhouette will tell you volumes about where you store your fat, but it's not always so straightforward. Modern technological wizardry has given us a tool to look within—computerized tomography, the CAT scan—that enables researchers to see in pictures where the fat deposits accumulate and how deceptive external appearances can be. But CAT scans are very expensive, so they're not a practical tool for gauging fat distribution in the general public. Although there is no method more accurate, there are many less costly, and later in this chapter, we give you a method that doesn't require expensive equipment or physician interpretation and doesn't carry the $1000 price tag of a CAT scan. For the purpose of illustration, however, we can use representative CAT scanning studies to help you better understand the various ways that fat can deposit. Refer to Figure 4.1. These figures are photo reproductions of four CAT photographs that show us what we would see if we could cut a person in half and look end on at the fat, the muscle, the bone, and the organs. Figure A represents an "average" healthy subject, figure B is a very lean trained athlete, figure C an apple-shaped person who stores fat inside the abdominal cavity, and figure D a pear-shaped person who lays down fat mainly in the hips and legs. In these instances the total body weight might be the same in subjects A and B and in subjects C and D, but as you can see, what makes up the weight can be vastly different. The body fat percentages may be identical in subjects C and D, but the location of the excess means that subject C, with the abdominal pattern, will have a higher risk for developing elevated blood pressure, cholesterol, triglycerides, and blood sugar.

To determine your own waist-to-hip ratio—a good estimate of storage pattern—you will need only a standard cloth tape measure, a pencil, and paper. Measure your waist at the level of your navel and your hips at their widest point. To ensure accuracy in measuring, measure directly on your skin, not over clothing. Also keep the tape level and snug, but not pinching your skin. Take each measurement three times and average the numbers. Hang on to these numbers; you'll need the measurements and averages again later, when you compute your body composition.

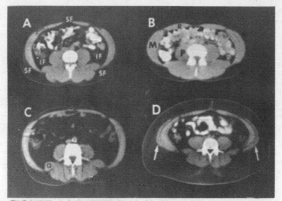

FIGURE 4.1 DIFFERENCES IN FAT DISTRIBUTION
(IF = intra-abdominal fat   SF = fat beneath the skin   M = muscles)

AVERAGE WAIST MEASUREMENT

Waist #1 _____ inches

Waist #2 _____

Waist #3 _____

Total ÷ 3 = _____ inches

AVERAGE HIP MEASUREMENT

Hip #1 _____ inches

Hip #2 _____

Hip #3 _____

Total ÷ 3 = _____ inches

With these two numbers you can easily determine your waist-to-hip ratio by dividing the average waist measurement by the average hip measurement.

avg. waist measurement ÷ avg. hip
measurement = _____

Refer to the following waist-to-hip ratio chart to determine your pattern.

WAIST-TO-HIP RATIOS		
Male	less than 1	hip and leg pattern
	1 or greater	abdominal pattern
Female	0.8 or less	hip and leg pattern
	greater than 0.8	abdominal pattern

If you find yourself (or your loved ones) among the apples, storing fat in the abdominal region, even if you are
not currently excessively overweight and do not yet suffer
from high blood pressure, elevated cholesterol or triglycerides, or blood sugar problems, you should consider
yourself at risk for these insulin-related disorders. Following this program now will help to ensure that you preserve
your health. If you already suffer from one or more of
these disorders, then reducing abdominal fat stores becomes even more important.

You can use this measurement tool to track your
progress as you proceed through the intervention phase.
Men should strive to bring their waist-to-hip ratio to 1 or
less, and women with apple shapes should aim for 0.8 or
less. If your shape is pearlike, while you will still want to
strive for a properly composed body to optimize your
health, your risk of serious metabolic disorders is lower.
Now that you've determined your pattern of storage, let's

take a look at an equally simple method for assessing what your weight is made of—the lean and fat of you. This method requires the pencil and cloth tape measure you used before, a reasonably accurate scale, and the charts and worksheets provided.

What's Your Body Composition?

DETERMINING YOUR BODY FAT

The first step in determining your composition is to calculate your body fat as a percentage of your total weight. Refer now to the worksheet for computing your percentage of body fat. (The calculations vary with gender, so make sure you're using the appropriate one for you and follow the instructions. We'll take each gender in turn.)

FOR WOMEN:

1. Measure your height in inches without shoes.

2. Using the measurements you made before, record your height, waist, and hip measurements in the labeled spaces on the worksheet on page 70.

3. Turn to the conversion constants chart for women and find each of these average measurements in the appropriate column. Record the adjacent constants (A for hips, B for abdomen, and C for height) on the worksheet where indicated. These constants have been derived experimentally and allow you to convert your measurements into a form that can be used to compute your body fat percentage.

WOMEN:
COMPUTING YOUR BODY FAT PERCENTAGE

First, find your average measurements IN INCHES:

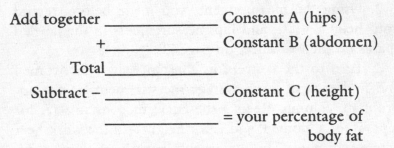

	Hips	Abdomen	Height
Measurement #1	_____	_____	_____
+			
Measurement #2	_____	_____	
+			
Measurement #3	_____	_____	
Total =	_____	_____	
Divide by 3 =	_____	_____	_____

4. Using the chart that follows, look up each of these average measurements and your height in the appropriate column. The numbers listed beside them will be constant A (hips), constant B (abdomen), and constant C (height). Use these constants below. Add constants A and B, then subtract constant C from their sum. Round your answer to the nearest whole number. This figure is your percentage of body fat.

Add together _____ Constant A (hips)

+_____ Constant B (abdomen)

Total_____

Subtract − _____ Constant C (height)

_____ = your percentage of
body fat

CONVERSION CONSTANTS TO PREDICT PERCENTAGE OF BODY FAT—WOMEN

HIPS		ABDOMEN		HEIGHT	
INCHES	CONSTANT A	INCHES	CONSTANT B	INCHES	CONSTANT C
30	33.48	20	14.22	55	33.52
30.5	33.83	20.5	14.40	55.5	33.67
31	34.87	21	14.93	56	34.13
31.5	35.22	21.5	15.11	56.5	34.28
32	36.27	22	15.64	57	34.74
32.5	36.62	22.5	15.82	57.5	34.89
33	37.67	23	16.35	58	35.35
33.5	38.02	23.5	16.53	58.5	35.50
34	39.06	24	17.06	59	35.96
34.5	39.41	24.5	17.24	59.5	36.11
35	40.46	25	17.78	60	36.57
35.5	40.81	25.5	17.96	60.5	36.72
36	41.86	26	18.49	61	37.18
36.5	42.21	26.5	18.67	61.5	37.33
37	43.25	27	19.20	62	37.79
37.5	43.60	27.5	19.38	62.5	37.94
38	44.65	28	19.91	63	38.40
38.5	45.00	28.5	20.09	63.5	38.55
39	46.05	29	20.62	64	39.01
39.5	46.40	29.5	20.80	64.5	39.16
40	47.44	30	21.33	65	39.62
40.5	47.79	30.5	21.51	65.5	39.77
41	48.84	31	22.04	66	40.23
41.5	49.19	31.5	22.22	66.5	40.38
42	50.24	32	22.75	67	40.84
42.5	50.59	32.5	22.93	67.5	40.99
43	51.64	33	23.46	68	41.45
43.5	51.99	33.5	23.64	68.5	41.60
44	53.03	34	24.18	69	42.06
44.5	53.41	34.5	24.36	69.5	42.21
45	54.53	35	24.89	70	42.67
45.5	54.86	35.5	25.07	70.5	42.82
46	55.83	36	25.60	71	43.28
46.5	56.18	36.5	25.78	71.5	43.43
47	57.22	37	26.31	72	43.89
47.5	57.57	37.5	26.49	72.5	44.04
48	58.62	38	27.02	73	44.50
48.5	58.97	38.5	27.20	73.5	44.65
49	60.02	39	27.73	74	45.11
49.5	60.37	39.5	27.91	74.5	45.26
50	61.42	40	28.44	75	45.72
50.5	61.77	40.5	28.62	75.5	45.87
51	62.81	41	29.15	76	46.32
51.5	63.16	41.5	29.33	76.5	46.47
52	64.21	42	29.87	77	46.93
52.5	64.56	42.5	30.05	77.5	47.08
53	65.61	43	30.58	78	47.54

53.5	65.96	43.5	30.76	78.5	47.69
54	67.00	44	31.29	79	48.15
54.5	67.35	44.5	31.47	79.5	48.30
55	68.40	45	32.00	80	48.76
55.5	68.75	45.5	32.18	80.5	48.91
56	69.80	46	32.71	81	49.37
56.5	70.15	46.5	32.89	81.5	49.52
57	71.19	47	33.42	82	49.98
57.5	71.54	47.5	33.60	82.5	50.13
58	72.59	48	34.13	83	50.59
58.5	72.94	48.5	34.31	83.5	50.74
59	73.99	49	34.84	84	51.20
59.5	74.34	49.5	35.02	84.5	51.35
60	75.39	50	35.56	85	51.81

Let's look at how one patient computed her body fat percentage. Lisa is 5′6″ and weighs 157 pounds. She measured her hips at 38.5″, 38″, and 38.5″. Her average hip measurement is 38.3 inches. (Calculate as follows: 38.5 + 38 + 38.5 = 115, and 115 ÷ 3 = 38.3.) Lisa should round the hip measurement down to 38. Her abdomen measurements are 27″, 26.5″, and 27.75″ for an average abdominal measurement of 27.08″, rounded to 27. Turning to the conversion constants chart, she will find her hip measurement (38) and to its right constant A (44.65), then her abdominal measurement (27) and to its right constant B (19.20), and finally her height (66 inches) and to its right constant C (40.23). Following the worksheet, she will now add constants A and B (44.65 + 19.20 = 63.85), and from that number she will subtract constant C (63.85 − 40.23 = 23.62). Lisa's body fat is 23.6 percent.

FOR MEN:

1. Measure your wrist at the space between your hand and your wrist bone, where your wrist bends. Keep the

tape snug, but do not compress the skin. Take three mea-surements for your wrist, record them on the worksheet, and compute the average.

2. Weigh yourself on a scale in pounds and record the weight in the appropriate space on the worksheet. Record the waist measurement you made earlier for the waist-to-hip ratio.

3. Subtract your average wrist measurement from your average waist measurement. Find this number listed as waist-minus-wrist across the top of the body fat calcula-tion chart for men. On the left side of this table, find your weight. Follow across from your weight and down from your waist-minus-wrist measurement. Where these two columns intersect, you will find your body fat percentage. Let's work through an example using these worksheets and charts.

Mark weighs 200 pounds. He takes the following wrist measurements: 6.5", 6.75", and 6.75" for an average wrist measurement of 6.67". (Calculate as follows: 6.5 + 6.75 + 6.75 = 6.7.) His waist (abdomen) measurements are 38", 37.75", and 38.25" for an average of 38 inches. (Compute as follows: 38 + 37.75 + 38.25 = 114, and 114 ÷ 3 = 38.) Mark will subtract his wrist measure from his waist (38 − 6.7 = 31.3) and round to the nearest one-half. Then he will find his waist-minus-wrist number (31) across the top of the conversion constants chart. Tracking down the left side of the chart, he will find his weight (200 pounds), and he will follow across to the column under his measure of 31 to find the number 22. Mark has a body fat per-centage of 22 percent.

MEN:
COMPUTING YOUR BODY FAT PERCENTAGE

First, find your average measurements IN INCHES or POUNDS:

	Wrist	Waist	Weight
Measurement #1	_____	_____	_____
Measurement #2	_____	_____	
Measurement #3	_____	_____	
Total =	_____	_____	
Divide by 3 =	_____	_____	_____

Waist
measurement _____

Minus wrist
measurement - _____

_____ = "waist minus wrist"

Using the waist-minus-wrist chart, find your weight in pounds in the left column. Find your "waist minus wrist" number across the top of the chart. Going across from the left and down from the top, find the point at which these two readings intersect. This figure represents your percentage of body fat:

_____ = percentage of body fat

Calculating Your Lean Body Weight

Now that you've got a good estimate of your body fat percentage, you can use this number to compute your lean body weight. Because the body is made of two basic segments—fat weight and lean weight—if you know how much you weigh and what percent of your weight is fat, you can determine how much your lean tissue weighs.

First, take your weight in pounds and multiply it by your percentage of body fat as a decimal (for example, if your body fat is 42 percent, you would multiply by 0.42 to get your answer):

total weight × % body fat = weight of fat in pounds

Once you know the weight of your body fat, you can subtract it from your total weight to get your lean body weight:

total weight − fat weight = lean body weight

For Lisa in our earlier example, the calculation would look like this: Her weight (157 pounds) times her body fat percentage as a decimal (23.6 percent becomes 0.236) equals the total number of pounds of fat she carries (157 × 0.236 = 37 pounds of fat). Her total weight (157) minus her fat weight (37) equals her lean weight (120 pounds).

Mark would figure his lean weight the same way. His weight (200 pounds) times his body fat percentage as a decimal (22 percent becomes 0.22) equals the total pounds of fat he carries (200 × 0.22 = 44 pounds of fat). His total weight (200) minus his fat weight (44) equals his lean weight (156 pounds).

Knowing your lean body weight is important for two reasons: it's the basis for determining your daily protein requirement (which you'll do in Chapter 5), and it allows you to calculate a *realistic* goal weight for yourself. Even though we stress to our patients as we have to you that we don't care what you weigh as long as it's composed prop-

WAIST-MINUS-WRIST
BODY FAT CALCULATION—MALE

WAIST MINUS WRIST (IN INCHES) Weight in lbs.	22	22.5	23	23.5	24	24.5	25	25.5	26	26.5	27	27.5	28	28.5	29	29.5	30	30.5	31
120 :	4	6	8	10	12	14	16	18	20	21	23	25	27	29	31	33	35	37	39
125 :	4	6	7	9	11	13	15	17	19	20	22	24	26	28	30	32	33	35	37
130 :	3	5	7	9	11	12	14	16	18	20	21	23	25	27	28	30	32	34	36
135 :	3	5	7	8	10	12	13	15	17	19	20	22	24	26	27	29	31	32	34
140 :	3	5	6	8	10	11	13	15	16	18	19	21	23	24	26	28	29	31	33
145 :	3	4	6	7	9	11	12	14	15	17	19	20	22	23	25	27	28	30	31
150 :	2	4	6	7	9	10	12	13	15	16	18	19	21	23	24	26	27	29	30
155 :	2	4	5	6	8	10	11	13	15	16	17	19	20	22	23	25	26	28	29
160 :	2	4	5	6	8	9	11	12	14	15	17	18	19	21	22	24	25	27	28
165 :	2	3	5	6	8	9	10	12	13	15	16	17	19	20	22	23	24	26	27
170 :	2	3	4	6	7	9	10	11	13	14	15	17	18	19	21	22	24	25	26
175 :	2	3	4	6	7	8	10	11	12	13	15	16	17	19	20	21	23	24	25
180 :	1	3	4	5	7	8	9	10	12	13	14	16	17	18	19	21	22	23	25
185 :	1	3	4	5	6	8	9	10	11	13	14	15	16	18	19	20	21	23	24
190 :	1	2	4	5	6	7	8	10	11	12	13	15	16	17	18	19	21	22	23
195 :	1	2	3	5	6	7	8	9	11	12	13	14	15	16	18	19	20	21	22
200 :	1	2	3	4	6	7	8	9	10	11	12	14	15	16	17	18	19	21	22

WAIST MINUS WRIST : (IN INCHES)

Weight in lbs.	22	22.5	23	23.5	24	24.5	25	25.5	26	26.5	27	27.5	28	28.5	29	29.5	30	30.5	31
205	1	2	3	4	5	6	8	9	10	11	12	13	14	15	17	18	19	20	21
210	1	2	3	4	5	6	7	8	9	11	12	13	14	15	16	17	18	19	21
215	1	2	3	4	5	6	7	8	9	10	11	12	13	15	16	17	18	19	20
220	0	2	3	4	5	6	7	8	9	10	11	12	13	14	15	16	17	18	19
225	0	1	2	3	4	6	7	8	9	10	11	12	13	14	15	16	17	18	19
230	0	1	2	3	4	5	6	7	8	9	10	11	12	13	14	15	16	17	18
235	0	1	2	3	4	5	6	7	8	9	10	11	12	13	14	15	16	17	18
240	0	1	2	3	4	5	6	7	8	9	10	11	12	13	14	15	16	17	18
245	0	1	2	3	4	5	6	7	8	9	10	11	12	13	14	15	16	17	17
250	0	1	2	3	4	5	6	6	7	8	9	10	11	12	13	14	15	16	17
255	0	1	2	3	4	5	6	6	7	8	9	10	11	12	13	14	15	16	17
260	0	1	2	2	3	4	5	6	7	8	9	10	11	12	13	14	14	15	16
265	0	1	1	2	3	4	5	6	7	8	8	9	10	11	12	13	14	15	16
270	0	0	1	2	3	4	5	6	7	7	8	9	10	11	12	13	14	15	15
275	0	0	1	2	3	4	5	5	6	7	8	9	10	11	12	13	13	14	15
280	0	0	1	2	3	4	4	5	6	7	8	9	10	11	11	12	13	14	15
285	0	0	1	2	3	4	4	5	6	7	8	8	9	10	11	12	13	14	15
290	0	0	1	2	3	3	4	5	6	7	7	8	9	10	11	11	12	13	14
295	0	0	1	2	2	3	4	5	6	6	7	8	9	10	10	11	12	13	14
300	0	0	1	2	2	3	4	5	5	6	7	8	9	9	10	11	12	12	13

WAIST MINUS WRIST (IN INCHES)	31.5	32	32.5	33	33.5	34	34.5	35	35.5	36	36.5	37	37.5	38	38.5	39	39.5	40	40.5
Weight in lbs.																			
120	41	43	45	47	49	50	52	54	56	58	60	62	64	66	68	70	70	74	76
125	39	41	43	45	46	48	50	52	54	56	58	59	61	63	65	67	69	71	72
130	37	39	41	43	44	46	48	50	52	53	55	57	59	61	62	64	66	68	69
135	36	38	39	41	43	44	46	48	50	51	53	55	56	58	60	62	63	66	67
140	34	36	38	39	41	43	44	46	48	49	51	53	54	56	58	59	61	63	64
145	33	35	36	38	39	41	43	44	46	47	49	51	52	54	55	57	59	60	62
150	32	33	35	36	38	40	41	43	44	46	47	49	50	52	53	55	57	58	60
155	31	32	34	35	37	38	40	41	43	44	46	47	49	50	52	53	55	56	58
160	30	31	33	34	35	37	38	40	41	43	44	46	47	48	50	51	53	54	56
165	29	30	31	33	34	36	37	38	40	41	43	44	45	47	48	50	51	52	54
170	28	29	30	32	33	34	36	37	39	40	41	43	44	45	47	48	49	51	52
175	27	28	29	31	32	33	35	36	37	39	40	41	43	44	45	47	48	49	51
180	26	27	28	30	31	32	34	35	36	37	39	40	41	43	44	45	47	48	49
185	25	26	28	29	30	31	33	34	35	36	38	39	40	41	43	44	45	46	48
190	24	26	27	28	29	30	32	33	34	35	37	38	39	40	41	43	44	45	46
195	24	25	26	27	28	30	31	32	33	34	35	37	38	39	40	41	43	44	45
200	23	24	25	26	28	29	30	31	32	33	35	36	37	38	39	40	41	43	44

WAIST MINUS WRIST (IN INCHES)	31.5	32	32.5	33	33.5	34	34.5	35	35.5	36	36.5	37	37.5	38	38.5	39	39.5	40	40.5
Weight in lbs.																			
205 ::	22	23	25	26	27	28	29	30	31	32	34	35	36	37	38	39	40	41	43
210 ::	22	23	24	25	26	27	28	29	30	32	33	34	35	36	37	38	39	40	42
215 ::	21	22	23	24	25	26	28	29	30	31	32	33	34	35	36	37	38	39	40
220 ::	20	22	23	24	25	26	27	28	29	30	31	32	33	34	35	36	37	38	39
225 ::	20	21	22	23	24	25	26	27	28	29	30	31	32	33	34	35	36	37	38
230 ::	19	20	21	22	23	24	25	26	27	28	30	31	32	33	34	35	36	37	38
235 ::	19	20	21	22	23	24	25	26	27	28	29	30	31	32	33	34	35	37	37
240 ::	18	19	20	21	22	23	24	25	26	27	28	29	30	31	32	33	34	36	36
245 ::	18	19	20	21	22	23	24	25	26	27	28	28	29	30	31	32	33	35	35
250 ::	18	18	19	20	21	22	23	24	25	26	27	28	29	30	31	31	32	34	34
255 ::	17	18	19	20	21	22	23	24	25	26	27	27	28	29	30	31	32	33	34
260 ::	17	18	19	19	20	21	22	23	24	25	26	27	28	29	30	30	31	33	33
265 ::	16	17	18	19	20	21	22	23	24	25	26	26	27	28	29	29	30	32	32
270 ::	16	17	18	19	19	20	21	22	23	24	25	25	26	28	29	29	30	31	31
275 ::	16	16	17	18	19	20	21	22	23	24	25	25	26	27	28	28	29	31	31
280 ::	15	16	17	18	19	19	20	21	22	23	24	24	25	27	28	28	29	30	30
285 ::	15	16	17	17	18	19	20	21	22	23	24	24	25	26	27	27	28	29	30
290 ::	15	15	16	17	18	19	20	20	21	22	23	23	24	26	26	27	27	29	29
295 ::	14	15	16	17	17	18	19	20	21	21	22	23	24	25	26	26	27	28	28
300 ::	14	15	16	16	17	18	19	19	20	21	22	22	23	24	25	26	26	27	28

WAIST-MINUS-WRIST
BODY FAT CALCULATION—MALE

WAIST MINUS WRIST (IN INCHES)	41	41.5	42	42.5	43	43.5	44	44.5	45	45.5	46	46.5	47	47.5	48	48.5	49	49.5	50
Weight in lbs. 120	77	79	81	83	85	87	89	91	93	95	97	99	99	99	99	99	99	99	99
125	74	76	78	80	82	84	85	87	89	91	93	95	96	98	99	99	99	99	99
130	71	73	75	77	78	80	82	84	86	87	89	91	93	94	96	98	99	99	99
135	68	70	72	74	75	77	79	80	82	84	86	87	89	91	92	94	96	98	99
140	66	68	69	71	72	74	76	77	79	81	82	84	86	87	89	91	92	94	96
145	63	65	67	68	70	71	73	75	76	78	79	81	83	84	86	87	89	91	92
150	61	63	64	66	67	69	70	72	74	75	77	78	80	81	83	84	86	87	89
155	59	61	62	64	65	67	68	70	71	73	74	76	77	79	80	82	83	85	86
160	57	59	60	61	63	64	66	67	69	70	72	73	75	76	77	79	80	82	83
165	55	57	58	60	61	62	64	65	67	68	69	71	72	74	75	76	78	79	81
170	54	55	56	58	59	60	62	63	64	66	67	69	70	71	73	74	75	77	78
175	52	53	55	56	57	59	60	61	63	64	65	66	68	69	70	72	73	74	76
180	50	52	53	54	56	57	58	59	61	62	63	65	66	67	68	70	71	72	74
185	49	50	51	53	54	55	56	58	59	60	61	63	64	65	66	68	69	70	71
190	48	49	50	51	52	54	55	56	57	58	60	61	62	63	65	66	67	68	69
195	46	47	49	50	51	52	53	55	56	57	58	59	60	62	63	64	65	66	68
200	45	46	47	48	50	51	52	53	54	55	57	58	59	60	61	62	63	65	66

WAIST MINUS WRIST : (IN INCHES)

Weight in lbs.	41	41.5	42	42.5	43	43.5	44	44.5	45	45.5	46	46.5	47	47.5	48	48.5	49	49.5	50
205	44	45	46	47	48	49	51	52	53	54	55	56	57	58	60	61	62	63	64
210	43	44	45	46	47	48	49	50	51	53	54	55	56	57	58	59	60	61	62
215	42	43	44	45	46	47	48	49	50	51	52	53	54	56	57	58	59	60	61
220	41	42	43	44	45	46	47	48	49	50	51	52	53	54	55	56	57	58	59
225	40	41	42	43	44	45	46	47	48	49	50	51	52	53	54	55	56	57	58
230	39	40	41	42	43	44	45	46	47	48	49	50	51	52	53	54	55	56	57
235	38	39	40	41	42	43	44	45	46	47	48	49	50	51	51	52	53	54	55
240	37	38	39	40	41	42	43	44	45	46	46	47	48	49	50	51	52	53	54
245	36	37	38	39	40	41	42	43	44	44	45	46	47	48	49	50	51	52	53
250	35	36	37	38	39	40	41	42	43	44	44	45	46	47	48	49	50	51	52
255	34	35	36	37	38	39	40	41	42	43	44	44	45	46	47	48	49	50	51
260	34	35	35	36	37	38	39	40	41	42	43	43	44	45	46	47	48	49	50
265	33	34	35	36	36	37	38	39	40	41	42	43	43	44	45	46	47	48	49
270	32	33	34	35	36	37	37	38	39	40	41	42	43	43	44	45	46	47	48
275	32	32	33	34	35	36	37	38	38	39	40	41	42	43	43	44	45	46	47
280	31	32	33	33	34	35	36	37	38	38	39	40	41	42	43	43	44	45	46
285	30	31	32	33	34	35	35	36	37	38	39	39	40	41	42	43	43	44	45
290	30	31	31	32	33	34	35	36	36	37	38	39	39	40	41	42	43	43	44
295	29	30	31	32	32	33	34	35	36	36	37	38	39	39	40	41	42	43	43
300	29	29	30	31	32	33	33	34	35	36	36	37	38	39	39	40	41	42	43

erly, if you're like most people, you have an "ideal" weight in your head that you'd like to reach and maintain. Based on how many pounds of lean body tissue you currently have, that may or may not be an attainable weight for you. If you have to sacrifice lean muscle weight to reach it, we encourage you to revise your goal. So what is a realistic "ideal" goal weight for you?

Your Ideal Body Weight

Refer to the next chart to find the body fat percentage range that is appropriate for your age and gender. Take the numbers at each end of the range and subtract each from 100 percent as we show with the following example. We'll need to use another subject, because Lisa is already within her ideal weight range.

> Example: Missy, age 35
>   Lean body weight = 96 pounds
>   Ideal body fat percentage = 21–27 percent
> Step 1: Subtract each of the ideal range numbers
>   from 100.
>   100% − 21% = 79% and 100% − 27% = 73%
> Step 2: Divide lean body weight by these numbers.
>   96 ÷ 79 = 1.22 and 96 ÷ 73 = 1.32
> Step 3: Multiply these numbers by 100.
>   1.22 × 100 = 122 and 1.32 × 100 = 132

This calculation gives an ideal body weight range of 122 to 132 pounds for Missy. These numbers are actually those of a patient in our practice. She is 5'3" tall, and the "ideal" weight charts doctors usually follow tell her she should weigh about 115 pounds. She has not weighed 115 since junior high school, and it's easy to see why she isn't likely ever to weigh so little. Were she to attempt to do so, she would have to dwindle her body fat percentage down below 16 percent (which is unlikely for a woman of her age unless she were a trained athlete, and from a hormonal standpoint would not be particularly healthy even if she could manage to do it). Or she would have to lose pounds of lean body mass from the 96 she currently carries, also not advisable. A better option is to keep every pound of metabolically active lean tissue she has, carry an appropriate amount of body fat for good health, and forget about what she weighs, because **what she weighs doesn't matter!** At 125 pounds, she's tight and lean and strong and healthy. To force herself toward an "ideal" of 115 is lunacy.

IDEAL BODY FAT PERCENTAGES

AGE	MALES	FEMALES
10–30	12–18%	20–26%
31–40	13–19%	21–27%
41–50	14–20%	22–28%
51–60	16–20%	22–30%
61 and older	17–21%	22–31%

Now it's your turn. Using the Ideal Body Weight Worksheet, on page 85, calculate your realistic ideal body weight. This weight will be the target that you aim for. Every pound of lost body fat takes you closer to it. Every inch lost in the waist reduces your apple shape and your risk for metabolic disorder. Great motivators will say that unless you know where you're going, you can't hope to get there. Now you've got a clear picture of your destination, and that will help you focus your efforts toward a specific goal.

The Well-Composed Body

Unless, like Lisa, you already fall well within the guidelines for a well-composed body, you're about to begin on a journey of self-improvement. After completing the worksheets, you may—like Missy—have found that you had an unrealistically low target weight in mind. Or you may have found that the 20 pounds you've been saying you needed to shed is really more like 40. Wherever you begin, keep reminding yourself that you're not out to lose weight. Your real goal is to develop a properly composed body— one supported by a lean healthy muscle mass, strong and vigorous, with enough fat for good health. Whatever weight that turns out to be is a perfect weight for you. We stress to our clinic patients that our program is not just a weight-loss diet—it's a prescription for reclaiming your health. Fat loss is only a small part of the overall benefit. That's why, when you've completed your intervention and you're ready to maintain your fitness for life, we want you to begin that new lifestyle fitter, leaner, and healthier, not just lighter.

IDEAL BODY WEIGHT WORKSHEET

Your calculated lean body weight = _____

Ideal body fat range percentage for your age and sex from charts on pages 71–72 and 76–81

_____% to _____%

Step 1: Subtract each of these percentages from 100:

100% – _____% = _____ and 100% – _____% = _____

Step 2: Divide your lean body weight by each of the numbers from step 1:

_____ / _____ = _____ and _____ / _____ = _____

Step 3: Multiply each of these answers from step 2 by 100:

_____ × 100 = _____

your ideal weight is in this range

_____ × 100 = _____

Part II

The Protein Power Plan

Chapter 5

Putting It All Together: Designing Your Food Plan

So it may be true after all; eating pasta makes you fat.

The New York Times
February 8, 1995

If you've been struggling with your weight, your blood pressure, your cholesterol, or your blood sugar on a diet of pasta and whole grains, living the fat-free, low-fat, no-fat way and failing, *stop blaming yourself!* You haven't failed; you've just been on the wrong diet. If you've been feeling discouraged because your doctor said, "Cut the fat to 30 grams a day or less and your weight will come down," and you did, but it didn't, don't despair. Help is here. If you suffer from elevated cholesterol and you've forgotten what it's like to eat a juicy steak for dinner and can't remember the last time you ate an egg, and your levels remain elevated, take heart. Changing your diet can and will help you regain control over these metabolic disorders. You can lose fat, you can reduce your cholesterol and triglycerides, you can lower your blood pressure, you can normalize your blood sugar by changing the way you eat—and you can maintain these benefits for a lifetime. Good health is within your grasp—all you need is the right information. This chapter will provide that information. Join us now, and we'll show you how to eat your way to good health and fitness, from the two-stage intervention process through transition and into maintenance.

Before you begin, a word of medical caution: if you are pregnant or are currently taking medications to control cholesterol, blood pressure, fluid retention, or blood sugar, do not begin this regimen without a physician's guidance.

The Program in a Nutshell

• Determine your protein needs (page 92) and plan your meals around the right number of grams of protein. Choose fish, poultry, red meat, low-fat cheese (cottage cheese, feta, mozzarella, muenster), eggs, tofu. Be sure you get enough protein (your body can't store it); if you're hungry, it's fine to go beyond your requirement. 1 ounce of protein = 7 grams.

• Add 30 carbohydrate grams or less divided throughout the day for Phase I Intervention—(if you need to lose a lot of fat and/or correct a health problem)—or 55 grams or less per day for Phase II—if you want to lose a little fat, recompose your body (your lean to fat ratio), or improve your general health. If you're taking medication for a serious health problem or you're more than 20 percent overweight, you should have medical supervision. Remember, you can subtract the fiber grams from the carbohydrate grams in commercial foods (check the labels) which means you can eat more carbs. The subtracting has already been done for you in the food charts in the book. Choose green leafy vegetables, tomatoes, peppers, avocados (yes!), broccoli, eggplant, zucchini, green beans, asparagus, celery, cucumber, mushrooms, and salads. Check the carb bargain lists on pages 111, 112, and 114.

• Aim for 25 grams of fiber each day.

• Don't worry about fat, but choose healthy fats: olive oil, nut oils, avocado, and butter (yes!). Your body can and will use incoming fat as fuel.

• Never let yourself get hungry—keep snacks on hand and eat regular meals.

• Drink at least 8 glasses of water a day.

• A glass of wine (3 grams of carbohydrate) or a Miller Lite beer (slightly over 3) is fine, but count the carbs.

• Take a high-quality vitamin supplement (page 184) plus at least 90 mg of potassium.

• Artificial sweeteners and diet sodas are fine, in moderation.

- You'll be (temporarily) cutting out sugar and starches, even potates and beans (except green beans) and corn. Dessert can be a low-carb fruit—berries, peaches, melon—or sugar-free Jell-O.
- If you snack, remember to subtract those carb grams from your next meal.
- Exercise!—resistance training (with weights) is best, but any activity that makes you sweat is fine.
- When in doubt, eat lean meat, fish, or fowl and salad.
- Be sure to see the sample menus on page 216.

How Much Protein Do You Need?

The cornerstone of any good nutritional program is an adequate amount of high-quality protein. Whatever stage of our nutritional program you're in, it is of paramount importance that you get adequate daily protein.

In Chapter 4 you learned how to calculate your lean body mass and percentage of body fat. If you have not already done so, do this now. Your lean body mass (LBM) is the metabolically active part of you, consuming most of the energy, repairing the daily wear and tear on vital body structures, and replacing vital fluids and body chemi-

---

[1] We say ideally you hope to keep every pound, but in point of fact, if you are significantly overweight, you will probably lose some lean body mass as your declining weight reduces the demand on those muscles that get you from place to place. If you are currently more than 40 percent above your ideal weight, your weight-bearing muscles do more than their share of

cals—in short, doing all the work of living. It's what gives you a reason to eat. Ideally, you want to keep all of it, every glorious pound, so you must feed it, love it, water it, exercise it, and be thankful for it.[1] On typical low-calorie, high-carbohydrate, low-fat diets, protein intake is often marginal, and as a result as much as 50 percent of weight lost can be muscle weight. Each pound of active muscle mass lost reduces your rate of metabolism. (You can offset this loss by exercising your muscle mass against resistance-weight training, resistance stair stepping, etc. See Chapter 7.)

The proper care of a lean body mass requires that every day you provide it with enough high-quality complete protein to carry out all its vital functions. Specifically, each and every pound of your LBM needs six-tenths of 1 gram (0.6 gram) of protein every day if you are a person of moderate physical activity and fitness—that is, you do modest exercise for 20 to 30 minutes a couple of times a week. That means 60 grams of protein per day for a person with a 100-pound LBM, 72 grams per day for a person with a 120-pound LBM, 90 grams for a 150-pound LBM, and 108 grams per day for someone with a 180-pound LBM. Your specific daily protein need will depend on how many pounds of LBM you have and how active you are. If you are 40 percent or more above your ideal weight, you should rate yourself one activity category higher (more active) than you actually are to account for

---

work and they beef up to meet the demand placed on them. As your weight declines, the demand goes down, and the muscles can taper too. When this happens, they can weigh less because their work is less. That's fine. We just don't want you to lose pounds of muscle because you starved the muscle to death.

the increased work you must do when you walk, run, climb stairs, etc., carrying the excess pounds along.

The activity categories are as follows:

1. *Sedentary.* If you get no physical activity whatsoever, your protein need will be 0.5 gram per pound of lean mass. Sedentary = 0.5

2. *Moderately Active.* If you are average in physical activity, devoting 20 or 30 minutes to exercise two or three times per week, your protein need is 0.6 gram per pound of lean mass. Moderately active = 0.6

3. *Active.* If you participate in organized physical activity for more than 30 minutes three to five times per week, your protein need is 0.7 gram per pound of lean mass. Active = 0.7

4. *Very Active.* If you engage in vigorous physical activity lasting an hour or more five or more times per week, your lean mass requires 0.8 gram per pound. Very active = 0.8

5. *Athlete.* If you are a competitive athlete in training, doing twice-daily heavy physical workouts for an hour or more, your protein need is 0.9 gram per pound of lean mass. Athlete = 0.9

To figure your own daily protein need, simply take your LBM (in pounds) and multiply it by the activity category number that most closely describes your current level.

_____ pounds of lean body mass
× _____ activity category number
_____ = daily minimum protein need

The answer will be your minimum protein requirement in grams per day. Divide this number by three to discover your own minimum protein intake per meal, based on three meals per day.

_____ ÷ 3 = _____ grams per meal

Ideally, each of your three meals per day should contain *at least* this amount of high-quality complete protein, no matter which phase of the program you're following. You can use any standard guide of food contents (*The Complete Book of Food Counts,* Corinne T. Netzer, Dell, 1994, is a good one) to select foods that will fulfill your protein requirement.

We've made this plan even easier to follow; we've done the calculations for you by breaking down the protein intake per meal into four general categories with serving sizes for the main food sources of lean protein in various combinations. Refer now to the protein equivalency charts at the end of this chapter (starting on page 154), where you will find these four basic levels of protein intake providing 20 grams per meal, 27 grams per meal, 34 grams per meal, and 40 grams per meal. Select the equivalency chart that meets *and exceeds* your protein need, and you will find the serving sizes of these foods alone and in combination sufficient to meet your needs. Don't worry about getting too much protein; concern yourself with making sure you don't get too little.

Let's run through an example of how to use these charts. Imagine your protein need is 70 grams per day. Your protein requirement per meal is 70 divided by 3, or 23 grams per meal. Now turn to the protein equivalency charts. Chart A, the 20-gram-per-meal level, would not provide enough protein for you, so you would have to step up to Chart B, the 27-gram-per-meal level. Scan

down the left-hand side of the table and across the bottom
to find entries for each of the major sources of complete
protein: meat, eggs, hard cheese, soft cheese, curd cheese,
and tofu or soy. Select a protein source from the left side
and one from the bottom (note that they could be the
same source or you could combine different sources). Follow the table across from the left choice and up from the
bottom choice, and where the two intersect you will find
the serving size for that source or combination of sources.
For example, if you wanted to eat an omelet made of eggs
and soft cheese, you would find egg on the bottom and
soft cheese on the left and follow them to their intersection, where you would find that you would require 2
whole eggs plus 2 egg whites plus 2 ounces of soft cheese
to fulfill your needs at that meal.

You should also note that 1 ounce of lean "meat" and
1 ounce of hard cheese are equivalent in protein content.
Therefore, if you wanted to prepare your omelet with
smoked turkey and Gouda cheese, you could substitute
turkey for half the cheese and create a delicious egg dish
with 2 whole eggs plus 2 egg whites plus ½ ounce of
smoked turkey ½ ounce of shredded Gouda cheese.

You will also note that with regard to its protein content any "meat" source provides very close to 7 grams of
protein to the ounce. Whenever we refer to "meat" in our
discussions of the protein equivalent listing labeled "meat,
fish, or poultry," we mean beef, chicken, tuna, pork,
salmon, shrimp, scallops, herring, turkey, rabbit, alligator,
rattlesnake, wild boar, bass, lobster, gazelle . . . you get
the idea—all protein from animal sources is "meat" to us.
And that means that in conjunction with any of a wide variety of cheeses, tofu, and egg protein, and within the
boundaries of what you can and will eat, you can create

endless combinations of protein varieties to meet your daily needs.

I *CAN* EAT RED MEAT AND EGGS?

Yes, you can. And no, your cholesterol will not go up because you eat red meat and egg yolk. Because you'll be carefully controlling your metabolic hormones, your liver will not take the incoming saturated fats and dietary cholesterol from these (or any) foods and turn them into excess blood cholesterol. (See Chapter 13 for details.) Does that mean you could have steak and eggs for breakfast again? Sure. Or pork ribs for lunch? Yes. What you absolutely *cannot* do, however, is eat all the red meat and egg yolks you want and at the same time load up on starch and sugar. That means you can't have biscuits and gravy and hash brown potatoes with your steak and eggs.

If you suffer from elevated blood pressure, elevated cholesterol, marked fluid retention, or inflammatory conditions such as arthritis, bursitis, asthma, allergies, or skin rashes, you may want to limit your intake of red meat and egg yolk somewhat. We suggest this not because of the cholesterol content but because these foods are also rich in arachidonic acid, one of the fatty acids that leads directly to the production of the "bad" eicosanoids that promote or worsen these conditions. (See Chapter 12.) If you suffer from these problems, eliminate red meat and egg yolk entirely from your regimen for a full three weeks to see if your symptoms improve. Then eat a hearty serving of them for a meal or two and see if your symptoms return or worsen. If so, you are a person sensitive to the arachidonic acid content of foods and should take care to indulge only occasionally in these foods—especially egg yolk, the most concentrated source of arachidonic acid. And when you choose to eat beef, follow the guidelines for preparation from Chapter 12.

BUT WHAT IF I'M A VEGETARIAN?

Strict vegetarianism can create a little monotony in protein provisioning since the only adequate sources not overly laden with carbohydrate come in the form of soy (as tofu or tempeh) and the algae spirulina. You may find you have to get very creative, because you'll need to eat quite a lot of these to meet your protein need. The most serious deficiency that vegetarians face is protein malnourishment. Your choice of an animal-free diet doesn't alter your human need for enough good-quality protein to nourish your lean body mass, nor does it spare you from the consequences of getting too little.*

For example, our patient Kathy, a strict vegetarian, came to us complaining that she was always tired. Upon examining her, we found her triglycerides and blood pressure mildly elevated and her blood count a little low. Kathy had been active in running and sports until chronic foot pain and fatigue caused her to quit running; as a result, she began to gain a little weight. Although Kathy occasionally ate tofu, she primarily followed a nearly all-carbohydrate, low-fat to no-fat diet of whole grains, pasta, potatoes, rice, salads, fruits, and juices. Our first order of business was to increase her protein and fat intake and then reduce her reliance on starches. With an 88-pound lean body mass,

---

* See appendix for information on *The Soya Bluebook*.

Kathy needed at least 60 grams of protein per day, which meant ½-cup serving of firm tofu or about 3 ounces of tempeh at every meal along with some olive oil in such dishes as tofu stir-fry or tempeh burgers—a much larger quantity than she had been consuming. Within a few weeks she not only began to feel more energetic, but her triglycerides and blood pressure quickly normalized and she began to feel like running again.

Ovolactovegetarians will enjoy much greater variety in their diets since an endless variety of cheeses, eggs, a little yogurt, and other milk products can augment the tofu, tempeh, and spirulina. Take note on the protein equivalency charts that firm tofu provides a generous 10 grams of protein per ¼ cup with only about 2 grams of carbohydrate, whereas tempeh is slightly lower in protein content and higher in carbohydrate. Like animal "meats," tempeh provides 7 grams of protein to the ounce or ¼ cup but also contains 7 grams of carbohydrate. And spirulina, in dried form, is very protein rich, providing about 15 grams per ounce, but also contains 7 grams of carbohydrate.

NOT JUST THREE MEALS A DAY

Whether you're vegetarian or omnivorous, you must eat breakfast, lunch, and dinner each day to ensure that you meet the minimum amount of protein required to protect and provide for your lean body mass and that you spread out your intake throughout the day. *But remember that these three servings provide your minimum intake.* You may add additional protein in several snacks (more about snacks a little later on) during the day if you're hungry. A good rule of thumb for portion size in protein snacking is an amount equal to about half a protein meal serving. And although this is the ideal to which you aspire, because protein has a balancing effect on the hormones of metabolism, you needn't limit your protein intake to these amounts. If you're hungry—especially in the early part of your nutritional rehabilitation—eat lean protein to your heart's content. Additional lean protein won't disrupt the metabolic harmony you're striving to achieve. Later, when you've moved into a dynamic phase of correction, instead of cravings and hunger haunting you, you will more often have to remind yourself to eat all your meals.

The other major component in constructing your new nutritional regimen will be to set your carbohydrate limits, but before we do, let's go over the other components: fluid intake, fat, and vitamin, mineral, and electrolyte needs. None of these plays a role in driving or disrupting the metabolic apple cart, but they're still important, and you need to understand how they fit into your plan.

Don't Forget Your Vitamins, Minerals, and Electrolytes

As we point out in Chapter 6, optimal metabolic function depends on your getting adequate amounts of all the important vitamins and minerals regularly. If you eat all the kinds of fruits, vegetables, meats, cheeses, and grains that are available to you—even at the most restrictive stages of this diet—you will get adequate amounts of every necessary vitamin and mineral. Unfortunately, most of us have food likes and dislikes. We eat the things we like in quantity and usually make little effort to eat those foods we're not so fond of, even though they might contain important micronutrients. For that reason we ask that you supplement your food intake with a daily complete multiple vitamin and chelated mineral supplement—for good measure. You will find a number of good complete ones listed in Chapter 6.

Even if there is no food that you don't like and eat regularly, the power of insulin control to signal your kidney to waste excess fluid will result in potassium loss in urine. You will need to replace potassium in the first few weeks of your intervention to keep your body from becoming depleted. You can augment your potassium intake through the regular use of Morton's Lite Salt or NoSalt brand salt substitute, which are pure potassium salts, or by taking any of the supplemental potassium replacements listed in Chapter 6. *Remember! If you are currently taking blood pressure medication, ask your physician before you take extra potassium. Some of these medications prevent potassium loss, and your potassium level could become dangerously high from supplementing potassium while you are on the medication.*

So How Much Fat Can I Eat?

In Chapter 12 you learn which fats are best and why. Here they are in brief.

The Good Fats and Oils

Olive oil: extra-virgin, virgin, or pure
Nut oils: walnut, macadamia, hazelnut
Peanut oil

Sesame seed oil (light)
Avocado and avocado oil
Unsalted butter or clarified butter (saturated source)

More important, however, you learn why *fat doesn't make you fat*. Don't worry about eating high-quality monounsaturated and naturally saturated fats as long as you follow the plan guideline with regard to carbohydrate intake. Most of the problems associated with "dieting"— dry skin, brittle nails, dull hair, hair loss, the development of gallstones, menstrual irregularities, susceptibility to colds and other infections—occur because the fat content of the diet is too low. Because humans need fat and use it quite well as fuel, we don't limit fat in our clinic patients. We allow them to set their own intake need, because fat intake is self-regulating. By that we mean that people have a built-in "off" switch for fat consumption. Few people would sit and eat a stick of butter, consume lard by the spoonful, or swig olive oil by the cup. Without carbohydrate to wrap the fat around, it's not very appealing. When you don't eat chips, french fries, baked potatoes, doughnuts, cakes, pies, pastries, cookies, and chocolate, you avoid a huge amount of incoming fat, even when you get a moderate amount in lean meats. Select fats from the "good fat" list and eat them responsibly as you feel the need.

Unless your body fat storage signal has been turned on—i.e., excess dietary carbohydrate has elevated your in-

---

[2] If you are trying to lose weight—especially if you are a small person—you may have to curb your fat intake somewhat. Otherwise you may have too much food coming in, so your body won't need to dip into your fat stores—see the questions and answers at the end of this chapter.

sulin level—*your body can and will use incoming dietary fat as fuel to burn to meet its energy needs.*[2] You must remember, however, that if the fat storage system *has* been turned on by excess insulin driven by too much dietary carbohydrate, the fat coming in via your diet will know right where to go to find a good home—straight to your fat cells to be stored or to your liver to be turned into cholesterol. If you hope to correct the metabolic disturbance from which you suffer—be it excess body fat, elevated blood pressure, deranged blood sugar, excessive cholesterol production, or some combination of these—you cannot eat a diet that is both high in carbohydrate *and* full of fat.

However, if you carefully follow the guidelines of this plan—which means keeping a weather eye on your carbohydrate intake—*don't worry about counting fat grams.*

Drink Till You Float

We tell our patients to drink till they float, and for two very important reasons we want you to do the same thing. When you burn body fat or dietary fat for fuel in the absence of an abundance of carbohydrate, some of the fat may be burned incompletely. These partially burned fat by-products are called *ketones.* Far from being the dangerous or detrimental substance some nutritional authorities would have you think, ketones are nothing more than the natural by-product of fat breakdown. Your body can and will burn them for energy, or, if there are too many to use, it will dispose of them in your breath or by passing them out in the stool or in the urine. And this is where water drinking becomes important: the more water you drink, the more urine you make, the more ketones will pass out in the urine, and the more fat you lose. So drink up!

A second reason for increasing your water intake is exercise. Because your body in its hormonally balanced state will not retain excess fluid, the increased water loss in exercise can leave you dehydrated. Especially if you engage in vigorous athletic competition, *you must increase your water intake by as much as 50 percent!*

And although we've said "water" here, in truth any water-based fluid will work (as long as it doesn't have carbohydrate or calories). You need to drink *at least* 2 quarts of noncaloric fluid daily. Your fluid intake could be water, mineral water, diet soda, coffee, tea, or herbal tea. Your coffee or tea can be artificially sweetened or unsweetened, and you can lighten it with a small amount of whole milk or half-and-half. Both these lighteners have fewer carbohydrates than skim milk or nondairy creamers.

You may drink your coffee, tea, or diet cola caffeinated or decaffeinated. Most people don't have any trouble with caffeine use. But a few people will be sensitive enough to insulin output that the caffeine in beverages will keep their insulin levels somewhat elevated. If you are doing everything else right, and you find yourself still hungry between meals, still retaining fluid, or not losing weight at the rate you would predict, you may be one of those caffeine-sensitive people, and you should try to decaffeinate yourself.

Most of your daily intake should occur between and before meals. What difference could it make to your nutritional well-being *when* you drink your daily fluid requirement? Why not drink it with meals?

Although some people say drinking with meals slows them down, we've come to the conclusion that the only function cold beverages serve during a meal is to allow you to eat much faster and consume larger quantities of food than you otherwise would. Without water or a big glass of iced tea, we eat more slowly, chew the food better, enjoy the meal more, and eat a lot less than before. Now, we'll frequently have just a glass of wine with our meal. Try it yourself, and see if you don't eat much less when your meal isn't accompanied by a large cold beverage. Even though you're eating less, you don't feel deprived.

Instead, *precede* every meal, even breakfast, with the large beverage. Research suggests that drinking a large glass of cold water 15 to 30 minutes before a meal tends to reduce hunger, and as a result you will eat less. You'll also get a head start on drinking enough water; it's sometimes easy to forget to drink the full amount during the day. So our best advice is that you drink, drink, drink—before meals, in between meals, but not while you eat. Limit your mealtime beverage to ½ to 1 cup in sips, not gulps!

Bottoms Up: Wine and Spirits

If you like, have a glass of *dry,* not sweet, white or red wine with one of your meals. Several recent studies have shown wine (particularly red wine) to be an effective agent for increasing the body's sensitivity to insulin—the main goal of this program. Since we are shooting for lower insulin levels, it not only doesn't hurt to add the wine to our regimen; it actually helps. In our research files we have the report of an old study done by a New York physician back in the early sixties in which he divided his dieting patients into three groups—wine drinkers, hard-liquor drinkers, and nondrinkers. He kept all groups on the same reducing diet and found that the wine drinkers lost the most weight. He had no idea why; he just reported his results. They make sense now because we understand that wine improves insulin sensitivity. Many researchers believe the disparity between the levels of heart disease found in France and other southern European countries and those of the United States and Britain—the so-called French paradox—can be laid at the doorstep of increased wine consumption. And so, like the French, Italians, and others living around the Mediterranean, we can increase our insulin sensitivity, decrease our insulin levels, and enjoy life more by adding a moderate amount of wine to our program.

Moderate means a glass of wine or two—no more—with one meal. Wine does have some carbohydrate content left in it after the fermentation process, so the drier the wine, the fewer grams of carbohydrate it will contain. A good rule of thumb is that *dry* white and red wines contain about 1 to 1.5 grams of carbohydrate per ounce; sweet dessert wines or sherries contain significantly more, too many more to enjoy them in the intervention phases of this program. If you choose to drink wine with your meals, remember to include these grams as a part of your daily carbohydrate allotment. More on that in the next section.

Distilled spirits, while they contain scant to no carbohydrates—it's all been turned to alcohol—tend to *raise* insulin and to impair insulin sensitivity if consumed in more than modest quantities. In general, avoid distilled alcohol during your intervention, except for an occasional cocktail containing a single ounce of distilled liquor, straight, on the rocks, or in a mixed drink (no sweet mixers allowed).

An occasional margarita is okay if you make your own without the sugar syrup most bars use. Forget about beer, except Miller Lite (3.2 grams of carbohydrate per can).

Controlling the Starches and Sugars

To achieve metabolic control, your tasks are simple—reduce the amount of insulin circulating in your blood during the day and restore the sensitivity of your tissues to insulin. The quickest—and actually the only—way to achieve metabolic control is to restrict the amount of metabolically active carbohydrate you put into the system. Does this mean that you can never enjoy fruit or bread or pasta again? No. But it does mean that you will at first need to lean toward the carbohydrate bargains in these food categories and exert some control over your intake. How much control? That depends on how out of kilter your system currently is, based on your medical history and/or laboratory evaluations. For that reason we have provided two levels of intervention. Select the protocol that most closely describes your own condition and begin there.

PHASE I INTERVENTION—30 GRAMS
CARBOHYDRATE OR LESS PER DAY

If you are overfat by 20 percent or more, have high blood pressure, elevated cholesterol and/or triglycerides, low HDL cholesterol, type II diabetes or glucose intolerance, or have any combination of these disorders, you need strong corrective action and must begin with this protocol. Phase I places the strongest rein on insulin output and will help you gain control of your insulin production quickly.

PHASE II INTERVENTION—55 GRAMS OF CARBOHYDRATE PER DAY

This phase also lowers insulin production but allows for a slightly richer carbohydrate intake. We offer this phase for people who need to reduce their body weight by less than 20 percent to reach ideal weight and have none of the metabolic conditions just mentioned, for people who are happy at their current weight but wish to reduce body fat and build lean muscle, and as an intermediate step for people who began with Phase I and have now normalized their blood pressure, blood lipids, and blood sugars.

COUNTING CARBS THE SMART WAY

You may refer to one of the standard reference guides such as *The Complete Book of Food Counts* to develop your own portions of vegetables, salads, fruits, and cereal grains to meet your carbohydrate quota. But remember in calculating your carbohydrate intake for these foods that the actual usable carbohydrate content of a given food is the total carbohydrate content minus the dietary fiber—what we call the *effective carbohydrate content* or *ECC* (see pages 158–168). In a nutshell, this means that you don't have to count the fiber grams in your daily carbohydrate total because the fiber doesn't act metabolically as a carbohydrate. *The usable carbohydrate per serving as given on a standard nutrition label for a food will be the total carbohydrate content listed, minus any dietary fiber listed.*

You don't have to calculate any portions if you don't want to. We've developed a list of the effective carbohydrate content for a wide range of everyday foods. Refer to the effective carbohydrate content charts, where we've given you specific tables listing the ECC for fruits, vegetables, and breads and cereal grains in usable portion sizes. The values are arranged in 5-gram increments, so you will find a 5-gram portion, a 10-gram portion, a 15-gram portion, a 20-gram portion, and a 25-gram portion for each food listed. All you have to do is decide what food you want to eat, and the list will automatically tell you how much of it you can have at that carbohydrate level. Next to the serving size you will see the actual number of grams of carbohydrate the serving contains (in most cases it will be equal to that gram level or slightly below it). You will see that the standard portion of some foods is actually considerably less than 5 grams—these entries represent real carbohydrate bargains. See our bargain boxes on pages 111, 112, and 114.

For example, on a Phase I diet, at breakfast you might choose to spend your 7 to 10 grams of carbohydrate as 1 cup of sliced strawberries or as a slice of buttered "light" wheat toast. Or at lunch you might like five saltine crackers with your tuna salad, or perhaps you'd prefer half an apple. For 7 grams in a carbohydrate meal or snack, you *could* eat any of the items in the box. Remember that once it is digested, your body turns all carbohydrate to sugar, so from that standpoint all these entries are equivalent. However, what's missing from the junk choices are the fiber, the vitamins and minerals, and the cancer-fighting phyto-

---

Carbohydrate Comparisons

7 Skittles = 1 marshmallow = 1 medium raw carrot = $1/3$ medium banana = $1/4$ very small potato = 1 caramel = $1/7$ Milky Way bar = $1/2$ Reese's peanut butter cup = 14 Reese's Pieces = 7 jelly beans = $1/3$ Hershey Bar = $1/2$ cup grapes = $1/2$ orange = $1/2$ cup melon = $1/2$ cup fresh berries = 1 Starburst fruit chew = 7 cups mushrooms = 14 cups fresh lettuce = $3^1/2$ cups fresh broccoli = 3 french fries

---

chemicals found in the fresh fruits and vegetables. The choice of what you eat is always yours, but so are the consequences of that choice. Choose wisely.

You'll quickly see that most of your foods at this level will be in their natural state.

You will also note that at the higher levels of carbohydrate per portion—where you will be in maintenance—a number of foods are listed as "unlimited." This means that reaching that carbohydrate level in a single serving would give you an amount too large for anyone to consume. In these cases, refer to the lower carbohydrate levels for that food to see how many grams a more realistically sized portion contains.

The ECC charts make it easy for you to ferret out those foods lowest in carbohydrate for Phase I, when your per-meal carbohydrate intake will be small, as well as to assemble combinations of carbohydrate foods when your per-meal carbohydrate intake increases as you move to Phase II or into maintenance. For example, in Phase II your total carbohydrate intake per meal will be 15 grams.

Carbohydrate Bargains Under 1 Gram of Carbohydrate

1 cup alfalfa sprouts (0.4)
$^1/_2$ cup arugula (0.4)
1 cup sliced bok choy (0.8)
1 celery rib (0.9)
1 tablespoon minced chives (0.1)
$^1/_2$ cup sliced endive (0.8)
1 cup shredded lettuce (0.4)
1 tablespoon chopped canned pimiento (0.6)
$^1/_2$ cup sliced raw radicchio (0.9)
5 radishes (0.8)
1 cup fresh spinach (0.6)

That means you could have one serving from the 15-gram-portion column for a single food or that you could have three servings from the 5 gram-portion column for three different foods—or one from the 10-gram-portion column and one from the 5-gram one. By the time you get to maintenance—where in a later section you will learn that your per-meal carbohydrate intake may be 20, 25, or more grams—you might be able to select five different carbohydrate foods and have the 5-gram portion for all of them at one meal! Or you could choose any combination—the total must simply add up to the amount you need at your meal or snack.

The ECC charts will take you effortlessly from early intervention all the way through maintenance and beyond, so make copies of these lists and tape them to the front of your refrigerator.

Carbohydrate Bargains of 3 or Fewer Grams of Carbohydrate

$^1/_4$ cup blackberries (2.9)
6 fresh asparagus spears (2.4)
$^1/_2$ cup canned asparagus (2.8)
4 frozen asparagus spears (2.9)
$^1/_2$ cup canned bamboo shoots (2.3)
1 cup chopped raw broccoli (2.2)
$^1/_2$ cup frozen broccoli/cauliflower florets (2.7)
$^3/_4$ cup frozen broccoli/pearl onions/red peppers (2.6)
$^1/_4$ cup cooked sliced carrots (3.0)
1 cup cauliflower florets (2.6)
$^1/_2$ medium cucumber (3)
$^1/_4$ cup chopped leeks (2)
$^1/_2$ cup raw mushroom pieces (1.1)
$^1/_2$ cup cooked mushroom pieces (2.3)
5 whole enoki mushrooms (2)
$^1/_2$ cup chopped raw scallions (2.5)
$^1/_2$ cup chopped parsley (1.9)
$^1/_2$ cup chopped sweet pepper (2.4)
1 tablespoon chopped raw shallot (1.7)
$^1/_2$ cup boiled sliced summer squash (2.6)
1 medium tomatillo (2)
1 cup raw turnip greens (1.8) (or $^1/_2$ cup cooked)

To Snack or Not to Snack?

If that is the question, in America the answer is usually "Snack!" But before you get the wrong idea, by *snack* we don't mean cupcakes and chips. We mean a well-composed small meal or a little meal on the run.

The crux of controlling your metabolism lies in controlling your metabolic hormones: insulin and glucagon. When you eat a meal (or snack) made up of the proper composition of protein and carbohydrate, you set the hormonal tone in your body for the next several hours. After that time you need to fine-tune the system again. In the course of a normal day that will mean eating four or more times a day, and for most of us that translates into breakfast, lunch, dinner, and a snack or two.

Quick snacks on the run should still ideally provide high-quality protein (a good rule of thumb is an amount equal to one-half your regular protein meal) with a controlled amount of carbohydrate. *Snack* is not a euphemism for junk, although as a country we've come to think so. Now you have to work a little to find commercially available snack foods that are not composed mainly of carbohydrate, but there are a few out there. Be patient. Remember how the food manufacturing industry quickly hopped on the low-fat bandwagon to bring us fat-free pretzels, fat-free cookies, fat-free coffee cake, ice cream, and potato chips? Well, as the tide of nutrition turns—and believe us, it is turning—we'll all soon be bobbing about in a sea of commercially packaged carbohydrate-restricted snacks. Until then, good snacks could include those in the box.

Remember that your three regular meals will provide your minimum daily protein need, so you don't ab-

Carbohydrate Bargains of 5 or Fewer Grams of Carbohydrate

$^1/_2$ medium avocado (3.7)
$^1/_4$ cup blueberries (4.3)
$^1/_2$ cup strawberries (3.3)
$^1/_2$ cup beet greens (3.9)
$^1/_2$ cup frozen Pillsbury broccoli/carrots (3.1)
4 brussels sprouts (3.4)
1 cup red or green cabbage (3.6)
1 medium carrot (5)
$^1/_2$ cup chopped Swiss chard (3.6)
$^1/_2$ cup chopped dandelion greens (3.3)
$^1/_2$ cup diced eggplant (3.2)
$^1/_2$ cup chopped fresh fennel (3.1)
$^1/_2$ cup sliced snap beans (3.8)
$^1/_4$ cup frozen Japanese-style vegetables (3.7)
1 cup mustard greens (4)
1 whole hot chili pepper (4.3)
$^1/_2$ cup chopped jalapeño peppers (4.2)
$^1/_2$ cup boiled unsweetened rhubarb (3.5)
1 cup frozen spinach (3.1)
$^1/_2$ cup spaghetti squash (5)
1 cup raw diced summer squash (4)
1 medium tomato (4.3)
1 cup boiled turnip pieces (4.4)
4 whole water chestnuts (4)
$^1/_2$ cup canned sliced water chestnuts (4.5)
$^1/_2$ cup sliced wax beans (4.5)

Snack Possibilities

Snack	Portion	Protein	Carb
Sunflower seeds	1 oz.	5	4
Walnuts	1 oz.	4	5
Macadamia nuts	1 oz.	3	4
Peanuts	1 oz.	7	5
Pork rinds	1 oz.	17	0
Lean meat slices	1 oz.	7	0–1
String cheese	1 oz.	6	1
Meat/cheese/cracker	½ oz each on 2 crackers	7	4
Homemade peanut butter crackers	1 T./2 crackers	4	5
Hard-cooked egg	1 large	6	0.6
Cottage cheese	¼ cup	7	2
Apple/cheddar slices	¼ apple/1 oz.	7	6
Jerky	1 oz.	7	1
Sandwich (light bread, 1 oz. meat)	½	7	7

solutely have to snack—it's optional. But if you choose to do so, especially during the first few weeks of the diet, while you're gaining corrective momentum (see the questions and answers at the end of this chapter for an explanation), you should stick carefully to the guidelines.

Phase I Intervention

BREAKFAST

1 protein meal serving*
7–10 grams carbohydrate†
2 cups noncaloric fluid
(1–1¹/₂ cups before meal, ¹/₂–1 cup during)
Multivitamin and mineral supplement
Potassium supplement or added potassium

OPTIONAL MORNING SNACK

¹/₂ protein meal serving
5 grams carbohydrate
1 cup noncaloric fluid

LUNCH

1 protein meal serving
7–10 grams carbohydrate†
2 cups noncaloric fluid
(1–1¹/₂ cups before meal, ¹/₂–1 cup during)
Potassium supplement or added potassium

OPTIONAL AFTERNOON OR BEDTIME SNACK

¹/₂ protein meal serving
5 grams carbohydrate
1 cup noncaloric fluid

---

* You must calculate *your* protein requirement, page 92.
† You should reduce your carbohydrate intake per meal to 7 grams if you choose to eat the optional snacks—unless they contain zero carbohydrate. You may combine the contents of one snack with a meal or have wine with dinner; however, *do not allow the total carbohydrate content of any meal to exceed 12 grams or the total for the day to exceed 30 grams.*

DINNER

1 protein meal serving
7–10 grams carbohydrate†
2 cups noncaloric fluid
(1–1¹/₂ cups before meal, ¹/₂–1 cup during)
Potassium supplement or added potassium

Phase I Worksheet

Record your values below:

Lean Body Mass = _____ pounds.

Protein requirement per day = _____ grams.

Protein requirement per meal = _____ grams.

   As ounces of lean meat = _____ ounces.

   As egg protein = _____ eggs + _____
egg whites.

   As curd cheese = _____ cup(s).

   As tofu = _____ ounce(s).

   Combined sources =

_____

_____

_____

Daily carbohydrate total = 30 grams.

Carbohydrate per meal = 7–10 grams.

Carbohydrate per snack = 5 or fewer grams.

Portion sizes for your favorite carbohydrate choices:

_____

_____

_____

_____

Phase II Intervention
BREAKFAST

1 protein meal serving*
15 grams carbohydrate
2 cups noncaloric fluid
(1–1¹/₂ cups before meal, ¹/₂–1 cup during)
Multivitamin and mineral supplement

OPTIONAL MORNING SNACK†

¹/₂ protein meal serving
5 grams carbohydrate
1 cup noncaloric fluid

LUNCH

1 protein meal serving
15 grams carbohydrate
2 cups noncaloric fluid
(1–1¹/₂ cups before meal, ¹/₂–1 cup during)

OPTIONAL AFTERNOON OR BEDTIME SNACK†

1/2 protein meal serving
5 grams carbohydrate
1 cup noncaloric fluid

---

* You must calculate *your* protein requirement, page 92.

† You may combine the two snacks to make a single larger one if you so desire, you may drop them entirely, you may use them following the meals as a dessert, or you may add the snacks to any two of the other three meals to make them slightly larger meals. *In no event should you allow your carbohydrate intake for any one meal or snack to exceed 20 grams or your daily total to exceed 55 grams.*

DINNER

1 protein meal serving
15 grams carbohydrate
2 cups noncaloric fluid
(1–1¹/₂ cups before meal, ¹/₂–1 cup during)
Potassium supplement or added potassium

Phase II Worksheet

Record your values below:

Lean Body Mass = _____ pounds.

Protein requirement per day = _____ grams.

Protein requirement per meal = _____ grams.

As ounces of lean meat = _____ ounces.

As egg protein = _____ eggs + _____ egg whites.

As tofu = _____ ounce(s).

As curd cheese = _____ cup(s).

Combined sources = _____

_____

_____

_____

Daily carbohydrate total = 55 grams.

Carbohydrate per meal = 15 grams.

Carbohydrate per snack = 5 grams.

Portion sizes for favorite carbohydrate choices: _____

_____

_____

_____

_____

Following the Plan

Now that you're acquainted with the diet plans, let us explain how to use them to reclaim your health, fitness, and vitality.

If your current state of health dictates that you should begin with Phase I—i.e., you need to lose more than 20 percent of your weight, you suffer from elevated blood pressure, cholesterol, or triglycerides or disturbances in blood sugar, or your laboratory evaluation (see Chapter 4 for complete recommendations) uncovered abnormalities such as elevation of your insulin or hemoglobin A_1c—you should remain in Phase I, adhering as strictly to the plan as you possibly can, until your abnormal laboratory values and/or blood pressure readings have stabilized in the normal range and have remained so for at least four weeks. By that time you should have developed a corrective momentum and the metabolic changes that have taken place should now permit you to slide up to Phase II and a slightly higher carbohydrate intake. If you are more than 20 percent above your ideal body weight remain on Phase II until you are near your goal.

If you are currently on medication to lower your blood pressure, blood sugar, or cholesterol, you should remain at Phase I, adhering as strictly as possible to the plan, until your medication doses are significantly reduced or eliminated *by your physician* and your readings have remained normal for at least four weeks. *This plan is so powerful in lowering blood pressure, blood sugar, and blood fats that you must under no circumstances attempt it without close supervision by a physician. You will not be able to remain on your current medications at your current doses safely. Your physician will need to taper and in all probability discontinue your medications for these problems once you begin Phase I. Do not make these changes on your own.* Once your medications have been tapered and your readings have remained stable for at least four weeks, you may move to the Phase II plan for the duration of your diet, just as we've described.

If you are not overweight and have used the diet only to reduce elevated blood fats, blood pressure, or blood sugar, when all your readings are stable you should move to Phase II for three to four weeks and then begin your transition to maintenance.

If you are overweight but have no other metabolic disturbances and are using the plan as a tool to reduce excess body fat and/or recompose your weight, begin on Phase I for four to six weeks, then move to the Phase II plan and remain there until you are near your goal.[3] Your goal should be to work toward an ideal body composition of under 20 percent body fat if you are an average male and approximately 20 to 25 percent if you are an average female.[4] We give you these ideal percentages as targets. Aim for them, and if you hit them, fantastic! Depending on where you've begun this journey toward fitness, getting there may take some time, but every percentage point closer that you come to that ideal is travel

---

[3] If you choose to remain in Phase I, you may do so. Some of our patients have found that remaining on the more restrictive plan lessens their cravings for carbohydrate foods. If you find that by moving to Phase II you seem hungrier, drop back to Phase I and remain there until you approach your goal.

[4] Competitive athletes will be leaner: 8 to 12 percent fat for men and low to mid-teens in percentage for women. We do not advise women to push their body fat percentages lower than this because of the increased risk for menstrual changes and infertility.

in the right direction—toward a leaner, healthier you. Take your time; you can safely stay on this plan as long as it takes to reach your health and fitness goals. How long is that? Read on.

Recomposing Your Body

If a part of your goal is to lose excess body fat—and for most people who suffer from insulin resistance, it is—this plan offers you the easiest and most effective system available for doing that quickly, safely, and permanently. The two questions most often asked by our clinic patients are "How fast can I lose and how long will it take me to get to my goal?" and "How many calories can I eat a day?" We've spent nearly a decade taking care of thousands of overweight people, and we have found that you don't usually have to worry about calories on this program.[5] The metabolic alterations that take place as your insulin falls and your sensitivity to it improves will increase the rate at which you use calories, and you will find that the standard calorie rules simply don't apply in predicting weight loss.

---

[5] When you're eating a diet structured to keep the metabolic hormones in balance, your caloric intake will pretty much take care of itself. Eat all your meals and snacks every day, and even if you're not especially hungry (this happens more often than you would imagine), be sure that your intake never falls below about 850 to 1,000 calories a day.

FAT LOSS VS. WEIGHT LOSS

You will note that we specifically said *fat loss*, not *weight loss*. From this moment forward, we ask that you divorce yourself from the notion that you want to lose **weight**. You don't. You want to lose **fat** and **size** and become lean and healthy again. You want to recompose your body by losing excess fat and maintaining your lean mass as closely as you can. And that's a very different proposition from merely losing weight. Weight includes everything. It's water; it's what's in your stomach or intestine or bladder; it's fat; it's muscle.

This plan is designed to help you lose fat and not muscle. When you follow it diligently, you will lose fat steadily. And remember, when fat is what you lose, size changes occur very quickly, because six pounds of fat takes up almost a gallon of space in volume!

Your weight on the scale may not always reflect an accurate loss of fat from week to week, again because everything has weight. Fluctuations in rate of scale weight loss occur especially with women who regularly experience fluid gains and losses with menstrual cycling. In a given week a woman might have lost 2 pounds of fat but retained 3 pounds of water. When she steps on the scale, all she sees is a 1-pound gain. For that reason we encourage our patients not to rely on the scale as a measure of progress except over the long haul. A much more reliable measure is your volume. Select an article of clothing—a pair of pants or jeans, a fitted skirt or dress—that you cannot currently wear. Each week, attempt to put it on and chart how close you come. Maybe the pants will come only to mid-thigh level. Fine. But in a few weeks you'll find that you can pull them all the way up. Not zip them, mind you, but get them on. Then the zipper gets closer to meeting week by week, until one day it will actually zip if you lie down across the bed and wrestle with it. Finally, it will zip easily.

That's how it was for our patient Wayne, who began his corrective regimen under our care at a weight of 326 pounds, suffering from high blood pressure and sleep apnea,[6] with a 56-inch waist. (Wayne had actually begun his own attempt to reduce at 340 pounds using a low-fat diet and heavy exercise. After a year, he'd lost only 14 pounds!) Wayne used his 56-inch belt as his gauge, making a new hole every inch along the way, until his waist measured 36 inches. Now—eight months since he began our diet—he's working to get back into his 34-waist blue jeans. Of course, he has also been able to track his progress in other ways: he no longer needs to take blood pressure medication, and the machine that he once depended on to help him breathe during sleep is gathering dust on a shelf.

This volume-measuring technique really gives you a true reflection of your progress—nothing has changed about the clothing; what's changed is your size. It also helps to take your focus away from the scale as an indication of how poorly or how well you've done. It helps to reinforce the important message that it's not what you weigh, but what your weight is made of that counts.

---

[6] Many excessively overweight people suffer from sleep apnea, which means that they quit breathing in their sleep many times during the night, rousing themselves almost awake but not quite. They sleep fitfully, restlessly, usually snore loudly, and toss about. They awaken fatigued and fall asleep easily during the day.

Put It in Writing

Make copies of the following worksheet entitled Daily Meal Outline and use it to design your daily meal plans. We encourage you to use it every day to plan for and think about what you are going to eat and where: Will you be eating breakfast at home? On the way to work? Grabbing something on the run? Sitting down with family? Will you dine at your desk at lunch, or do you need to meet with clients or friends and dine out? What will you eat? Where? When you plan ahead, you will find you won't very often get caught in that well-known spot where there's simply nothing for you to eat but a honey bun and a soft drink!

Try to be as honest with your records as you can. A common finding by garbologists is that most Americans eat much more junk food than they admit to, and they admit to a fair amount. One such study in Arizona a few years ago reported that residents ate 20 times more chocolate and 15 times more pastries than they reported having eaten in a consumer survey.

Try to make it a habit to keep good records of what you're eating, how much you exercise, and how you feel. Having an accurate written record also gives you some hard data to look at if you hit a plateau (see Questions Commonly Asked About the Program, page 138) or don't lose fat at your predicted rate. Are you simply eating too much? Have you missed exercising regularly? Are you drinking your fluid and taking your vitamins? Drinking a lot of caffeine? Eating more carbohydrate than you realized? Having a journal to review will help you answer those questions honestly.

Make the commitment that if it goes into your mouth

it goes into your journal. Studies have shown that people who will commit to keeping an honest and accurate diary of nutrition and exercise are as much as four times more successful than people who will not. So plan for success and you will succeed!

Daily Meal Outline

BREAKFAST

(Protein source)_____

(Carb source)_____

(Fluid)_____

MORNING SNACK (?)

(Protein source)_____

(Carb source)_____

(Fluid)_____

LUNCH

(Protein source)_____

(Carb source)_____

(Fluid)_____

AFTERNOON OR BEDTIME SNACK (?)

(Protein source)_____

(Carb source)_____

(Fluid)_____

DINNER

(Protein source)_____

(Carb source)_____

(Fluid)_____

Restaurant Dining Guide

For those of you who eat out often and get most of your nutrition either on the run or on the road, this dining guide will help you make selections in keeping with your *Protein Power* prescription. Even if you don't own a skillet, you can successfully restore your health, fitness, and metabolism dining out.

*Alcohol: A single 3-ounce glass of dry red or white wine or a Miller Lite will add 3 to 4 grams of carbohydrate to your meal.

*Beverages: diet soda, water, mineral water, tea or coffee without sugar.

*Desserts: Fresh berries or fresh fruit salad will work. Avoid cakes, cookies, custards, pies, pastries, and ice cream.

American Grill or Bistro

*Grilled meat, fish, or fowl, a large green salad with ranch, blue cheese, or olive oil vinaigrette dressing; steamed or sautéed vegetables in place of the usual potatoes, pasta, or rice. Hold the bread and crackers.

*Chef's salad or grilled chicken Caesar salad. Beware the croutons and crackers—limit to four or five of either on maintenance.

*Quiche and green salad or small fresh fruit salad. Eat only the quiche filling, scooping it out of the crust.

*Tomato stuffed with chicken, tuna, or crab

salad, or cottage cheese. Keep crackers to a limit of three or four, none on intervention.

Barbecue Joint

*Sliced beef, pork, chicken, or dry rub ribs with cole slaw and tossed salad. Deviled eggs are fine. Ask for barbecue sauce on the side and limit it to a tablespoon, none on intervention. Hold the beans, fries, or other potatoes and Texas toast, bread, or biscuits.

Fast Foods/Burger Joints

*Grilled chicken sandwich or burger (with cheese and bacon if you like) along with a side salad, ranch, blue cheese, or Italian dressing. Remove one or both buns and eat with a knife and fork. Avoid the fries, baked potatoes, pasta bar, pies, and sundaes.

*Grilled chicken salad with ranch or Italian dressing.

*Sub-sandwich-style (but no bread), deli meats and cheeses on salad greens with ranch or Italian dressing.

Chinese Restaurant

*Soups: Egg drop or hot and sour soup.

*Appetizers: Skewered beef or chicken.

*Beef, chicken, pork, shrimp (or combinations) with broccoli or assorted mixed Chinese vegetables.

Avoid: Egg roll, noodles, mu shu pancakes, and limit rice to about $1/8$ to $1/4$ cup. Read your fortune, give away the cookie!

French Restaurant

*Clear soups and fresh green salads.

*Medallions of beef or pork finished with butter sauces, green peppercorn sauce, or Choron sauce.

*Roasted lamb, duck, quail, game hen.

*Grilled or poached fish.

*Sauté of vegetables (squashes, carrots, onion, cauliflower, asparagus).

Avoid: bread, potatoes, rice, and heavy cream sauces, which may contain significant carbohydrate from flour.

Indian Restaurant

*Tandoori chicken or lamb; chicken, beef, or lamb curry; chicken tikka or chicken masala.

*Tossed green salad, tomato and cucumber salad, pickled onion, *zukeni bhaghi* (stewed zucchini and yellow squash), *saag panir* (creamy spinach).

Avoid: The breads, breaded and fried vegetables, potato dishes, and limit rice to a tablespoon or two.

Italian Restaurant

*Sautéed (not breaded) calamari or antipasto appetizers.

*Chicken or veal piccata, grilled fish or pork cutlet, or rotisserie or grilled chicken with tossed salad and any sautéed or steamed vegetables available to substitute for pasta.

Avoid: The pasta dishes and bread. Even a single piece of garlic bread can contain 14 or more grams of carbohydrate.

Japanese Sushi/Teriyaki Restaurant

*Sushi or sashimi. Beware of overeating the rice.

*Miso soup (seaweed, broth, and bean curd).

*Teriyaki chicken, beef, or fish with salad. Avoid tempura, which is breaded and fried.

Mexican Restaurant

*Chicken or beef fajitas, minus the tortilla wrappers. Eat the garnishes: lettuce, chopped tomato, guacamole, sour cream, pico de gallo.

*Grilled chicken, fish, beef, beef or pork medallions, or shredded beef, pork, or chicken with *insalata mista* (tossed salad).

*Taco salad—but leave the shell uneaten.

Avoid (for intervention) or strictly limit: rice and beans (no more than 1 tablespoon of either), tortilla wrappers (one half), shells (one half), or chips (3 or 4).

Pizza Parlor

*Pizza and a tossed salad with ranch, blue cheese, or Italian dressing. Load up the toppings you like: the trick is to eat only the toppings and leave the crust uneaten.

Avoid: breadsticks, garlic toast, spaghetti or other pasta dishes.

Transition and Maintenance

When are you ready to make the transition from intervention to maintenance?

1. When you have reduced or eliminated any medicines you took to lower blood pressure, blood sugar, or blood fats with Phase I and normalized your readings for at least four weeks and these values have remained stable in Phase II for an additional three to four weeks.

2. When you have recomposed your weight to your desired lean and fat percentages on Phase II.

3. When you are within 5 percent of your ideal body weight if you're using the plan to lose body fat.

4. When you must leave the plan for some reason—such as surgery, pregnancy, severe injury, or illness. You should not place yourself in a reduced-calorie state in any of these circumstances, and you should, if they arise, quickly move to controlled maintenance at sufficient calories to meet their high energy demands even if you have not reached your ultimate goal. Because these kinds of situations often occur without warning, you will need to hasten your transition to a maintenance level. If you have even a few days, follow the step-by-step instructions outlined here as day-by-day increases in intake instead of week by week. It's not the best solution, but it will suffice in an emergency. Once the situation resolves and you have healed completely, you can resume your Phase I or Phase II diet as before—with all the same caveats.

The Smooth Transition

The next several weeks are the most important of the entire regimen, so take great care to follow the guidelines strictly. For some time your body has been in a controlled slide, a state of corrective momentum. It's now time to gently slow and then stop the momentum of those changes and equilibrate and stabilize at your new leaner, healthier level.

The changes that you've wrought occurred because you harnessed your rampaging insulin and kept it under tight rein. Your job now is to slowly and carefully let out some slack. You will accomplish this by gradually increasing your per-meal carbohydrate level until you reach a daily total carbohydrate gram intake roughly equal to or slightly more than your daily protein intake. It's important that you make this transition to maintenance slowly and methodically (except in the face of emergencies). Moving in one big leap from the controlled carbohydrate level that's kept you in a state of hormonal balance to your maintenance level will stimulate a sudden big release of insulin with all the attendant potential for adverse consequences.

Move from Phase II to maintenance according to the following guidelines: Increase your daily carbohydrate intake in 10-gram increments until you reach an amount approximately equal to your daily protein intake—e.g., if your daily protein intake is 75 grams, increase your daily carbohydrate gram total from 55 grams (the Phase II level) to 65 grams and finally to 75 grams. Remain at each new higher intake level for five to seven days to stabilize your insulin production before advancing again. This slow upward climb will allow you to ease the reins on your insulin production and prevent rebound weight gain, fluid retention, or blood pressure increases that could occur by turning insulin loose all at once.

If you are active or very active physically, or if you continue to lose weight while consuming protein and carbohydrate in equal amounts, you may continue to increase your carbohydrate grams in 10-gram jumps (again, stabilizing after each jump for five to seven days) until your carbohydrate intake exceeds your protein intake by 30 percent. For a daily protein intake of 75 grams, you would multiply 75 by 1.3 for a total carbohydrate intake of 97.5 grams (which you could round up to 100 grams) per day. A few people might even be able to go to a little higher carbohydrate intake, but in general your maintenance carbohydrate level should be equal to or up to about 30 percent more than your protein intake.

If weight reduction was a part of your goal, *slowly* increase your carbohydrate intake as outlined until your carbohydrate intake equals your protein intake or until you stop losing weight. Remain at that daily total carbohydrate level for two months to allow your fat cell activity to stabilize.[7] Then slowly—in 10-gram jumps followed each time by a five- to seven-day stabilization period—continue to increase your daily carbohydrate intake. Weigh yourself (a poor measurement, we know, but the handiest one for this purpose) at the end of each stabilization period, and when you first see a gain, drop back to the last carbohydrate gram intake at which your weight remained stable and stay there.[8]

Refer to your ECC charts for fruits, vegetables, and bread and cereal grains. You can enjoy these 10-gram jumps by selecting servings of those higher-carbohydrate goodies you've been missing. For example, you might add a peach at breakfast if you love fruit; an extra half pita pocket at lunch, a small serving of pasta, or a small biscuit

---

[7] The very act of weight loss causes your fat cells to *want* to store fat. This heightened storage activity falls back to normal after several months. This is another reason why it's in your best interest to get focused on the program and lose all your excess at once, not stop-start.

[8] Your weight will be a reflection of appropriate carbohydrate intake only if you've actually adhered to that daily gram total. If you intentionally or inadvertently exceed your prescribed carbohydrate total, you will retain fluid quickly, which will cause a gain in scale weight. It's important that you be very careful to follow your plan during this period.

with your dinner if you've missed starches; or a small frozen yogurt as a snack to satisfy your sweet tooth. Ideally, try to spread your added carbohydrate intake throughout the day instead of piling it all onto one meal, because *the more carbohydrate you eat at a sitting, the bigger insulin response you'll stir up.* (Although it's better not to do so, if you do plan to bank your carbohydrates to eat a bigger serving—for example, you've planned a "night on the town"—scale back the carbohydrate portion of the remaining meals or snacks throughout the day so that your total intake doesn't exceed your allotment. And remember, it's better *not* to do this!)

In our years of practice we've seen people who would begin to lose their metabolic control on fewer than 60 grams per day and others who had to push their carbohydrate intake above 150 grams per day to stop weight loss. Each of us is a little different, and what you will discover through your diligent upward creep in making this transition from intervention to maintenance is your own tolerance level for carbohydrate intake. The key to maintaining your correction is keeping your daily intake of carbohydrate at or very near this level most of the time. Now we'll show you how to develop a realistic strategy for maintaining your achievement and still enjoying your life.

YOU *CAN* MAINTAIN FOR LIFE

You've worked hard to reclaim your health, to reduce or recompose your weight, and to restore your body to balance. Now the work of living within the system begins. With your new understanding of how food influences the hormones of metabolism you have the key to maintaining your health and fitness for the rest of your life. The choice of whether to eat a well-composed meal or a poorly com-posed one will always be yours, and therefore the respon-sibility for maintaining your balance and health is yours alone. You've got the tools and information to do so, and you should endeavor to do so *most of the time.*

Good things have happened to you metabolically that will help you maintain more easily. One of the benefits of going through Phases I and II of this plan is that you re-store your insulin receptors to a level of better sensitivity, which allows you to *occasionally* "blow it out" dietarily on foods you love without suffering long-term damage.

In our clinical practice this is the advice we give to our patients as they go into the phase of maintenance: there is no food you can't have—in some quantity at some time. There will be foods, however, that are so rich in sugars and starches, such potent unbalancers of your metabolic hor-mones, that you cannot have unlimited amounts of them anytime you want unless you are willing to accept the con-sequences of that action. The inescapable consequences of a return to your old dietary habits will be to disrupt your metabolic balance and send you hurtling pell-mell back to your previous weight and beyond, back to taking daily medications to lower your blood pressure, cholesterol, or blood sugar to curb the skyrocketing values.

Nutritional maintenance of your health requires vigi-lance and effort most of the time interspersed with occa-sional brief vacations from the straight and narrow. Let's see how this works.

The Nutritional Vacation

Our society—like most—celebrates by feasting. Think of any joyous holiday celebration, and the first thing that will likely come to your mind is some favorite or traditional family dish associated with it. In our family, Thanksgiving just wouldn't be complete without a turkey stuffed with Granny Eades's cornmeal stuffing. And we wouldn't recognize Christmas Eve without homemade eggnog and decorated sugar cookies or Christmas dinner without mincemeat pie. And a Fourth of July picnic without traditional strawberry shortcake? Not at our picnic table. Celebration by feasting traces its origins as far back as mankind has kept written records, and as long as humans gather together in joy or thanks, food will play a big role. It does in our family, and it will in yours.

The fact that you have inherited a tendency for metabolic disturbance doesn't mean you must forever forfeit your right to join in the celebrations. We urge you to take a look at the celebrations and food traditions that are most meaningful in your life, whatever they may be. Select several times a year—perhaps your birthday, anniversary, holidays traditionally celebrated in your family or faith, a romantic getaway, a long-planned trip, or those once-in-a-lifetime events, such as weddings or class reunions—and *plan to enjoy them.* The key is to plan for it, look forward to it, enjoy it, and then, using the Recovery Guidelines outlined in the next section, recover from it and return to maintenance until the next planned vacation. Knowing that you have planned a vacation from maintenance somehow makes the idea of maintaining more tolerable and the small sacrifices you make day by day less burdensome. By choosing when and how you vary, you free yourself from anxiety and guilt that you might otherwise associate with breaking from your maintenance plan. You planned it, you knew in advance what the short-term consequences would be, and you had a prearranged plan of action to get back on the track immediately. It's not uncommon for a day or two of dietary debauchery to leave you four, five, six, even seven pounds heavier with retained fluid—and feeling lousy. So the purpose of this brief phase of recovery is to quickly drop your elevated insulin levels that the vacation inspired, waste off that fluid excess, get your eicosanoids (see Chapter 12) flowing back in the right direction, get you feeling chipper again, and slide you back onto your maintenance intake.

Recovery Guidelines

1. Return to Phase I for three days or until you have lost any weight you gained during your vacation (most of which will be from fluid retention).
2. Move to Phase II for the remainder of the week.
3. Return to your maintenance level and keep on living in metabolic equilibrium.

Although we want you to live happily and enjoy life to the fullest in your maintenance, we'd be remiss in not reminding you that the fewer variances the better. Our own experience—personally and with thousands of our patients—is that the longer you adhere to this biochemically correct lifestyle, the less appealing dietary indiscretion becomes. When you're in balance, you feel so good—mentally sharp, physically strong and well, emotionally stable—and when you vary from balance you feel so lousy that you will ask yourself, as we often have, "Why did I eat that?"

Questions Commonly Asked About the Program

Q. *Won't eating all this protein harm my kidneys?*

A. No, not if your kidneys are normal to begin with. People who restrict their carbohydrate intake seem to believe they are following a "high-protein" diet. On this program you calculate your *minimum* protein requirements—the amount of protein you would need no matter what kind of diet you followed. Even if you exceed this amount substantially—as long as your kidneys function normally—you should have no ill effects. A number of researchers have studied this exact question and, in fact, an impeccable 1995 study from Germany demonstrated that kidney function actually improved with increased protein consumption.

Q. *What should I do if I feel dizzy or light-headed?*

A. If you feel like you're going to pass out, or especially if you feel this sensation immediately upon standing up from a chair or bed, you probably need to increase your salt intake. This regime packs a potent diuretic force. As you progress on the program, your lowered insulin begins to allow your kidneys to release their retained fluid. You will notice how much more time you spend in the rest room as you rid yourself of this excess fluid. Unfortunately the kidneys also get rid of sodium and potassium along with this excess fluid, often leading to a sodium and/or potassium deficit and a little dehydration. The lowered sodium along with the dehydration causes the light-headedness. Increase your salt intake by adding regular table salt to your foods, eating a dill pickle, or drinking bouillon, and you should find your problem solved in short order.

Q. *I used to be able to lose weight easily, but now I have a difficult time even getting the first few pounds off. Why?*

A. Because you must first overcome what we call the inertia of weight loss. If you have dieted repeatedly, you are going to have more trouble getting into gear than someone who has never dieted. With repeated dieting your body gets more adept at squeezing out every ounce of energy from each bit of food as it is given smaller and smaller amounts. Your metabolism has an internal computer that has served our species well over eons of evolutionary time that resets your metabolic response to food depending on how much it gets. If you are used to eating large amounts of food, your metabolic rate is probably pretty high because the computer knows your body has fuel to waste. When you diet—or if you were somehow stranded in the Arctic or suffered a famine—your metabolic computer rapidly decreases your metabolic rate to conserve stored energy (fat) and wring the last dollop of energy out of any food coming in (all for survival reasons; your computer doesn't know you're dieting—it thinks you're starving, and it wants you to survive the lean time ahead). Not only is this computer exquisitely sensitive, but unfortunately for repeat dieters, it has a memory. If you have been through Jenny Craig twice, the Diet Center several times, Nutri/System and Optifast a time or two, not to mention Weight Watchers every other year, your computer has it all stored. And when you start on the next diet, it immediately adopts a bunker mentality and signals the entire metabolic system to go into conserve mode, making it progressively more and more difficult to lose. One of the nicest features of this program is that the large amount of food it provides begins to reprogram the computer and gradually brings it out of the fear-of-famine mode that is such an obstacle to weight loss. It will take a few weeks of diligent work, but you'll finally break free and begin to lose easily—a phase we call *dynamic weight loss* in which the fat reduction takes on a life of its own.

Q. *I have hit a plateau. What can I do to get things going?*

A. Plateaus are the purgatory of dieting. Everyone seems to experience them, hate them, and become frustrated by them. There are a few things you can do to get beyond the plateau, but before you do them, make sure you're on a true plateau. If you are just monitoring your weight on the scales and you seem stuck, you may be recomposing your body by gaining muscle weight as you lose fat. If you gain several pounds of muscle because you're exercising while at the same time you lose several pounds of fat, your weight on the scales doesn't change, but your size sure does. People who have been on a low-fat diet for a long time and who are protein deficient sometimes gain a few pounds of muscle simply from the decent amounts of protein they begin eating. If either of these situations describes you, you're not on a plateau; you're simply building muscle and/or rebuilding your lean body mass. You should notice a significant decrease in size even though you're not losing any scale weight.

If you truly are on a plateau, you can try several things. First, make absolutely certain you're following the program correctly. The most common mistake we see in our clinic with patients on plateaus is that they are not following their plan. That's one reason we have patients keep diaries and recommend that you keep a diary. Go back and *count* the number of grams of carbohydrate consumed—don't guess. It takes a while to get used to counting carbohydrates, and it can be disastrous to your success to assume or to guess. Until you get it down pat, always look it up before you eat it. We can't tell you how many patients we have who, when we discuss their "plateaus" with them, tell us, "Well, I did just like you told me except I ate a bagel on this day, and I had a banana on that day, and . . ." A bagel can contain anywhere from 30 to 50 grams of carbohydrate, a banana about 30. Fifty grams of carbohydrate—from whatever source—is the equivalent of $1/4$ cup of pure sugar. If you add this to your regimen every day or so, we can guarantee that you'll have plenty of plateaus.

If you absolutely are sticking to the plan and are still plateauing, try reducing your overall intake of food. Keep your protein intake at the minimum for your lean body mass, keep your carbohydrates at the level recommended for your phase, and lower your fat intake a little. That should do the trick, and when your weight loss starts picking back up, you can start increasing your intake a little. You can also cut your carbohydrate intake down to about 10 to 20 grams per day for a few days to get things going. Another thing you can do is to try some of the pre-packaged nutritional products we've used in our clinic for years with great success. (See appendix.)

Finally, make sure your fluid intake is sufficient. We have found often that a simple increase in fluids gets the weight coming off again in a hurry.

Q. *I've read a lot lately about "good" carbohydrates and "bad" carbohydrates, and I don't really understand the difference. Should I try to eat only the good ones? Or does it matter?*

A. The notion of "good" versus "bad" carbohydrates stems from the concept of the glycemic index developed by researcher David A. Jenkins and his group in Toronto in the early 1980s. Dr. Jenkins gave subjects 100 grams of pure glucose, then measured the amount of blood sugar rise this glucose produced. He then gave the same subjects various kinds of food containing the same 100 grams of carbohydrate, measured their blood sugar responses, and compared them with the blood sugar rise stimulated by the pure glucose. If the blood sugar rise was the same as glucose, then the food in question was said to have a glycemic index of 100. The lower the glycemic index, the less blood sugar response the particular food caused. Dr. Jenkins and others have continued to refine and improve on his early work, and the idea that low glycemic index foods are good carbohydrates and high glycemic index foods are bad has taken root.

The only problem with the whole concept is that the glycemic index doesn't compare apples to apples. It compares apples to glucose. Apples contain the whole complicated mélange of pectins, lignins, celluloses, hemicelluloses, and all the other substances that are collectively known as fiber along with the pure carbohydrate. Fiber slows the absorption of the pure carbohydrate, causing a lower blood sugar response, and probably has other independent actions on blood sugar and insulin as well. So the glycemic index of the apple is a function not of the specific carbohydrate it contains, but of the actions on this carbohydrate by the rest of the apple. In developing our ECC charts, we have removed the fiber component and left only the pure, *metabolically* active carbohydrate for you to count so that the whole concept of good and bad carbohydrates becomes meaningless *metabolically*. We emphasize the word *metabolically* because we're talking only about the blood sugar and insulin response to the food in question, not its overall nutritional worth.

For example, if you eat 5 grams of carbohydrate in a piece of candy, you will get about the same insulin response as you would if you ate 5 grams of carbohydrate in broccoli—not much. But what a difference nutritionally, not to mention in volume. The broccoli would be much more filling. The beauty of the ECC charts is that by using them you tend to gravitate toward foods that are more nutritionally dense and filling, and you never really have to worry about what is a good or a bad carbohydrate. Simply stay within your carbohydrate limits, select them from the ECC charts, and you will find that you probably have more food than you can eat.

Once you're on maintenance, you may want to remember that rice causes a lower blood sugar rise than potatoes, corn, and wheat. Next in line are beans and oats. But in the end the body receives it all as glucose—sugar—and you'll always need to watch your carbs.

Q. *Will I be constipated on this program, and if so, what can I do about it?*

A. You shouldn't be constipated for a number of reasons. First, if you select your carbohydrates from the ECC charts, you will tend to select foods with a high fiber content, which will help prevent constipation. Second, by reducing your insulin levels you will begin to make more good eicosanoids, which will increase the water content of your colon contents and prevent constipation. If you do experience a little constipation, it should be short-lived, but until it resolves you may want to use some of the fiber supplements described in the box at the end of Chapter 13, increase your fluid intake, and perhaps add one or two capsules of fish oil. (One good choice is MaxEPA-1000; another is Eico Marine from Eicotec, Inc., 21 Tioga Way, Marblehead, MA 01945.)

Q. *What if I have diarrhea?*

A. Surprisingly, this is a more common complaint on this regime than constipation. Usually loose stools, and occasionally diarrhea, start a few days into the program and resolve a few days later as the body adjusts to its new diet. If it doesn't resolve, you need to be checked for an infection—nothing to do with your new diet, just a possible coincidence. If that test is negative, reduce your intake of fish oil capsules, if you're taking them, reduce your intake of high-fiber foods, and, finally, make sure you don't have an allergy or sensitivity to one or more of the new foods you're consuming.

Q. *I've just started the program, and I feel extremely fatigued. Why?*

A. This is a common experience with our new patients. All of life is catalyzed by enzymes. If it weren't for enzymes, we would just be piles of nonreactive chemicals instead of the living, breathing beings we are. Our DNA codes for millions of enzymes, but we make and have circulating at any given time only those we need. If you have been on a low-fat, high-complex-carbohydrate diet, you have all the enzymes circulating around that deal with storing, breaking down, and retrieving carbohydrates as needed for energy. When you drastically change your diet, all these enzymes are then running around with nothing to do because they're so specific to their function that they can't work on your new diet. It takes a few days for your body to produce the new enzymes to deal with the composition of your new diet. After a couple of days of a little tiredness, however, your energy levels should rise considerably, and you should actually end up with a lot more energy than you had before you started the diet.

Q. *I have been on the diet for a couple of weeks now. I felt a little tired at first, then I felt fabulous, and now, all of a sudden, I feel exhausted, and my legs ache.*

A. You have described a textbook case of hypokalemia, or low blood potassium. Because the diet has such a diuretic effect on the kidneys, it often gets rid of enough potassium along with the excess fluid that some people become potassium deficient. Low potassium can cause all kinds of different symptoms such as tingling, light-headedness, fatigue, muscle aches, and especially deep muscle fatigue and cramps. We recommended that you use Morton's Lite Salt or NoSalt because these are pure potassium salts and usually will compensate for the potassium lost through the kidneys. If you aren't using these, start now. If you are, then get one of the potassium supplements listed on page 184 and start taking it. If your symptoms are from potassium deficiency, they should resolve in a matter of hours after beginning potassium supplementation. *If you are taking blood pressure medicines or diuretics, you must check with your physician or pharmacist before taking potassium supplements because* *some of these medicines prevent the body's release of potassium, and taking extra can cause serious problems.* If you are not taking any of these medications and have normal kidney function, it is virtually impossible to overdose on potassium taken as the salt substitute or as a supplement from a health food store.

Q. *Do I have to spread my carbohydrates around throughout the day, or can I save them up and eat them all at once?*

A. You will do better if you divide your carbohydrates into approximately equal portions and eat them throughout the day. If you have a special occasion coming up and you know you will overindulge, then save your carbohydrates and eat them all at once. We have had several patients who found some sort of carbohydrate treat they enjoyed immensely that they would save up for and eat once during the day. One patient was losing weight by leaps and bounds and lowering his dangerously elevated cholesterol on the Phase I Intervention, when he found a candy he liked that contained 17 grams of carbohydrate. He would eat one of these candies every afternoon. He then spread his remaining 13 grams of carbohydrate around the rest of his meals. He continued to lose and told us that the pleasure he got from that one piece of candy more than offset the reduction in carbohydrate the rest of the day. If you decide to pursue this line of dieting, remember to cut back during the rest of the day, or your progress will slow.

Q. *I have suffered with indigestion and reflux for years and take medication every day to stop the burning. Since I've been on this diet, I've forgotten to take my medicine several times and I've had no indigestion. Could the diet have done this?*

A. Yes. In fact the disappearance of gastritis, reflux, and indigestion on our Protein Power plan is one of its most predictable beneficial effects. This diet improves the quality of protective mucus in the stomach lining and normalizes muscular control˙ of the esophageal sphincter to prevent reflux and spasm. Eicosanoid modulation is the reason (see Chapter 12) for this dramatic response, working in the same way as the newest ulcer and reflux medications, but without the considerable expense and unpleasant side effects.

Q. *I've heard that diets high in protein can cause osteoporosis. Is this true?*

A. No. In the first place this diet is *not* a high protein diet, it is an *adequate* protein diet. Second, even a high protein diet doesn't cause an overall loss of calcium. The notion that high protein diets cause calcium loss is a persistent rumor—even among those who should know better—that no amount of scientific research (and there's plenty) seems to be able to dispel. Diets high in meat protein have been consumed for millennia by people the world over without harm, so don't worry about osteoporosis.

Q. *If I make some of the changes you recommend—for example, cutting back some on my carbohydrate intake—will I see improvement, or do I need to follow the program exactly to get results?*

A. If you are overweight or have any of the other problems we have been discussing, cutting back a little on your carbohydrates won't accomplish much. If you indeed have one of these disorders, you have damaged insulin receptors. The only way to repair them is to get your insulin level down and let them heal. A little bit of carbohydrate cutting won't do that—it has to be fairly drastic, as in the Phase I Intervention. Only then can you expect the long-term benefits you really want.

Q. *Will I lose weight faster if I cut out all carbohydrates? Would it be dangerous?*

A. Cutting your carbohydrate below the level of Phase I (7 to 10 grams per meal) probably won't speed your loss, so there's little point in going lower. Each gram of carbohydrate provides only about 4 calories, so you can see that you're saving only about 100 calories in the day (eating three meals each containing 28 to 40 calories in carbohydrate). As to the danger of it, traditional Eskimos, living above the Arctic Circle, eat virtually no carbohydrate and do fine. Refer to the study undertaken by Vilhjalmur Stefansson (see footnote 2, Chapter 1) for more details.

Q. *Won't this diet put me into ketosis?*

A. If you're very much overweight, Phase I will almost certainly put you into ketosis, but there's nothing wrong with that. It simply tells you that you're burning fat. If you're not much overweight, the diet will probably put you right on the cusp of ketosis, which is where you want to be. Ketosis is a much-misunderstood subject, so let's go into it in a little detail. Ketones (ketone bodies, the actual scientific name) are made when fat breaks down. As you read the words on this page you are producing ketones, but unless you're on this diet or have been fasting, you're probably not in ketosis—the state of having a measurable level of ketones in your blood. Ketones are an intermediate stage of fat breakdown, and not only are they not poison as described by several health writers, but they're used as fuel by most of the body's tissues including the brain. The heart, in fact, prefers ketones to all other fuel. The body must have sufficient carbohydrate to completely burn for energy all the ketones produced. The diet causes the breakdown of fat, producing an abundance of ketones—especially in the overweight person—but the intervention diets don't provide enough carbohydrate to burn all of them. These excess ketones circulate in the blood and must be gotten rid of in other ways. The body releases them via the urine, the stool, and the breath. Since ketones are incompletely burned fat, any that you get rid of without actually using them for energy means you are ditching unwanted fat without having to actually burn it off.

Q. *But aren't ketones and ketosis dangerous?*

A. Unless you're a type I diabetic, not at all. You might think so, however, because some health writers such as Jane Brody of *The New York Times,* a major proponent of the low-fat, high-complex-carbohydrate diet, say that ketones are "toxic compounds that can damage the brain and cause nausea, fatigue, and apathy." She goes on to tell you that ketones are "fat waste products" that "pollute" the blood. But Dr. Lubert Stryer, Professor of Biochemistry at Stanford University and the author of the biochemistry textbook used in most medical schools, says ketones are "normal fuels of respiration and are quantitatively important as sources of energy." "Indeed," Dr. Stryer continues, "heart muscle, and the renal cortex [kidney] use [ketones] in preference to glucose." Drs. Donald and Judith Voet, authors of another popular medical biochemistry textbook, say that ketones "serve as important metabolic fuels for many peripheral tissues, particularly heart and skeletal muscle." So if you believe Ms. Brody, you would think that ketones poison you; if you trust the consensus among medical experts and scientists, you will understand that ketones are a perfectly normal fuel used preferentially by most of the tissues in the body for their energy needs. In fact—except for type I diabetics—there is no evidence for the opinion that ketones are dangerous.

Q. *Why do I sometimes get a funny taste in my mouth or bad breath on this diet?*

A. Ketones released through the lungs can cause an unpleasant odor (acetone breath) and/or a funny taste in the mouth. The best thing to do for this is to drink plenty of fluids. If you make a lot of urine, most of the ketones will escape that way. If not, about the only way out they have is through the breath. Breath sprays and sugar-free gum can help, but beware of overusing the gum. Sugar-free means *sucrose* (table sugar)-free, not necessarily carbohydrate-free.

Q. *Why have I had trouble sleeping since starting the diet?*

A. Heavy ketosis can cause sleeplessness. If you are producing and releasing a lot of ketones,[9] you may be able to increase your carbohydrates a little or move ahead to Phase II Intervention.

Q. *I don't have any trouble getting to sleep, but I wake up in the middle of the night starving. I raid the refrigerator and eat whatever is at hand before I can get back to sleep. Will the diet do anything to stop these cravings?*

A. Yes. This is not the typical description of a food craving but sounds more like an ulcer or gastritis problem—

---

[9] You can check your ketone production status by purchasing Ketostix from any drugstore. These little coated plastic sticks, when dipped into a sample of your urine, will change color. By comparing the color on the stick to the chart on the jar they came in, you can determine your ketone status.

both of which are common to insulin-resistant people on high-carbohydrate diets. The body naturally releases a surge of stomach acid in the wee hours of the morning that doesn't bother anyone with a normal stomach lining. But in people who have either ulcers or gastritis (inflammation of the stomach lining), this surge of acid often produces enough pain and discomfort to awaken them. They typically don't have a sense of actual stomach pain but instead feel a kind of gnawing hunger that begs to be relieved. Consuming a large portion of food neutralizes this excess acid, they feel better, and they go back to sleep. On our program the reduction in carbohydrate intake begins immediately to allow most ulcers and gastritis to heal. Most of these problems are caused by an eicosanoid imbalance that is quickly normalized as soon as insulin levels fall. A few days after starting the program these episodes should begin to become much less frequent and finally go away. If you do awaken, however, make sure you eat according to your intervention plan, and *don't overeat carbohydrates* or you will perpetuate the problem.

Q. *What about artificial sweeteners? Are they dangerous?*

A. Our own preference is to avoid artificial sweeteners as much as possible simply because no one knows the very long-term effects of them. We try to eat as few unnatural products as possible, but we don't completely avoid artificial sweeteners because they are found in too many good low-carbohydrate foods. Are they dangerous? That depends. Compared to what? Compared to an equivalent sweetening amount of sugar, they are innocuous. If all you consumed was 1 teaspoon of sugar per day in your morning coffee, we would say go ahead and use the sugar. But, if you're talking about a soft drink, that's a different story. A 12-ounce can of most soft drinks contains about 4 tablespoons of pure sugar, $^1/_4$ cup, which calculates to 48 grams, more than your whole day's allotment on Phase I. In the case of soft drinks the sugar poses much more of a health risk than the artificial sweetener that replaces it in the diet version.

Aspartame, the artificial sweetener in NutraSweet, passed more than one hundred FDA tests before it was approved. On the horizon is left-handed sugar, a molecular manipulation of real sugar that is not metabolized by the body—no calories, almost no carbohydrates. The FDA is still testing, but this sugar is available in Canada, where it's called Splenda and has been in general use for more than six years.

You can ruin your diet by overindulging in artificial sweeteners, as one of our patients did. It turned out she was using some 50 teaspoons of Equal a day—and those little fractions of carbohydrate added up to big trouble.

Q. *What about my "sweet tooth"? Because of the carbohydrate restriction, this program doesn't have any really sweet foods, so I can't indulge my cravings for sweets.*

A. Believe it or not, your craving for sweets will diminish with time. Just as insulin receptors become resistant to the stimulation of insulin over time, requiring much more insulin to make them work, your sweet receptors (taste buds) do the same. With chronic stimulation by a sweet, sugary diet your taste buds become resistant to the stimulation of sweets, requiring more and more to give you the pleasant sensation you desire. As you destimulate them by removing the refined carbohydrate from your diet, your sweet receptors will regain their sensitivity. At that point foods that you previously would have eaten by the plateful to get your sweet fix will provide the same sensation in much smaller amounts. In fact, if you try to eat the amounts you did before, you will pay the price in the way you feel later. A few such experiences and your sweet-consumption habits will have changed for good.

Q. *I understand about calculating protein, carbohydrate, and all that, but what does that mean in real food? What would a day of eating look like?*

A. Let's suppose your protein need is 27 grams per meal and set up a typical day on Phase I.

For breakfast, you might enjoy a ham-and-cheese omelet, a slice of "light" sourdough toast with a pat of sweet butter, half a cup of sliced fresh strawberries with cream, and a cup of coffee.

At lunch, you might dine with friends at a local restaurant, where you could have a grilled-chicken Caesar salad (hold the croutons) with sliced fresh peaches and cream for dessert, with coffee. Or if you're on the run, and the only thing available is the local burger joint, you could dash in for a double cheeseburger with everything—hold the buns—a salad, and a big glass of iced tea—remember to drink most of the tea *before* you eat.

In the afternoon, for a snack, you might eat some slices of hard salami with sharp cheddar cheese and a glass of mineral water or a diet soda.

For dinner you could grill a juicy steak, with sautéed mushrooms, fresh asparagus in a vinaigrette dressing, sliced fresh tomatoes, and a large green salad. Accompany the meal with a glass of dry red wine if you like, or have just a little water and coffee or tea, and save room for a little sliced melon.

PROTEIN EQUIVALENCY CHART A

TOTAL PROTEIN INTAKE ≤60 GRAMS PER DAY (20 GRAMS PER MEAL)

	Meat, fish, poultry	Egg	Hard cheeses	Soft cheeses	Curd cheeses	Tofu
Meat, fish, poultry	3 oz.					
Eggs	1 egg + 2 whites + 1 oz. "meat"	2 eggs + 2 whites				
Hard cheeses	2 oz. "meat" + 1 oz. cheese	1 egg + 2 whites + 1 oz. cheese	Unacceptable*			
Soft cheeses	2 oz. "meat" + 2 oz. cheese	1 egg + 2 whites + 2 oz. cheese	Unacceptable	Unacceptable		
Curd cheeses	2 oz. "meat" + 1/4 cup cheese	1 egg + 1 white + 1/4 cup cheese	1/2 cup curd + 1 oz. hard cheese	1/2 cup curd + 2 oz. soft cheese	3/4 cup curd	
Tofu	1/4 cup tofu + 1.5 oz. "meat"	1 egg + 1 white + 1/4 cup tofu	1/4 cup tofu + 1 oz. cheese	1/4 cup tofu + 2 oz. cheese	1/4 cup curd + 1/4 cup tofu	1/2 cup tofu

"Meat" = 7 grams per ounce
Eggs + 6 grams whole, 4 grams white
Hard cheese = 6–7 grams per ounce

Soft Cheese = 3–4 grams per ounce
Curd Cheese = 7 grams per 1/4 cup
Tofu = 10 grams per 1/4 cup

*Because of the high fat content, the number of calories consumed to make these an adequate sole protein source would be too high for most people.

PROTEIN EQUIVALENCY CHART B

TOTAL PROTEIN INTAKE 61–80 GRAMS PER DAY (27 GRAMS PER MEAL)

	Meat, fish, poultry	Egg	Hard cheeses	Soft cheeses	Curd cheeses	Tofu
Meat, fish, poultry	4 oz.					
Eggs	2 eggs + 2 whites + 1 oz. "meat"	2 eggs + 4 whites				
Hard cheeses	3 oz. "meat" + 1 oz. cheese	2 eggs + 2 whites + 1 oz. cheese	Unacceptable*			
Soft cheeses	3 oz. "meat" + 2 oz. cheese	2 eggs + 2 whites + 2 oz. cheese	Unacceptable	Unacceptable		
Curd cheeses	3 oz. "meat" + 1/4 cup cheese	2 eggs + 1/2 cup cheese	3/4 cup curd + 1 oz. hard cheese	3/4 cup curd + 2 oz. soft cheese	1 cup curd	
Tofu	1/2 cup tofu + 1 oz. "meat"	1 egg + 3 whites + 1/4 cup tofu	1/2 cup tofu + 1 oz. cheese	1/2 cup tofu + 2 oz. cheese	1/2 cup tofu + 1/4 cup curd	3/4 cup tofu

"Meat" = 7 grams per ounce
Eggs + 6 grams whole, 4 grams white
Hard cheese = 6–7 grams per ounce
Soft Cheese = 3–4 grams per ounce
Curd Cheese = 7 grams per 1/4 cup
Tofu = 10 grams per 1/4 cup

*Because of the high fat content, the number of calories consumed to make these an adequate sole protein source would be too high for most people.

PROTEIN EQUIVALENCY CHART C

TOTAL PROTEIN INTAKE 81–100 GRAMS PER DAY (34 GRAMS PER MEAL)

	Meat, fish, poultry	Egg	Hard cheeses	Soft cheeses	Curd cheeses	Tofu
Meat, fish, poultry	5 oz.					
Eggs	2 eggs + 2 whites + 2 oz. "meat*"	3 eggs + 4 whites				
Hard cheeses	4 oz. "meat**" + 1 oz. cheese	2 eggs + 4 whites + 1 oz. cheese	Unacceptable*			
Soft cheeses	4 oz. "meat***" + 2 oz. cheese	2 eggs + 4 whites + 2 oz. cheese	Unacceptable	Unacceptable		
Curd cheeses	3 oz. "meat*" + 1/2 cup cheese	2 eggs + 2 whites + 1/2 cup cheese	1 cup curd + 1 oz. hard cheese	1 cup curd + 2 oz. soft cheese	1¼ cups curd	
Tofu	1/2 cup tofu + 2 oz. "meat"	2 eggs + 1/2 cup tofu	scant 3/4 cup + 1 oz. cheese	3/4 cup + 1 oz. cheese	1/2 cup tofu + 1/2 cup curd	heaping 3/4 cup tofu

"Meat" = 7 grams per ounce
Eggs = 6 grams whole, 4 grams white
Hard cheese = 6–7 grams per ounce
Soft Cheese = 3–4 grams per ounce
Curd Cheese = 7 grams per ¼ cup
Tofu = 10 grams per ¼ cup
*Because of the high fat content, the number of calories consumed to make these an adequate sole protein source would be too high for most people.

PROTEIN EQUIVALENCY CHART D

TOTAL PROTEIN INTAKE 101–120 GRAMS PER DAY (40 GRAMS PER MEAL)

	Meat, fish, poultry	Eggs	Hard cheeses	Soft cheeses	Curd cheeses	Tofu
Meat, fish, poultry	6 oz.					
Eggs	2 eggs + 4 white + 2 oz. "meat"	3 eggs + 6 whites				
Hard cheeses	5 oz. "meat" + 1 oz. cheese	2 eggs + 5 whites – 1 oz. cheese	Unacceptable*			
Soft cheeses	5 oz. "meat" + 2 oz. cheese	2 eggs + 5 whites + 2 oz. cheese	Unacceptable	Unacceptable		
Curd cheeses	4 oz. "meat" + ½ cup cheese	2 eggs + 3 whites + ½ cup cheese	1¼ cups curd + 1 oz. hard cheese	1¼ cups curd + 2 oz. soft cheese	1½ cups curd	
Tofu	½ cup tofu + 3 oz. "meat"	2 eggs + 2 whites + ½ cup tofu	¾ cup tofu + 1 oz. cheese	¾ cup tofu + 2 oz. cheese	¾ cup tofu + ½ cup curd	1 cup tofu

"Meat" = 7 grams per ounce
Eggs + 6 grams whole, 4 grams white
Hard cheese = 6–7 grams per ounce
Soft Cheese = 3–4 grams per ounce
Curd Cheese = 7 grams per ¼ cup
Tofu = 10 grams per ¼ cup
*Because of the high fat content, the number of calories consumed to make these an adequate sole protein source would be too high for most people.

EFFECTIVE CARBOHYDRATE CONTENT OF FRUITS

FOOD	5-GRAM PORTION	10-GRAM PORTION	15-GRAM PORTION	20-GRAM PORTION	25-GRAM PORTION
Apple—Raw	1/4 apple (4.5)	1/2 apple (9)	3/4 apple (13.5)	1 apple (18)	1 1/4 apples (22.5)
Microwave-cooked	1/4 cup (5)	1/2 cup (10)	3/4 cup (15)	1 cup (20)	1 1/4 cups (25)
Applesauce—unsweetened	1/8 cup (3)	1/4 cup (6)	1/2 cup (12)	3/4 cup (18)	1 cup (24)
Apricots—raw	1 1/2 med.	3 med. (10.4)	4 med. (14)	5 med. (17.5)	7 med. (24.5)
canned (water)	4 halves (5)	8 halves (10)	12 halves (15)	16 halves (20)	20 halves (25)
Avocado (California)	3/4 med. (5.4)	1 med. (7.3)	2 med. (14.6)	2 1/2 med. (18.3)	3 med. (21.9)
Banana—raw	*	1/3 med. (8.3)	1/2 med. (12.5)	2/3 med. (16.7)	1 med. (25)
Blackberries—raw	1/2 cup (5.9)	3/4 cup (8.9)	1 1/4 cups (14.7)	1 1/2 cups (17.8)	2 cups (23.6)
Blueberries—raw	1/3 cup (5.7)	1/2 cup (8.6)	3/4 cup (13)	1 cup (17.2)	1 1/2 cups (25.8)
Boysenberries—frzn/unsweet	1/4 cup (4)	1/2 cup (8)	1 cup (16)	1 1/4 cups (20)	1 1/2 cups (24)
Cantaloupe—raw pieces	1/2 cup (5.7)	3/4 cup (8.6)	1 cup (11.4)	1 3/4 cups (20)	2 cups (22.8)
Cherries—sour canned (water)	1/4 cup (5.4)	1/2 cup (10.9)	3/4 cup (15.7)	1 cup (21)	1 1/4 cups (26.4)
—sweet raw	5 whole (5.1)	10 whole (10.2)	15 whole (15.3)	20 whole (20.4)	25 whole (25.5)
—sweet canned (water)	*	1/4 cup (7.3)	1/2 cup (14.6)	2/3 cup (19.5)	3/4 cup (22)
Crabapples—raw slices	1/3 cup (4)	1/4 cup (8.3)	1/2 cup (11)	3/4 cup (16.5)	1 cup (22)
Cranberries—raw	*	3/4 cup (8)	1 cup (12)	1 1/2 cups (16)	2 cups (24)
Cranberry sauce, jellied	2 tsp (4.6)	1 Tblsp (7)	2 Tblsp (14)	*	*
Currants—black raw	1/2 cup (5.6)	3/4 cup (8.4)	1 cup (11.2)	1 1/2 cups (16.8)	2 cups (22.4)
Dates—dried whole	*	1 whole (6)	2 whole (12)	3 whole (18)	4 whole (24)
Figs—raw whole	1/2 med. (4.8)	1 med. (9.6)	1 1/2 med. (14.4)	2 med. (19.2)	2 1/2 med. (24)
—dried whole	*	*	1 whole (12.2)	1 1/2 whole (18.3)	2 whole (24.4)
Fruit cocktail—canned, water	1/4 cup (5.2)	1/2 cup (10.4)	3/4 cup (15.6)	1 cup (20.8)	1 1/4 cups (26)
Fruit salad—canned, juice	*	1/3 cup (10.6)	1/2 cup (16)	1 cup (16)	3/4 cup (24)
Grapefruit—raw	1/4 whole (4.4)	1/2 whole (8.8)	3/4 whole (12.4)	1 whole (17.6)	1 1/2 whole (26.4)
—canned, juice	1/4 cup (5.5)	1/3 cup (7.4)	2/3 cup (14.8)	3/4 cup (16.7)	1 cup (22.2)
Grapes—seedless	1/3 cup (5.3)	1/2 cup (7.6)	1 cup (15.8)	1 1/3 cups (21.1)	1 1/2 cups (23.4)
Guava—raw	1/2 med. (5.3)	1 med. (10.7)	1 1/2 med. (16)	2 med. (21.4)	2 1/2 med. (25.7)

Honeydew—raw, pieces	1/4 cup (3.9)	1/2 cup (7.8)	1 cup (15.6)	1 1/4 cups (19.5)	1 1/2 cups (26.5)
Kiwifruit—raw	1/2 med. (4.4)	1 med. (8.7)	1 1/2 med. (13)	2 med. (17.4)	2 1/2 med. (21.7)
Lemon peel	*	*	*	*	*
Lemon—raw	1 med. (5.4)	2 med. (10.8)	3 med. (16.2)	4 med. (21.6)	5 med. (27)
Lime—raw	1/2 med. (3.5)	1 med. (7.1)	2 med. (14.2)	*	*
Mandarin orange—juice-packed	*	1/3 cup (8)	1/2 cup (11.9)	3/4 cup (17.9)	1 cup (23.8)
Mango—raw, pieces	*	1/4 cup (8.3)	1/2 cup (16.5)	2/3 cup (21.1)	3/4 cup (24.8)
Nectarine—raw	*	1/2 med. (6.9)	1 med. (13.8)	1 1/2 med. (20.7)	2 med. (27.6)
Orange, Valencia or navel—raw	1/2 med. (5.5)	3/4 med. (8.6)	1 med. (11.5)	1/2 med. (17)	2 med. (23)
Papaya—raw	*	1/2 med. (6.8)	1/2 med. (13.5)	3/4 med. (20)	1 med. (27)
Passionfruit, purple—raw	1 med. (4.2)	2 med. (8.4)	3 med. (12.6)	5 med. (21)	6 med. (25.2)
Peach—raw	1/2 med. (4.2)	1 med. (8.3)	1 1/2 med. (12.5)	2 med. (16.6)	3 med. (25)
—canned, water	1/3 cup (5)	3/4 cup (11.1)	1 cup (14.9)	1 1/3 cups (20)	1 3/4 cups (26)
—dried, halves		1 half (8)	1 1/2 halves (12)	2 halves (16)	3 halves (24)
Pear—raw	1/4 med. (5.2)	1/2 med. (10.4)	3/4 med. (15.6)	1 med. (20.8)	1 1/4 med. (26.4)
—canned, water	1/4 cup (4.8)	1/2 cup (9.5)	3/4 cup (14.3)	1 cup (19.1)	1 1/4 cups (23.8)
—dried, halves	*	1/2 half (6.1)	1 half (12.2)	1 1/2 halves (18)	2 halves (24.4)
—Asian	1/4 med. (3.3)	3/4 med. (9.9)	1 med. (13.1)	1 1/2 med. (19.6)	2 med. (26.2)
Persimmon—raw	*	1 med. (8.4)	1 1/2 med. (12.6)	2 med. (16.8)	3 med. (25.2)
Pineapple—raw, pieces	1/4 cup (4.3)	1/2 cup (8.7)	3/4 cup (13)	1 cup (17.3)	1 1/2 cups (26)
—canned, juice	*	1/4 cup (9.3)	1/3 cup (12.4)	1/2 cup (18.6)	2/3 cup (24.8)
Plum—raw	1/2 med. (4.3)	1 med. (8.6)	1 1/2 med. (12.9)	2 med. (17.2)	3 med. (25.8)
Pomegranate—raw	*	1/4 med. (6.6)	1/2 med. (13.2)	3/4 med. (19.8)	1 med. (26.4)
Prunes—dried	1 whole (5.3)	2 whole (10.6)	3 whole (15.9)	4 whole (21.2)	5 whole (26.5)
Quince	*	1/2 med. (7)	1 med. (14)	1 1/2 med. (21)	1 3/4 med. (24.5)
Raisins		*	1/8 cup (13.9)	1/8 cup (13.9)	1/4 cup (27.8)
Raspberries—raw	1/2 cup (4.2)	1 cup (8.4)	1 3/4 cups (14.7)	2 cups (16.8)	3 cups (25.2)
Strawberries—raw	3/4 cup (5)	1 1/2 cups (9.9)	2 cups (13.2)	3 cups (19.8)	4 cups (26.4)
—frozen, unsweet	1/3 cup (4.5)	1/2 cup (6.8)	1 cup (13.6)	1 1/2 cups (20.4)	2 cups (26.2)
Tangerine—raw	1/2 med. (4.7)	1 med. (9.4)	1 1/2 med. (14.1)	2 med. (18.8)	2 1/2 med. (23.8)
Watermelon—raw, pieces	1/2 cup (5.5)	3/4 cup (8.3)	1 cup (11)	1 1/2 cups (165)	2 cups (22)

EFFECTIVE CARBOHYDRATE CONTENT OF BREADS, CEREALS, AND GRAINS

FOOD	5-GRAM PORTION	10-GRAM PORTION	15-GRAM PORTION	20-GRAM PORTION	25-GRAM PORTION
Bagel	*	*			1 small (27)
Biscuit—small (³/4 oz.)	1/2 small (4.8)	1 small (9.7)	1 1/2 small (14.5)	2 small (19.4)	2 1/2 small (24.2)
—med. (1 oz.)	*	1/2 med. (6)	1 med. (12)	1 1/2 med. (18)	2 med. (24)
—large (2 oz.)	*	*		1/2 large (16)	1/2 large (16)
Boston brown bread—canned	*	1/2 slice (10)	3/4 slice (15)	1 slice (20)	1 slice (20)
Bread, pita pocket	*	1/2 pocket (10.1)	1/2 pocket (10.1)	1 pocket (20.3)	1 pocket (20.3)
Bread, raisin, regular—sliced	*	1/2 slice (6.3)	1 slice (12.6)	1 1/2 slices (18.9)	2 slices (25.2)
Bread, sandwich, regular—sliced	*	1/2 slice (6)	1 slice (12)	1 1/2 slices (18)	2 slices (24)
light—sliced	1/2 slice (3.5)	1 slice (7)	2 slices (14)	2 1/2 slices (17.5)	3 slices (21)
Breadstick, sesame (Keebler)	2 sticks (5.3)	4 sticks (10.6)	5 sticks (13)	7 sticks (18.2)	9 sticks (23.4)
Breadstick, soft (Pillsbury)	*	1/2 stick (8.3)	3/4 stick (12.5)	1 stick (16.6)	1 1/2 sticks (24.9)
Bun, hamburger or hot dog— regular	*	1/2 bun (10)	1/2 bun (10)	1 bun (20.1)	1 bun (20.1)
—light	*	1/2 bun (7)	1 bun (14)	1 1/2 buns (21)	1 1/2 buns (21)
Couscous—cooked	*	1/4 cup (10)	1/3 cup (13.6)	1/2 cup (20.5)	scant 2/3 cup (26)
Crackers (saltine, club, Ritz-style, melba)	2 regular (4)	4 regular (8)	6 regular (12)	10 regular (20)	12 regular (24)
(oyster type)	10 (5.3)	20 (10.6)	25 (13.3)	35 (18.6)	45 (23.9)
(Triscuits)	1 cracker (3)	3 crackers (9)	5 crackers (15)	6 crackers (18)	8 crackers (24)
(Sociables, Nabisco)	3 crackers (4.5)	6 crackers (9)	10 crackers (15)	12 crackers (18)	15 crackers (22.5)
(Wasa, Sesame Rye)	2 pieces (4)	5 pieces (10)	7 pieces (14)	10 pieces (20)	12 pieces (24)
Cheez-It (Sunshine)/ Cheese Nips (Nabisco)	8 Nips (4.8)	15 Nips (9)	25 Nips (15)	30 Nips (18)	40 Nips (24)
Flours					
cornmeal—whole-grain	*	2 Tblsp (10)	3 Tblsp (15)	4 Tblsp (20)	5 Tblsp (25)
oat bran—raw	*	4 Tblsp (11.7)	5 Tblsp (15)	6 Tblsp (18)	8 Tblsp (24)

rice flour—brown	*	1 Tblsp (7.5)	2 Tblsp (15)	2 Tblsp (15)	3 Tblsp (22.5)
rye flour	*	2 Tblsp (10)	3 Tblsp (15)	4 Tblsp (20)	5 Tblsp (25)
soy flour—roasted, full-fat	scant 1/4 cup (5.5)	1/3 cup (8.3)	1/2 cup (12.5)	2/3 cup (16.6)	1 cup (25)
wheat germ	1/8 cup (5.3)	1/4 cup (10.6)	1/3 cup (14)	1/2 cup (21.2)	scant 2/3 cup (26)
white flour—all-purpose	*	2 Tblsp (10.5)	3 Tblsp (15)	4 Tblsp (20)	5 Tblsp (25)
whole-wheat flour	*	2 Tblsp (9)	3 Tblsp (13.5)	4 Tblsp (18)	5 Tblsp (24)
Grain cakes—pressed (rice, oats, wheat, popcorn, sesame, barley)	1/2 cake (3.5)	1 cake (7)	2 cakes (14)	3 cakes (21)	3 cakes (21)
Melba toast	2 pieces (4)	5 pieces (10)	7 pieces (14)	10 pieces (20)	12 pieces (24)
Muffin—English (plain)	*	1/2 muffin (10)	1/2 muffin (13)	3/4 muffin (19.5)	1 muffin (26.2)
—Corn (small)	*	1/2 muffin (7.5)	3/4 muffin (15)	1 muffin (20)	1 muffin (20)
—Oat bran (Estee from mix)	*	*	1 muffin (15)	1 muffin (15)	1 1/2 muffins (22.5)
—Oat bran (General Mills from mix)	*	*	1/2 muffin (12.5)	3/4 muffin (19)	1 muffin (25)
Oatmeal—cooked, plain	*	*	scant 1/2 cup (15)	1/2 cup (16.5)	2/3 cup (22)
Pancake (from mix, 4" diameter)	*	1/2 cake (6)	1 cake (12)	1 1/2 cakes (18)	2 cakes (24)
(frozen Aunt Jemima, plain)	*	1/2 cake (6)	1 cake (12)	1 1/2 cakes (18)	2 cakes (24)
Pancake—Fluffy (our recipe)	*	1 serving (10)	1 1/2 servings (15)	2 servings (20)	2 1/2 servings (25)
Pasta (egg noodles, spaghetti, macaroni—cooked)	*	1/4 cup (10)	1/3 cup (13)	1/2 cup (20)	3/4 cup (26.6)
(chow mein noodles)	*	1/3 cup (8.7)	1/2 cup (13)	3/4 cup (20)	1 cup (26)
(noodles w/rice—LaChoy)	*	1/4 cup (10)	1/3 cup (13)	1/2 cup (21)	3/4 cup (26)
(lasagne—dry uncooked)	*	1/2 oz. (10)	2/3 oz. (13)	1 oz. (20)	1 1/4 oz. (25)
Piecrust (Keebler, Pillsbury All Ready, 9" dia.)	*	*	1/8 crust (15)	1/6 crust (20)	1/5 crust (24)
Pizza crust (small, thin-crust 9" diameter)	*	*	1/8 crust (15)	1/6 crust (20)	1/5 crust (24)
Popovers—homemade, small	1/2 small (5.1)	1 small (10.3)	1 1/2 small (15.4)	2 small (20.6)	2 small (20.6)

EFFECTIVE CARBOHYDRATE CONTENT OF BREADS, CEREALS, AND GRAINS

FOOD	5-GRAM PORTION	10-GRAM PORTION	15-GRAM PORTION	20-GRAM PORTION	25-GRAM PORTION
Rice—brown, cooked	1/8 cup (5.2)	1/4 cup (10.4)	1/3 cup (13.5)	1/2 cup (20.9)	scant 2/3 cup (25)
—white, long grain, cooked	1/8 cup (5.3)	1/4 cup (10.5)	1/3 cup (14)	1/2 cup (21)	scant 2/3 cup (25)
—wild, cooked	1/8 cup (4.4)	1/4 cup (8.8)	scant 1/2 cup (15)	1/2 cup (17.5)	scant 3/4 cup (26)
Rice—fried	1/8 cup (5.2)	1/4 cup (10.5)	1/3 cup (14)	1/2 cup (21)	1/2 cup (21)
Risotto—cooked	*	1/8 cup (6)	1/4 cup (12)	1/3 cup (16)	1/2 cup (24)
Rolls—crescent (Pillsbury, canned), small	1/2 roll (5.4)	1 roll (10.8)	1 roll (10.8)	1 1/2 rolls (16.2)	2 rolls (21.6)
—dinner, small	*	1/2 roll (7)	1 roll (14)	1 1/2 rolls (21)	1 1/2 rolls (21)
Stuffing, corn bread or bread	*	1/4 cup (10.5)	1/3 cup (14)	1/2 cup (21)	1/2 cup (21)
Tortillas (corn—tostada, taco shell, small)	*	1 shell (7)	2 shells (14)	3 shells (21)	3 shells (21)
(flour—fajita, small)	*	1/2 small (7.5)	1 small (15)	1 small (15)	1 1/2 small (22)
Waffle—plain, homemade 7" diameter	*	*	1/2 waffle (13)	3/4 waffle (19.5)	1 waffle (26)
—frozen, small	*	1/2 waffle (7)	1 waffle (14)	1 1/2 waffles (21)	1 1/2 waffles (21)

EFFECTIVE CARBOHYDRATE CONTENT OF VEGETABLES

FOOD	5-GRAM PORTION	10-GRAM PORTION	15-GRAM PORTION	20-GRAM PORTION	25-GRAM PORTION
Alfalfa sprouts—raw	*	*	unlimited	unlimited	unlimited
Amaranth—boiled	1 cup (5.4)	2 cups (10.8)			
Artichoke—boiled	*	1/2 med. (6.7)	1 med. (13.4)	1 1/2 med. (20.1)	2 med. (26.8)
Artichoke hearts—boiled	1/4 cup (4.4)	1/2 cup (8.7)	3/4 cup (13)	1 cup (17.4)	1 1/2 cups (21.7)
—marinated, oil	1/4 cup (3.5)	1/2 cup (6.9)	1 cup (13.8)	1 1/2 cups (20.7)	1 3/4 cups (24)
Arugula—raw	unlimited	unlimited	unlimited	unlimited	unlimited

Asparagus—boiled	10 spears (4)	20 spears (8)	30 spears (12)	unlimited	unlimited
—canned	1 cup (5.6)	1 1/2 cups (8.4)	2 1/2 cups (14)	3 cups (16.8)	4 cups (22.4)
—frozen, boiled	6 spears (8.2)	13 spears (9.5)	20 spears (14.6)	unlimited	unlimited
Bamboo shoots—raw	1 cup (4)	2 cups (8)	3 cups (12)	5 cups (20)	6 cups (24)
—canned	1 cup (4.6)	2 cups (9.2)	3 cups (13.8)	unlimited	unlimited
Bean salad (Pillsbury)—canned	1/8 cup (3.6)	1/4 cup (7.3)	1/2 cup (14.5)	2/3 cup (19.3)	3/4 cup (21.8)
Beans, chili (Hunt's)—canned	scant 1/4 cup (5)	1/3 cup (8)	1/2 cup (12)	3/4 cup (18)	1 cup (24)
(Joan of Arc, Caliente) —canned	1/4 cup (5.4)	1/2 cup (10.8)	2/3 cup (14.4)	3/4 cup (16.2)	1 cup (21.6)
Beans, w/pork&tom (Joan of Arc)—can	1/8 cup (4.4)	1/4 cup (8.7)	1/3 cup (11.6)	1/2 cup (17.4)	2/3 cup (23.2)
Beans, refried (Rosarita) —canned	1/8 cup (3.5)	1/3 cup (9.3)	1/2 cup (14)	2/3 cup (18.7)	3/4 cup (21)
Beet greens—boiled	2/3 cup (5.2)	1 cup (7.8)	2 cups (15.6)	2 1/2 cups (19.5)	3 cups (23.4)
Beets—boiled, sliced	1/2 cup (5.7)	3/4 cup (8.5)	1 cup (11.7)	1 1/2 cups (17.1)	2 cups (23.4)
—Harvard, canned	*	1/4 cup (11.2)	1/3 cup (14.9)	1/3 cup (14.9)	1/2 cup (22.4)
—pickled, canned	1/8 cup (4.7)	1/4 cup (9.3)	1/3 cup (12.4)	1/2 cup (18.6)	2/3 cup (24.8)
Black beans—boiled	1/8 cup (4.2)	1/4 cup (8.4)	1/3 cup (11.1)	1/2 cup (16.8)	3/4 cup (25.2)
Black turtle beans—canned	1/8 cup (4.9)	1/4 cup (9.9)	1/3 cup (13.2)	1/2 cup (19.8)	2/3 cup (26.4)
Broccoli—raw, chopped	2 cups (4.4)	unlimited	unlimited	unlimited	unlimited
—boiled, chopped	1 cup (4)	2 cups (8)	3 cups (12)	5 cups (20)	unlimited
—frozen, chopped or spears	3/4 cup (4.4)	1 1/2 cups (8.7)	2 1/2 cups (14.5)	3 cups (17.4)	4 cups (23.2)
Broccoli/carrots (Pillsbury) —frozen	3/4 cup (4.7)	1 1/2 cups (9.3)	2 cups (12.4)	3 cups (18.6)	4 cups (24.8)
Broccoli/cauliflower—frozen	1 cup (5.4)	2 cups (10.8)	2 1/2 cups (13.5)	3 cups (16.2)	4 cups (21.6)
Broccoli/corn/red pepper—frozen	1/3 cup (5)	2/3 cup (10.1)	1 cup (15.2)	1 1/3 cups (19.8)	1 1/2 cups (22.8)
Broccoli/peppers/bamboo shoots/mushrooms—frozen	1 cup (3.5)	2 cups (7)	4 cups (14)	5 cups (17.5)	6 cups (21)
Broccoli/pearl onions/ red peppers—frozen	1 cup (3.5)	2 cups (7)	4 cups (14)	5 cups (17.5)	6 cups (21)

EFFECTIVE CARBOHYDRATE CONTENT OF VEGETABLES

FOOD	5-GRAM PORTION	10-GRAM PORTION	15-GRAM PORTION	20-GRAM PORTION	25-GRAM PORTION
Brussels sprouts—boiled	5 sprouts (4.3)	11 sprouts (9.4)	15 sprouts (12.8)	17 sprouts (14.5)	25 sprouts (21.3)
with cheese—frozen	*	*	1/2 cup (12.5)	3/4 cup (18.8)	1 cup (25)
Butter beans—canned		1/3 cup (8)	1/2 cup (12.2)	2/3 cup (16)	1 cup (24.4)
Cabbage, Chinese (bok choy)					
—raw	3 cups (2.4)	unlimited	unlimited	unlimited	unlimited
Cabbage, green or red—raw	1 1/2 cups (4.5)	2 cups (6)	5 cups (15)	6 cups (18)	6 cups (21.6)
—boiled	1 1/2 cups (5.4)	2 cups (7.2)	3 cups (10.8)	5 cups (18)	5 med. (25)
Carrots—raw	1 med. (5)	2 med. (10)	3 med. (15)	4 med. (20)	5 med. (25)
—boiled, sliced	*	1/2 cup (6.7)	1 cup (13.4)	1 1/2 cups (20.1)	2 cups (26.8)
—canned, slices	3/4 cup (4.5)	1 1/2 cups (9)	2 cups (12)	3 cups (18)	4 cups (24)
—frozen, slices	1/2 cup (4.7)	1 cup (9.4)	1 1/2 cups (14.1)	2 cups (18.8)	2 1/2 cups (23.5)
Cauliflower—raw/boiled/frozen,					
pieces	2 cups (5.2)	4 cups (10.4)	5 cups (13)	unlimited	unlimited
Celery—raw	4 stalks (3.6)	unlimited	unlimited	unlimited	unlimited
—boiled, diced	3/4 cup (4.5)	1 1/2 cups (9)	2 cups (12)	3 cups (18)	4 cups (24)
Chard, Swiss—boiled, chopped	3/4 cup (5.4)	1 cup (7.2)	2 cups (14.4)	2 1/2 cups (19.8)	3 cups (21.6)
Chickpeas—boiled	*	1/4 cup (10)	1/3 cup (13.3)	1/2 cup (20)	2/3 cup (26.6)
—hummus	*	*	1/4 cup (12.5)	1/3 cup (16.6)	1/2 cup (25)
Chives—raw	unlimited	unlimited	unlimited	unlimited	unlimited
Coleslaw—homemade	1/3 cup (5)	1/2 cup (7.5)	1 cup (15)	1 1/3 cups (20)	1 2/3 cups (25)
Collard greens—boiled, chopped	1/2 cup (3.9)	1 cup (7.8)	2 cups (15.6)	2 1/2 cups (19.5)	3 cups (23.4)
—frozen, chopped	1/3 cup (4)	3/4 cup (9)	1 cup (12)	1 1/2 cups (18)	2 cups (24)
Corn, white—frozen or canned	*	1/4 cup (8)	1/3 cup (10.6)	1/2 cup (16)	3/4 cup (24)
Corn, yellow—boiled	*	1/4 cup (8.5)	1/3 cup (11.3)	1/2 cup (17)	2/3 cup (22.6)
—frozen, boiled	*	1/3 cup (10)	1/2 cup (15.1)	2/3 cup (20)	3/4 cup (22.5)
—on the cob	*	*	1/2 ear (12)	1/2 ear (12)	1 ear (24)
Cowpeas (black-eyed peas)					

—canned	*	1/3 cup (10.9)	1/3 cup (13)	1/2 cup (16.4)	2/3 cup (21.8)
—frozen, boiled	*	1/4 cup (10)	1/3 cup (13)	1/2 cup (20)	2/3 cup (26.6)
Cucumber—raw	1/2 med. (3)	1 med. (6)	2 med. (12)	3 med. (18)	4 med. (24)
Dandelion greens—raw	1 cup (5.2)	2 cups (10.4)	3 cups (15.6)	4 cups (20.8)	5 cups (26)
—boiled, chopped	1/2 cup (3.3)	1 cup (6.6)	2 cups (13.2)	3 cups (19.2)	4 cups (26.4)
Eggplant—raw pieces	1 cup (5)	2 cups (10)	3 cups (15)	4 cups (20)	5 cups (25)
—steamed, pieces	3/4 cup (4.8)	1 cup (6.4)	2 cups (12.8)	3 cups (19.2)	4 cups (25.6)
Endive, raw	2 cups (3.2)	4 cups (6.4)	unlimited	unlimited	unlimited
Fava beans—canned	1/8 cup (3.9)	1/4 cup (7.8)	2/3 cup (15.5)	2/3 cup (20.6)	3/4 cup (23.3)
Fennel—fresh	3/4 cup (4.7)	1 cup (6.3)	2 cups (12.6)	3 cups (18.9)	4 cups (25.2)
Garlic, raw	3 cloves (3)	unlimited	unlimited	unlimited	unlimited
Ginger—raw, sliced	1/4 cup (3.6)	1/2 cup (7.2)	unlimited	unlimited	unlimited
Great Northern beans—boiled	*	1/3 cup (10.4)	1/2 cup (15.6)	2/3 cup (20.8)	3/4 cup (24)
(Joan of Arc)—canned	*	1/3 cup (8.2)	1/2 cup (12.3)	2/3 cup (16.4)	3/4 cup (18.5)
Green beans (snap beans)					
—boiled	1/2 cup (3.8)	1 cup (7.6)	2 cups (15.2)	2 1/2 cups (19)	3 cups (22.8)
—canned	1 cup (4.4)	2 cups (8.8)	3 cups (13.2)	4 cups (17.6)	5 cups (22)
—frozen, whole	1/2 cup (4.2)	1 cup (8.4)	1 1/2 cups (12.6)	2 cups (16.8)	3 cups (25.2)
Hominy, canned	*	1/4 cup (7.5)	1/2 cup (15)	2/3 cup (20)	3/4 cup (22.5)
Italian-style vegs—frozen	1/3 cup (7.3)	1/2 cup (11)	2/3 cup (14.6)	3/4 cup (16.5)	1 cup (22)
Japanese-style vegs—frozen	1/3 cup (6.6)	1/2 cup (10)	3/4 cup (15)	1 cup (20)	1 1/4 cups (25)
Kale—boiled, chopped	1/2 cup (3.7)	1 cup (7.4)	2 cups (14.8)	2 1/2 cups (18.5)	3 cups (22.2)
Kelp—raw	1/4 cup (5.5)	1/2 cup (11)	2/3 cup (14.6)	3/4 cup (16.5)	2 cups (22)
Kidney beans, red—boiled	*	1/4 cup (8.4)	1/3 cup (11.2)	1/2 cup (16.8)	2/3 cup (22.4)
—canned	1/8 cup (5)	1/4 cup (10)	1/3 cup (13.3)	1/2 cup (20)	2/3 cup (26.6)
Leeks—boiled, chopped	1/2 cup (4)	1 cup (8)	1 1/2 cups (12)	2 cups (16)	3 cups (24)
Lentils—boiled	*	1/4 cup (8)	1/3 cup (10.6)	1/2 cup (16)	3/4 cup (24)
Lettuce, butterhead or iceberg					
—raw	unlimited	unlimited	unlimited	unlimited	unlimited
romaine—shredded	unlimited	unlimited	unlimited	unlimited	unlimited
Lima beans—boiled	1/8 cup (3.3)	1/3 cup (8.6)	1/2 cup (12.9)	3/4 cup (19.4)	1 cup (25.8)
—canned	1/8 cup (4.5)	1/4 cup (9)	1/3 cup (12)	1/2 cup (18)	2/3 cup (23.9)

EFFECTIVE CARBOHYDRATE CONTENT OF VEGETABLES

FOOD	5-GRAM PORTION	10-GRAM PORTION	15-GRAM PORTION	20-GRAM PORTION	25-GRAM PORTION
Mushrooms—raw, pieces	1 cup (2.2)	unlimited	unlimited	unlimited	unlimited
—steamed or canned, pieces	1 cup (4.6)	2 cups (9.2)	3 cups (13.8)	4 cups (18.4)	5 cups (23)
(enoki)—raw, whole	unlimited	unlimited	unlimited	unlimited	unlimited
(straw)—canned	1 cup (5.6)	unlimited	unlimited	unlimited	unlimited
(shiitake)—whole, broiled	2 whole (5.1)	4 whole (10.3)	5 whole (15.4)	8 whole (20.6)	
—dried, whole	2 whole (5.6)	3 whole (8.4)	5 whole (14)	7 whole (19.6)	8 whole (22.4)
Mustard greens—boiled, chopped	1 1/2 cups (4.5)	3 cups (9)	unlimited	unlimited	unlimited
—frozen, chopped	1 cup (4.6)	2 cups (9.2)	3 cups (13.8)	4 cups (18.4)	unlimited
Navy beans—boiled	*	1/4 cup (10.4)	1/3 cup (13.8)	1/2 cup (20.7)	2/3 cup (27.5)
—canned	*	*	1/4 cup (13.4)	1/3 cup (17.8)	1/2 cup (26.8)
Okra—boiled, slices	1/2 cup (5.8)	3/4 cup (8.7)	1 cup (11.6)	1 1/2 cups (17.4)	2 cups (23.2)
—frozen, slices	1/3 cup (5)	1/3 cup (7.5)	1 cup (15)	1 1/3 cups (20)	1 1/2 cups (22.5)
Onions—raw, chopped	1/2 cup (5.6)	3/4 cup (8.4)	1 cup (11.2)	unlimited	unlimited
—boiled, chopped	1/4 cup (5.3)	1/2 cup (10.7)	3/4 cup (15.9)	1 cup (21)	1 1/4 cups (26.3)
—dehydrated, flakes	1/8 cup (5.9)	1/4 cup (11.7)	1/3 cup (15.6)	1/3 cup (15.6)	1/2 cup (23.4)
Onions, green (spring)—raw, chopped	1 cup (5)	unlimited	unlimited	unlimited	unlimited
Parsley—raw, chopped	unlimited	unlimited	unlimited	unlimited	unlimited
—freeze-dried	unlimited	unlimited	unlimited	unlimited	unlimited
Parsnips—boiled, slices	*	1/3 cup (8.7)	1/2 cup (13.1)	2/3 cup (17.5)	1 cup (26.2)
Peas, green—boiled	1/4 cup (5.1)	1/2 cup (10.3)	3/4 cup (15.5)	1 cup (20.6)	1 1/4 cups (25.8)
—canned	1/3 cup (5.2)	1/2 cup (7.8)	1 cup (15.6)	1 1/3 cups (20.8)	1 1/2 cups (23.4)
Peas, split—boiled	*	1/4 cup (10)	1/3 cup (14)	1/2 cup (21.2)	1/2 cup (21.2)
Peas, sweet—canned	1/4 cup (4.2)	1/2 cup (8.4)	3/4 cup (12.6)	1 cup (16.8)	1 1/2 cups (25.2)
Peppers, hot chili—raw	1 whole (4.3)	2 whole (8.6)	3 whole (12.9)	4 whole (17.2)	6 whole (25.8)
—canned, chopped	1/2 cup (4.2)	1 cup (8.4)	1 3/4 cups (14.7)	2 cups (16.8)	unlimited

Food					
Peppers, jalapeño—canned, chopped	½ cup (3.3)	1 cup (6.6)	unlimited	unlimited	unlimited
Peppers, sweet—raw, chopped	1 cup (4.8)	2 cups (9.6)	unlimited	unlimited	unlimited
—freeze-dried, chopped	1 cup (4.4)	unlimited	unlimited	unlimited	unlimited
Peppers, sweet, yellow—raw, whole	½ large (5.9)	¾ large (8.9)	1 large (11.8)	1¾ large (20.7)	2 large (23.6)
Pimientos—canned	unlimited	unlimited	unlimited	unlimited	unlimited
Pinto beans—boiled	⅛ cup (4.7)	¼ cup (9.3)	⅓ cup (12.4)	½ cup (18.6)	⅔ cup (24.8)
—canned	⅛ cup (4.4)	¼ cup (8.7)	⅓ cup (11.6)	½ cup (17.5)	⅔ cup (23.3)
(Joan of Arc, Picante Style)	⅛ cup (3.7)	⅓ cup (9.7)	½ cup (14.6)	⅔ cup (19.5)	¾ cup (21.9)
Potato, sweet—baked, skin eaten *	*	¼ med. (6)	½ med. (12)	¾ med. (18)	1 med. (24)
—boiled, mashed	*	*	*	¼ cup (19.9)	⅓ cup (25.9)
Potato, white—baked, skin eaten *	*	*	¼ med. (12.8)	⅓ med. (17)	½ med. (25.5)
—baked, no skin	*	¼ med. (7.8)	⅓ med. (10.4)	½ med. (15.7)	¾ med. (23.4)
—boiled, no skin	*	¼ med. (6.3)	½ med. (12.5)	⅔ med. (16.7)	1 med. (25)
Potato, new—canned, whole	*	⅓ cup (10)	½ cup (15)	⅔ cup (20)	¾ cup (22.5)
Potatoes—french fried, drained	*	5 fries (10)	7 fries (14)	10 fries (20)	12 fries (24)
Potatoes, white—mashed	*	¼ cup (7.5)	½ cup (15)	⅔ cup (20)	¾ cup (22.5)
Pumpkin—boiled, mashed	¼ cup (3)	½ cup (6)	1 cup (12)	1½ cups (18)	2 cups (24)
—canned, solid pack	¼ cup (2.2)	½ cup (6.3)	1 cup (12.6)	1½ cups (18.9)	2 cups (25.2)
Radicchio—raw, shredded	unlimited	unlimited	unlimited	unlimited	unlimited
Radishes, red—raw	unlimited	unlimited	unlimited	unlimited	unlimited
Radishes, white—raw, sliced	unlimited	unlimited	unlimited	unlimited	unlimited
Red beans—canned	*	⅓ cup (8)	½ cup (12)	⅔ cup (16)	1 cup (24)
Rhubarb—boiled	½ cup (3.5)	1 cup (7)	2 cups (14)	3 cups (21)	3½ cups (24.5)
Rutabaga, boiled, sliced	⅓ cup (4.4)	½ cup (6.6)	1 cup (13.2)	1½ cups (19.8)	1¾ cups (23.1)
Sauerkraut—bottled or canned	½ cup (5.1)	¾ cup (7.6)	1 cup (10.2)	2 cups (20.4)	2½ cups (26.5)
Shallots—raw, chopped	3 Tblsp (5.1)	unlimited	unlimited	unlimited	1.4 grams per cup
Spinach—raw, chopped	unlimited	unlimited	unlimited	unlimited	unlimited
—frozen, boiled	1 cup (3.1)	3 cups (9.3)	5 cups (15.1)	unlimited	unlimited
—canned	3 cups (3.6)	unlimited	unlimited	unlimited	unlimited

EFFECTIVE CARBOHYDRATE CONTENT OF VEGETABLES

FOOD	5-GRAM PORTION	10-GRAM PORTION	15-GRAM PORTION	20-GRAM PORTION	25-GRAM PORTION
Squash, summer varieties (crookneck, scallop, zucchini)					
—raw, pieces	1 cup (4)	2 cups (8)	4 cups (16)	5 cups (20)	6 cups (24)
—boiled	1 cup (5.2)	2 cups (10.4)	3 cups (15.6)	4 cups (20.8)	5 cups (26)
Squash, winter varieties (acorn, butternut, Hubbard)					
—raw, pieces	1/2 cup (5.1)	1 cup (10.2)	1 1/2 cups (15.3)	2 cups (20.4)	2 1/2 cups (25.5)
—baked	1/3 cup (4)	2/3 cup (8)	1 cup (12)	1 1/2 cups (18)	2 cups (24)
(spaghetti variety)—baked or boiled	1/2 cup (5)	1 cup (10)	1 1/2 cups (15)	2 cups (20)	2 1/2 cups (25)
Succotash—boiled	*	*	1/4 cup (11.7)	1/3 cup (15.6)	1/2 cup (23.4)
—canned or frozen	*	*	1/3 cup (11.3)	1/2 cup (17)	3/4 cup (25.5)
Tomatillo—raw, whole	2 med. (4)	5 med. (10)	7 med. (14)	10 med. (20)	12 med. (24)
Tomato, green—raw, whole	1 med. (4.1)	2 med. (8.2)	3 med. (12.5)	5 med. (20.5)	6 med. (24.6)
red—raw, whole	1 med. (4.1)	2 med. (8.2)	3 med. (12.5)	5 med. (20.5)	6 med. (24.6)
red—canned	1/2 cup (5)	1 cup (10)	1 1/2 cups (15)	2 cups (20)	2 1/2 cups (25)
red with green chilies—canned	1/2 cup (4.3)	1 cup (8.6)	1 1/2 cups (12.9)	2 cups (17.2)	2 1/2 cups (21.5)
Tomato—sun-dried	1/8 cup (3.8)	1/4 cup (7.5)	1/2 cup (15)	2/3 cup (20)	3/4 cup (22.5)
Turnips—boiled, pieces	1 cup (4.4)	2 cups (8.8)	3 cups (13.2)	4 cups (17.6)	5 cups (22)
Turnip greens—boiled, chopped	2 cups (3.6)	4 cups (7.2)	unlimited	unlimited	unlimited
—canned, chopped	2 cups (5.6)	3 cups (8.4)	5 cups (14)	unlimited	unlimited
Water chestnuts—raw, sliced	1/8 cup (3.7)	1/4 cup (7.4)	1/2 cup (14.8)	2/3 cup (19.7)	3/4 cup (22.2)
—canned, whole	5 whole (5)	10 whole (10)	15 whole (15)	unlimited	unlimited
—canned, sliced	1/4 cup (4)	1/2 cup (8)	3/4 cup (12)	1 cup (16)	1 1/2 cups (24)
Wax beans—canned	1/2 cup (4.5)	1 cup (9)	1 1/2 cups (13.5)	2 cups (18)	2 1/2 cups (22.5)
White beans—boiled	*	1/4 cup (11.3)	1/3 cup (15)	1/3 cup (19)	1/2 cup (22.5)
—canned	*	1/8 cup (7.2)	1/4 cup (14.4)	1/3 cup (19)	1/2 cup (22.5)
Yams—baked or boiled, pieces	*	1/4 cup (9.4)	1/3 cup (12.5)	1/2 cup (18.8)	2/3 cup (25)

Chapter 6

Vitamins, Mi
Potassium

170 PROTEIN POWER

health practitioners
physicians to snake
nutritional guru
for that "ma
leviate hu
rages,
fuse
m

Nicotinic acid cures pellagra, but a beefsteak prevents it.

HENRY E. SIGERIST, medical historian

For your body to function optimally, your diet must include sufficient amounts of micronutrients—vitamins, minerals, and potassium. In this chapter you will learn what they are and how much of which ones you need for good health.

More than 4,000 years ago the Chinese recognized that people became ill with a disease called *beriberi* when they relied on a diet of polished rice. Some substance, they didn't know what, in the rice husks prevented this illness. We now understand that polishing the husks away removes all the thiamine (vitamin B$_1$) from the rice, and thiamine deficiency causes beriberi. From this early discovery of vitamin deficiency's role in causing disease to the recent studies showing the power of antioxidants and phytochemicals to protect us against cancer and heart disease,

of every stripe, from mainstream
oil salesmen, patent medicine peddlers,
s, and scientific researchers, have searched
ic bullet" cure-all micronutrient that will al-
han suffering and disease. As this vitamin debate
t has often left the health-conscious public con-
. Should you supplement your diet with vitamin and
ineral tablets or rely on the micronutrients in the foods
you eat? If you do supplement, what should you take and
how much? Is the RDA (Recommended Dietary Allowance) enough to promote optimal health, or should
you take more? Which vitamins and minerals, in particular, might be beneficial in the metabolic disorders related
to insulin resistance?

First, the RDA for vitamins and minerals: we speak from
the camp of those researchers, clinicians, and scientists
who feel that although a diet that provides the RDA of all
essential vitamins and minerals will certainly keep most
people from developing serious deficiency diseases, these
levels are woefully inadequate to ensure optimal health
and peak performance. For example, the RDA of vitamin
E is about 10 milligrams per day, but several recent studies have shown this antioxidant to be protective against
heart disease (and a number of other diseases of aging)
only if taken at doses six, ten, even *forty* times the RDA.

Rest assured that our program—even in its strictest
phases—provides you ample opportunity to consume
every essential vitamin, mineral, and nutrient in quantities
that meet or exceed the RDA, but whether you do so will
depend on your own taste preferences. Like George Bush
and his aversion to broccoli, we all tend to consume the
foods we like in quantity and avoid those we aren't quite
so fond of even though they might be rich in beneficial

micronutrients. Because our purpose here is to help you regain your health and overcome the problems that "civilized" eating has inflicted on you, we ask that you ensure the micronutrient adequacy of your diet by supplementing it with a complete general multiple vitamin and mineral tablet and potassium.

For good general health you need adequate amounts of all the vitamins and minerals. Certain vitamins and minerals, however, have a special bearing on insulin resistance and the disorders caused by it.[1]

The Vitamins

In general, vitamins function in your body as facilitators in certain chemical reactions. For example, your body must have vitamin C (ascorbic acid) to build strong collagen, the main structural protein in the body that makes the framework for bone, muscle fiber, tendon, ligament, skin, hair, and scar tissue to heal wounds. Without adequate vitamin C the collagen that's made is weak and of poor structural quality. It tears easily. When people become deficient in vitamin C, they bruise easily, their teeth loosen and fall out, they lose their hair, their gums bleed, their wounds don't heal well, their joints weaken, and finally they usually hemorrhage (from weak blood vessel walls) and die. The disease this vitamin deficiency causes is called

---

[1] To answer your questions about using vitamin and mineral supplementation to prevent or treat conditions other than insulin-related ones, look for *The Doctor's Complete Guide to Vitamins and Minerals* by Mary Dan Eades, M.D. (New York: Dell, 1994).

scurvy, and it nearly destroyed the navies of many countries until the British recognized that they could prevent it by making sure their sailors ate plenty of limes and lemons while at sea.

This preventive measure created a popular misconception that citrus fruits are the only good dietary source of vitamin C, but Arctic explorer Vilhjalmur Stefansson conclusively proved that wrong in the late 1920s. Fresh, lightly cooked meat and fish, he found, contain enough of a vitamin C–like substance (as well as all other critical micronutrients) to prevent scurvy and other deficiency diseases. The *Journal of the American Medical Association* documented that Stefansson, who spent one full year on a drastic diet of nothing but fresh meat and water not only did not die as predicted but emerged fitter, leaner, with lower cholesterol counts (about the only laboratory marker for heart disease available in the late 1920s), and healthier in every regard.

However, unless you can obtain a steady supply of very fresh meat and you like to eat it cooked rare, you will need to get your vitamin C from other sources. According to the RDA, your daily intake of vitamin C should be a modest 60 milligrams per day, about the amount contained in a medium orange. For most people that will be enough to prevent the development of scurvy. But that's just one side of the equation. What amount of vitamin C would it take to optimize health? That's the question that occupied Nobel Prize laureate Dr. Linus Pauling for the last four decades of his illustrious career. Reasoning that since humans are one of only four species (along with other primates, guinea pigs, and the fruit-eating bat) that have lost the ability to make vitamin C, we ought to obtain from our diets at least as much as other species make on their

own—and he concluded that the RDA is pitifully inadequate. We need not 60 milligrams but more on the order
of 6,000 to 20,000 milligrams. Based on body size, Dr.
Pauling calculated his own daily dose at 20,000 milligrams
(20 grams), which he took religiously. And during the last
decades of his life—he died recently at age ninety-three—
he devoted his resources and time to an intense study of
this vitamin's role in prevention and treatment of diseases
ranging from the common cold to atherosclerosis to cancer. We recommend that you supplement your diet with a
daily intake of at least 1 gram (1,000 mg) of vitamin C
and along with it vitamin E and beta-carotene, forming
the group called the *antioxidants*. Vitamin C stays in the
body for only twelve hours, so if you want to go beyond
the 1-gram recommendation, split your dose and take it
morning and night.

The Antioxidants

All day, every day, this modern world assaults us with
harmful substances—air pollution in the form of smog
and industrial toxins, secondhand cigarette smoke, addi-
tives and other chemicals in our food and water, pharma-
ceuticals, radiation—but the commonest and potentially
most damaging of all is a substance we must have for life:
oxygen. While you may not be accustomed to thinking of
oxygen as harmful—and rightly so since it's generally beneficial—you should also remember that exposure to oxygen can turn a pickup truck into a rusty heap of iron, a
succulent apple slice into an ugly piece of brown mush,
and a tiny spark into a raging inferno. There is a duality in
this substance; it can both create and destroy. Oxygen fuels the metabolic fire that burns within us and gives us life,

but it can also cause widespread damage—by a process called, naturally enough, *oxidation* (the same process that rusts out the truck) and through the formation of reactive substances called *free radicals*. What does all this have to do with the metabolic mayhem of insulin resistance?

It's oxidation of cholesterol molecules that renders them more reactive and more likely to lie down in the artery walls, forming plaque and causing heart attacks. Oxidation of essential fats alters their structure and disrupts their entry into and flow along the eicosanoid pathway, leading to the overproduction of "bad" eicosanoid messengers, leading to blood clotting for heart attack and stroke or to inflammatory messengers causing painful joints or to allergy messengers that promote asthma or hives. It's oxidation of other body tissues that ages them, leading to the development of arthritic damage, wrinkled skin, and cataracts, and it's oxidation that damages the cells, promoting the development of cancers.

How does oxidation do these things? The human body is made up of billions of cells, and those cells are made up of billions of atoms, and those atoms are composed of charged particles called *protons* and *electrons*. The positively charged protons exist in the middles (or nuclei) of the atoms, with the negatively charged electrons whirling in pairs in orbit around the middle. Normally all the positive and negative charges balance, all the electrons are happily paired, and the atom exists in a state of electrical neutrality. But to function, to create energy for life, we must upset this balance by shuffling these electrons from atom to atom in a controlled way. When an atom loses one of its electrons, it becomes electrically unbalanced, with more positives than negatives. When it takes on this charge, we call it a *free radical*—one of its electrons is alone, or free, in its orbit. This free radical becomes very reactive, on the prowl for an electron to replace the one it lost, potentially setting off a chain reaction of electron robbing. As long as the process remains controlled, all is well. But the uncontrolled development of too many of these free radicals—from toxins, cigarette smoke, pollution, and the like—can lead to cell damage, promoting the development of disease and accelerating the aging process.

Antioxidants, as their name implies, help to prevent the damaging effects of oxygen and other free-radical-forming substances on your body's tissues, and thus they reduce your risk of disorders ranging from heart disease to cancer. For example, recent medical research has shown that deficiencies of the antioxidants vitamin C and beta-carotene (the vitamin A forerunner) may contribute to the development of high blood pressure and that vitamins C and E help to reduce the risk of heart disease caused by atherosclerosis in the blood vessels supplying the heart (and elsewhere).

You will find vitamin C in foods such as sweet peppers, broccoli, citrus fruits, melons, strawberries, tomatoes, raw cabbage, leafy greens (spinach, mustard, and turnip greens), and fresh meat and liver. Good sources of beta-carotene are carrots, cantaloupe, spinach, broccoli, winter squash, and apricots. Seeds, nuts, and the oils derived from them, especially sunflower seeds and almonds, are the richest food sources of vitamin E. Following our dietary guidelines, you will gravitate naturally toward these kinds of foods since they are also the vegetable and fruit sources with the lowest carbohydrate content and the most fiber. If you like these foods and eat them often, wonderful. You should always get plenty of the antioxidants, other vitamins, and minerals you need from food.

Don't worry about getting too much vitamin C; the more the better because you can't store it and it won't hurt you. If—like a few of our patients over the years—you prefer such "vegetables" as ketchup, potatoes, corn, dried beans, rice, and pasta, don't let a day pass without supplementing your intake of all the antioxidants—beta-carotene and vitamins C and E. These foods may be vegetables, but in the main they are starches, just like bread and cereal—and you know by now that they're to be severely restricted. Remember the Egyptians?

THE ESSENTIAL B VITAMINS

In addition to the critical antioxidants, your diet must include all the other vitamins, but especially those in the B group. To make optimal use of the protein, carbohydrate, and fat in the foods you eat, to turn these raw materials into muscle, blood, enzymes, and energy, your body must have a steady supply of all the vitamins that make up the B vitamin complex. This group—niacin, thiamine, riboflavin, and vitamins B_5, B_6, and B_{12}—works interdependently, so when you supplement one of them, you should supplement *all* of them; take B complex, not just vitamin B_{12} or B_6. For the B vitamin group to function efficiently, you must also have plenty of folic acid. Like vitamin C, the B vitamins and folic acid are water-soluble, so you must replace them daily, either in the foods you eat or in supplement form.

You will find the richest food sources for B vitamins in meats: in organ meats, such as liver and kidney; in muscle meats, such as beef, pork, veal, and chicken; in seafood, especially oysters and clams, but also in ocean fish, such as tuna and salmon; in egg yolk; and in cheese and milk, es-

Barnes & Noble Bookseller
515 Opry Mills Drive
Nashville, TN 37214
(615) 514-5000
02-11-02 S02016 R004

CUSTOMER RECEIPT COPY

Art of Teaching Words o	9.95
0740719122	
Words of Encouragement	4.95
0880881186	
Protein Power	14.00
0553380788	

SUB TOTAL	28.90
SALES TAX	2.38
TOTAL	31.28

AMOUNT TENDERED

AMEX	31.28
CARD #:	***************3008
AMOUNT	31.28
AUTH CODE	582125

TOTAL PAYMENT   31.28

Thank you for Shopping at
Barnes & Noble Booksellers
Shop online 24 hours a day www.bn.com
#73775 02-11-02 08:00P AMES

Booksellers since 1873

Full refund issued for new and unread books and unopened music within
14 days with a receipt from any Barnes & Noble store.
Store Credit issued for new and unread books and unopened music after
14 days or without a sales receipt. Credit issued at lowest sale price.

Full refund issued for new and unread books and unopened music within
14 days with a receipt from any Barnes & Noble store.
Store Credit issued for new and unread books and unopened music after
14 days or without a sales receipt. Credit issued at lowest sale price.

pecially dry milk.
clude walnuts, pea
avocados.

FOLIC ACID

Folic acid, wl
etables, and
and blood,
mass. You
able to at
pletes the folic ac
who use this form of contu
is important to healthy fat loss and
tion.

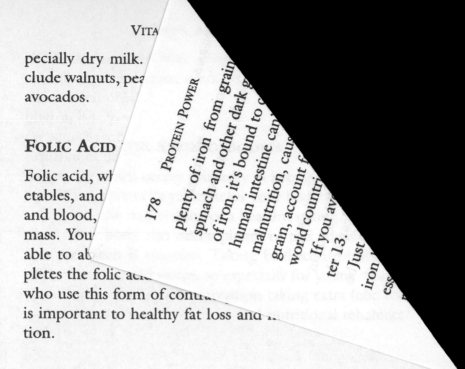

178   PROTEIN POWER

plenty of iron from grain
spinach and other dark g
of iron, it's bound to c
human intestine can
malnutrition, caus
grain, account f
world countri
If you av
ter 13.
Just
iron
ess

The Minerals

IRON: THE CASE FOR EATING RED MEAT

If you've been avoiding eating red meat, not for philosophical or religious reasons but because you've been told
it's not good for you, rejoice! Not only does red meat provide you with lots of high-quality protein and an abundance of every member of the B vitamin complex, but it's
also a rich source—perhaps the best source—of iron. The
iron in red meat, called *heme iron,* is bound to protein, a
form the human gastrointestinal tract can absorb more
easily and completely. For this reason vegetarians and others who do not eat red meat tend to develop iron deficiencies and anemia even though their diets may contain

and vegetable sources. While
_____en leafy vegetables contain a lot
_____ompounds (called *phytates*) that the
_____t absorb. Iron deficiency and protein
_____ed by a meatless diet and a reliance on
_____or widespread mental retardation in third-
_____es and developing nations around the world.
_____id red meat for cholesterol reasons, see Chap-

_____as the intestine will absorb protein-bound heme
_____better than other forms, so will it absorb other nec-
_____ary minerals when they are combined with protein. The
_____eason for this better absorption lies in how minerals en-
ter the intestine.

Make Ours Chelates, Please

Most minerals—particularly those in many inexpensively
manufactured vitamin and mineral tablets—occur as salts.
In a salt the mineral combines with other elements; for
example, iron as ferrous sulfate combines with sulfur and
oxygen. When these mineral salts enter the stomach, the
salts break apart into individual elements called *ions*.[2] The
mucous coating of the stomach lining is slightly charged,
and it attracts these positively and negatively charged ions
in much the same way that opposite poles of magnets at-
tract. Beneath the mucous coating each of the cells of the

---

[2] Don't be confused by our recommendation of taking potassium as a
salt. The electrolytes—potassium, sodium, and chloride—function as
ions.

lining of the stomach has a tiny channel—called the *ion channel*—that will admit a single ion at a time. Because the ions compete with each other for entry into the channel, the amount of any mineral that gets through depends on how much of it is in the stomach at the time and whether anything else is in the stomach.

Technology has offered us a way to bypass the bottleneck of the single ion channel. The process, called *chelation,* wraps each mineral ion in a jacket of amino acids, the building blocks of protein. The disguise works; the stomach lining absorbs these amino acid–chelated minerals as if they were protein. They don't have to stand in line to be admitted through the single ion channel. By using mineral chelates, you can completely and efficiently absorb all the minerals necessary for optimal health in much the same way your intestine will better absorb the heme form of iron. For this reason we ask that when you choose a vitamin and mineral supplement, you look carefully to be certain that it contains minerals as amino acid chelates. That way you'll know you will get—and get the benefit of—what you've paid for. You'll find several vitamin and chelated mineral supplements recommended at the end of this chapter.

THE OTHER MINERALS

Iron is only one of many minerals your diet should include. While all the trace minerals—particularly boron, iodine, molybdenum, and zinc—are important to your general health, of special importance to the metabolic disorders related to insulin resistance are the following minerals.

Chromium

The insulin receptor, the structure on the surfaces of your cells that actually becomes resistant to insulin, requires chromium to function properly. Deficiency of chromium is rampant—it affects 90 percent of the American population—because a diet high in starch and sugar puts a heavy demand on the insulin system to handle the incoming carbohydrate load, and that high demand depletes chromium. Restoring your chromium levels to normal will almost certainly require you to take a supplement since it will take a daily dietary intake of 200 micrograms to do the job and even the richest source, brewer's yeast, contains a meager 2 micrograms to the gram (liver and black pepper provide even less). Strenuous exercise also causes a chromium drain, so your need to replace this mineral will be especially high if you've been carbo-loading pasta, potatoes, and fat-free bagels before you run, bike, or swim.

Chromium's crucial role in maintaining proper insulin function makes it an important component in helping you recompose your body to a healthier, leaner state. Sufficient chromium will help you build lean muscle pounds and, through interaction with the thyroid hormone system, help you burn fat more efficiently.

If you've got a sweet tooth, chromium deficiency may be at the root of the problem. Because chromium deficiency intensifies sugar cravings, it can spur a vicious cycle: chromium deficiency stimulates your sweet tooth and drives you to eat sugary foods, which further depletes your chromium, which aggravates your sugar cravings, and on and on. By following our macronutrient prescription and supplementing with chelated or niacin-bound chromium, you should begin to find your intense craving for sweet foods diminishing in the first few weeks.

You may add supplemental chromium to your vitamin regimen if your multivitamin and mineral does not contain at least 200 micrograms. Although you will have replenished depleted chromium stores in a few weeks or months, you should continue to take this mineral every day to keep your stores full, especially if you exercise.

Calcium and Magnesium: More Than Just Bone Builders

You may think of calcium as a bone-building mineral, and indeed 99 percent of your body's calcium is stored in your skeletal framework. What you may not know, though, is that calcium and its mineral partner, magnesium, also play important roles in the transmission of nerve signals and in the contraction of muscle fibers and are involved in the development of high blood pressure. Deficiencies of these two minerals can contribute to elevating pressure, and correcting those deficiencies can bring the pressure down. Our program encourages you to eat foods that will provide plenty of dietary calcium and magnesium: nuts, legumes, green vegetables, seafood, liver, beef, egg yolks, cabbage, cauliflower, and dairy products. Especially if you do not regularly eat these foods, you should supplement calcium and magnesium in your diet as described in the list of general vitamin and mineral supplement products at the end of this chapter.

Eating a diet richer in protein and fat increases your ability to absorb calcium and to some extent magnesium, and that is fortunate; as you exercise on this nutritional regimen to build your lean body mass, your demand for these minerals will increase.

Selenium: Powerful Immune Booster

This mineral antioxidant works in conjunction with the antioxidant vitamin E to produce the body's own natural free-radical scavenger and potent protective antioxidant, glutathione. This body chemical promotes a healthy immune system to defend you from infection, may protect you from the development of cancers, and helps to slow down the aging process. Deficiency of selenium may also contribute to elevated cholesterol.

Our program provides you with the opportunity to eat plenty of the best dietary sources of selenium: seafood, organ meats, and muscle meats. Seeds may contain selenium, but it depends on the selenium content of the soil where they grew. Fruits and vegetables contain little of it. And that means, again, that vegetarians using our program to correct their insulin-related disorders (especially elevated cholesterol) will have to rely on supplemental selenium.

Potassium: Another Balancing Act

When you begin our program, your insulin will fall quickly, and perhaps the first corrective phenomenon you will notice is water loss. The metabolic changes will send a strong signal to your kidneys to release excess sodium and water. Although sodium release is the main goal, another salt, potassium, gets caught in the cross fire. During

the initial phases—especially the first few weeks and especially on Phase I—your loss of potassium in urine will ac-
celerate dramatically. If you engage in vigorous physical
exercise and sweat profusely, you will lose additional
potassium. If your potassium levels fall too low, you can
suffer from weakness, muscle cramping, fatigue, and
breathlessness.

The potassium level in your blood must stay within a
fairly narrow range for potassium to play its crucial role in
the passage of nerve impulses, in muscle contraction, and
in maintaining normal blood pressure. It exists mainly inside the cells of your body, and this huge reservoir acts as
a buffer to keep the amount in your blood relatively constant under normal circumstances. But the rapid loss of
excess fluid you will experience during the early phase of
the program is not a normal circumstance. Even eating
foods rich in potassium—such as cantaloupe, avocado,
broccoli, liver, dairy products, and citrus fruits—may not
sufficiently replace your losses. For this reason we ask that
you take one or two capsules of any of the products in the
following list or any commercially available product that
will provide at least 90 mg of potassium salts. You can also
use the over-the-counter salt substitutes (Morton's Lite
Salt or NoSalt brand, both of which are potassium salts)
to ensure you get plenty.

*If you currently take medication for high blood pressure or
fluid retention, be certain to check with your physician or
pharmacist before you supplement potassium. Certain of the
newer medications on the market for these conditions actually prevent potassium loss and could cause your potassium
level to rise too much. Just as too low a potassium level can
cause problems, so can a level that's too high. Once the pro-*

gram does its work, you may not have to take blood pressure medication any longer, but wait until your physician tells you it's safe to stop. And remember to check for a possible interaction.

Acceptable Products Include:

Twinlab—Potassium Aspartate (99 mg)
Twinlab—Liquid K Plus (99 mg)
Source Naturals K-Mag Aspartate (99 mg)
Alacer—The K Factors (92 mg)
KAL—KCL (99 mg)

In Search of an Excellent Vitamin and Mineral Supplement

When we looked for a high-quality complete multiple vitamin and mineral supplement to recommend to our patients, we wanted a supplement combination that would—even in the face of finicky eating, unusual taste preferences, or philosophical or religious restrictions—provide sufficiently for all of our patients' micronutrient needs. If you're searching for one on your own, look for one that approximates this list:

The Vitamins

Beta-carotene (for vitamin A)	25,000 IU
Vitamin D_3	50 IU
Ascorbic acid (vitamin C)	1,000 mg
Thiamine (vitamin B_1)	100 mg

Riboflavin (vitamin B_2)	10 mg
Niacin (vitamin B_3)	30 mg
Niacinamide	130 mg
Pantothenic acid (vitamin B_5)	450 mg
Pyridoxine (vitamin B_6)	15 mg
Cobalamin (vitamin B_{12})	250 mcg*
Folic acid	2 mg
D-alpha tocopherol (vitamin E)	200 IU

---

*Micrograms (1/1,000 of a milligram)

The Minerals

(These should be as amino acid chelates; look for the minerals bound to picolinate, citrate-maleate, aspartate, etc.) A typical example might look as follows:

Calcium (citrate-maleate)	500 mg
Magnesium (citrate-maleate)	250 mg
Potassium (citrate-maleate)	90 mg
Zinc (picolinate)	15 mg
Manganese (picolinate)	15 mg
Boron (picolinate)	3 mg
Copper (picolinate)	1 mg
Chromium (niacin bound)	200 mcg*
Selenium (picolinate)	200 mcg
Molybdenum (picolinate)	100 mcg
Vanadium (picolinate)	100 mcg

---

*Micrograms (1/1,000 of a milligram)

Acceptable Products Include:

KAL—High-Potency Soft Multiple Vitamin

Twinlab—Dual Tab Sustained-Release Mega Vitamin and Mineral Formula

Mega Food Multiple Vitamin and Mineral

Thorne Research Laboratories—Basic Nutrients V capsules (available only through medical professionals)

The Bottom Line

Your body relies on certain vitamins and minerals to work properly, to lose fat and build muscle effectively, and to remain healthy. To ensure that your diet always meets or exceeds these requirements, we encourage you to take a vitamin and chelated mineral supplement similar to the products we described here every day.

Chapter 7

The Antiaging Formula: Exercise

Exercise is the goddamn key. The more I do, the better I get.

TED WILLIAMS

Here, more than elsewhere, I saw multitudes to every side
of me; their howls were loud while, wheeling weights, they
used their chests to push.

You stumbled into the fourth circle of Dante's hell? Nah,
you just walked through the door of your local health
club. Everywhere you look people are groaning, sweating,
straining, flexing, posing, and pumping. You see fitness
buffs of all descriptions from the archetypal 90-pound
weaklings to guys who could give Arnold Schwarzenegger
a run for his money. All these disparate people have their
own pet theories on how to maximize their fitness gains
from exercise, and they have their own ideas of the best
nutritional strategy to help them along the way. The only
unifying factor in all this chaos is that 99.9 percent of
these nutritional ideas are incorrect. In this chapter you

will learn the role proper nutrition plays in physical development. You will learn the best exercise for turning back the clock on aging while at the same time increasing your lean body mass and burning off your excess body fat.

Exercise is absolutely essential to milking all the pleasure you can from a long and healthy life. Sure it's hard, and sure it takes time and effort, and sure we often dread it ourselves. But when we don't want to get up off our duffs and go do it, we usually remind each other of one of our favorite quotes: "The only time you can coast in life is when you're going downhill" (A. Roger Merrill).

The goals of any physical exercise are to increase muscular strength and endurance and to enhance performance. Muscles increase strength by enlarging, becoming more dense, and more efficiently tapping into their fuel supply. They become more conditioned by increasing their blood supply so that they can better access oxygen to burn this fuel. And stronger, more conditioned muscles lead to better performance in all athletics and in most of life. To put the time spent in exercise to most efficient use in achieving these goals, the body's metabolic biochemistry has to do its part by creating the proper conditions for muscle growth and repair. Let's start by looking at a hormone we haven't yet discussed that comes closer to being an elixir of youth than anything known.

The Youth Hormone

Have you ever had this experience? You get up early and work out, go to your job and put in a full day, watch your diet and deny yourself virtually everything that sounds good to eat, then come home to find your teenager sprawled half asleep in front of the TV amid a jumble of empty pizza boxes, soft drink cans, and candy wrappers. As he (or she) comes to life and asks, "What's for supper?" you do a slow burn. You've worked hard all day, exercised, and dieted, and you still have a roll around your middle that you can't get rid of. Your kid, on the other hand, lies around all day, gets up only to eat, eats three times the calories you do, yet is slender, muscular, and, if forced, could run circles around you. What gives?

One of the major factors causing this unfair disparity between them and us is an almost magical substance called *human growth hormone*. They have a lot; we don't have much. And it makes an enormous difference. (Actually we have as much as they do, but sadly, we just can't get to it nearly as well.) Fortunately the nutritional program in this book helps you increase your growth hormone levels better than any way we know short of injecting it.

Human growth hormone is a profound anabolic, or tissue-building, hormone produced in the pituitary, a small gland located at the base of the skull, and secreted at intervals throughout the day. It causes growth, repairs tissue, mobilizes fat stores, and shifts the metabolism to the preferential use of fat. Like human insulin, human growth hormone is produced commercially by recombinant DNA, and doctors use it extensively to treat a variety of disorders. Severely burned patients and those with massive soft tissue injuries or those recovering from major surgery all benefit from growth hormone therapy. Children with growth hormone deficiency who would otherwise be doomed to a life of dwarfism achieve normal growth with the administration of recombinant growth hormone. In the July 5, 1990, issue of the *New England Journal of*

Medicine, Daniel Rudman, M.D., and his research group at the Medical College of Wisconsin reported the results of their study on the effects of growth hormone administered to elderly males. Dr. Rudman's group showed that tiny amounts of growth hormone injected just beneath the skin of sixty-one- to eighty-one-year-old males produced almost unbelievable results in only six months: lean body mass increased by 8.8 percent, body fat decreased by 14.4 percent, bone density increased in the lumbar spinal bones, and skin thickness increased by 7.1 percent (thin, brittle skin is one of the consequences of aging). All these changes were a result of the growth hormone increase—the subjects didn't change their diet or exercise. After only six months' therapy with minuscule amounts of this extremely potent substance the more youthful changes these men exhibited were, in Dr. Rudman's words, "equivalent in magnitude to the changes incurred during 10 to 20 years of [reverse] aging." It's no wonder growth hormone clinics are popping up all over Mexico and other less medically regulated countries.

Another study, performed at the University of New Mexico, demonstrated that weight lifters injected with growth hormone for only six weeks lost four times more body fat and gained four times more lean body mass compared to those who received only placebo. These studies and others like them leave little doubt scientifically that growth hormone truly is the elixir of youth—it fosters a kind of regeneration of youth.

Jump-Starting Your Youth Hormone

The growth hormone difference between adults and adolescents isn't a disparity in amount but in release. Teenagers are much more sensitive to all the factors that stimulate the release of growth hormone, whereas adults are less sensitive and become even less so with increasing age. In truth, teenagers typically have more stimulating factors present than do adults. So if you want more growth hormone—and who doesn't?—you need to increase and intensify those factors that stimulate its release from the pituitary gland.

Factors That Stimulate the Release of Growth Hormone[1]

Decreased blood glucose levels
Increased blood protein levels
Carbohydrate-restricted diet
Fasting
Increased protein diet
Free fatty acid decrease
PGE_1 (a "good" eicosanoid)
Stage IV sleep
Exercise

Carbohydrate restriction, increased protein, good eicosanoids . . . hmmmm, sounds a lot like the nutritional regimen described in this book. That's not really so surprising, because if we've been programmed to perform

---

[1] These are the factors stimulating growth hormone release that you can actually do something about; there are others, but they are predominantly drug-induced.

optimally on this dietary structure by millions of years of evolution, it ought to exert positive effects throughout all parameters of our biochemistry.

Our nutritional plan will give you plenty of protein, keep your carbohydrates restricted, your blood glucose lowered, and your free fatty acids to a minimum and will induce the production of lots of good eicosanoids. As a result you should be stimulating the release of a fair amount of growth hormone. But you can get even more. Along with proper nutrition, sleep and exercise also stimulate the release of growth hormone—but not just any sleep and exercise; they must be the right kind.

It turns out Mom was right all those times she urged you to get to sleep early so you'd grow. Growth hormone is secreted in a pulsatile surge in stage III and stage IV sleep, the first hour or two after reaching deep sleep. So to maximize growth hormone release you need to make certain that you get deep, sound sleep every night.

Exercise stimulates the release of a powerful surge of growth hormone, which promotes repair and rebuilding of the muscle broken down during the workout. But the exercise must be strenuous and done until muscle exhaustion almost to the point of failure for maximum results. A few jumping jacks or a brisk stroll around the block will provide some cardiac benefit, but it won't stimulate the release of growth hormone. Although all strenuous exercise stimulates the release of growth hormone, resistance training (weight lifting) seems to stimulate the most. As you lift weights, your straining muscle develops microscopic tears. These minuscule injuries apparently call forth the growth hormone that then repairs them and, in addition, actually stimulates the growth of new muscle fibers to augment those with the microscopic damage. All the while this repair and tissue building are going on the growth hormone converts the muscles into little fat-burning machines and promotes the release of fat from adipose tissue to ensure them a steady supply of fuel.

As with almost every system in the body, there are two sides to this equation. Just as a number of factors stimulate the pituitary to give up its growth hormone, other factors inhibit this process. Since our sensitivity to all those release-stimulating factors diminishes with age, it becomes critical that we not only do everything we can to stimulate growth hormone release but also work to avoid those things that inhibit it.

Factors That Inhibit the Release of Growth Hormone

Increased blood glucose levels
Increased blood free fatty acids
Obesity
Pregnancy

Once again our regimen comes up a winner, pregnancy excepted. A couple of important points need to be made, however. First, since increased glucose levels inhibit the release of growth hormone, it behooves us to avoid anything sweet, starchy, or otherwise carbohydrate laden before we go to bed. Any of these substances will give us an elevation of blood glucose that will inhibit the normal shot of growth hormone released an hour or so after our falling asleep. See what all those snacks of milk and cookies at bedtime have been doing to you!

Second, the pulse of growth hormone released by exercise generally hits the circulation toward the end of the workout and immediately after. If you want to inhibit this growth hormone surge, all you have to do is to eat a power bar or a candy bar or drink fruit juice, as trainers often advise you to do before, during, and right after workouts in the mistaken notion that you need "explosive, high-carbo energy" as one of these products advertises. What you're really getting is no growth hormone. Always work out on an empty stomach, don't consume anything except water during the workout, and don't eat until an hour or so after. Then make sure it's a protein-rich meal—you need plenty of amino acids for the growth hormone to use to repair and rebuild your muscles.

Now that you've been introduced to the wonders of growth hormone, let's see how you can put it to work.

The Path of Most Resistance

The single best exercise you can do to improve your health is to lift weights. Yes, aerobic exercise is good, but it won't deliver the extra benefits of resistance training. And lifting weights is the best resistance training of all. Every day it seems a new medical study surfaces showing the efficacy of resistance training in improving the health of seniors, juniors, and all those in between. Working out with weights strengthens joints, increases the density of your bones to prevent osteoporosis, increases your muscle mass, improves your endurance if done correctly, *decreases* your insulin levels, and, as we've already seen, stimulates the release of growth hormone, which improves just about everything.

Each pound of muscle mass you pack on becomes a fat-burning dynamo, allowing you to increase your food intake without fear of fat gain. As your muscle mass continues to build, your body will begin to resculpt itself. You will lose all the little handles and bulges of fat you could never get rid of before, no matter how hard you dieted. Best of all, once that new muscle is there, and as long as you continue to work it, your metabolic rate will increase, allowing you to eat more than you can imagine—even of carbohydrate foods—without negative consequences. No more working hard to lose your weight only to watch it balloon back up as soon as you start eating normally again. You will actually be able to eat more than when you started and continue to lose fat. Sounds impossible, but it works like a charm—if you do.

If you're female, you may be thinking that this sounds great, but you're really not all that keen to look like the Incredible Hulk. Not to worry. Your female hormones and lack of male hormones will keep you unhulklike even if you train extensively. The women you see in bodybuilding magazines who *do* look like well-developed males usually have had a little help from their friends the anabolic steroids. Your friends—work, sweat, and your own growth hormone—will slim you down by decreasing your body fat. The muscle growth you experience will be in the filling-out of muscle tissue in places it has atrophied from underuse and in increasing the density of the rest of your muscles. When you start, your muscles will look like a piece of choice steak with fat marbled throughout. As you work out and follow this nutritional plan you will quickly begin to replace this intramuscular fat with more muscle, making your muscle not necessarily larger but denser.

A word of caution: if you're trying to lose weight, you may be disappointed if you follow the scales too closely, because as your muscles become more dense, they become heavier. The new muscle you add weighs more than the fat it replaces, but its increased metabolic requirement that is stoked by the fat stored elsewhere on your body ends up making you much smaller, not to mention better proportioned, than before, regardless of what the scales say. It's much better to measure your progress by the way your clothing fits than by the bathroom scale.

How Do I Start?

There are any number of good books available on weight training. Just remember when you get one of these manuals, read and follow only the instructions on the exercise part—ignore any nutritional advice. We recommend *Dr. Bob Arnot's Guide to Turning Back the Clock* (Little, Brown and Company) by Robert Arnot, M.D., which has an excellent section on weight training, especially for men. It's easy to read, has good illustrations showing the various exercises, and describes a number of different workouts designed to fit your time constraints while helping you achieve your particular fitness goals. Another option is a television program, *The Body Electric*, a half-hour show produced by WFSV-TV in Tallahassee, Florida. *The Body Electric* works several muscle groups on each program and uses weights. It's broadcast all over the country and in Canada.

When you begin your resistance training program, you need to follow a few basic guidelines:

1. Start with light weights first to strengthen the ligaments, tendons, and connective tissue around your joints, which are the weakest link when you begin and are the most prone to injury and discomfort. Only after your

joints have been stabilized and strengthened with several weeks of light weights should you begin your serious muscle building.

2. To achieve the quickest results, work your biggest muscles first. Do pushups, for instance. You're looking for the increased metabolism and fat burning you get from increased muscle mass, and working your biggest muscle groups—thighs, shoulders, butt, and chest—gives you more growth faster. A 5 percent increase in size and density of large muscle groups provides a lot more metabolic firepower than the same percentage increase in small muscle groups or individual muscles. Work on the size and definition of these smaller muscle groups later.

3. Use perfect form. The idea is to work and strengthen the particular muscle groups you are working on, not to lift a specific amount of weight. If you have to arch your back and change your position to complete your sets, go to a lesser amount of weight. As long as you keep your back straight, you will go a long, long way toward avoiding injury.

4. Don't forget to recalculate and increase your protein intake if you originally determined it based on a more sedentary level of activity. To make maximal gains and minimize the potential for injury, you must consume adequate protein, the stuff all that new muscle is made of.

5. To maximize growth hormone release, always perform your workouts on an empty stomach. Don't consume any carbohydrate snacks anywhere near the time of your workout, or you can kiss your growth hormone good-bye.

6. Work to increase *power*, not just strength. Strength is how much you can lift; power is how fast you can lift it. Power is strength divided by time and is a measure of what

your muscles can do for you. Athletic performance and defensive living rely on power for optimal performance; whether you're trying to rifle a tennis serve or leap out of the way of an oncoming car, you depend on the power and quickness of your muscles, not just their strength. You develop power by increasing the speed with which you lift the weights first, then increase the weight. If, for instance, you are doing four sets of ten repetitions with a particular weight, perform them slowly and with perfect form. With subsequent workouts, increase your speed with the same weight until you are snapping that weight up briskly through all the sets—then move to a higher weight and start again slowly and perfectly, then work on increasing speed.

7. Make your workouts aerobic so that you get the benefit of both weight training and endurance exercise. You do this by following guideline 5 and by not slowing down and resting between sets. If you have to decrease your weights to keep from becoming exhausted, do so. As you follow your new diet, you will build endurance as quickly as you build strength and power, because the foods you eat will actually increase the amount of oxygen transported to and released in your exercising muscles. How can your diet increase the amount of oxygen delivered to the tissues?

Oxygen is carried to the tissues in the red blood cells and released. To increase the delivery of oxygen, we need to get more red blood cells to the oxygen-deprived tissues—in this case our working muscles. We can do this in two ways: first by increasing the number of red blood cells, which our new diet does nicely thanks to its high content of readily absorbable iron, the element that drives the production of red blood cells; second by delivering more of these red blood cells to the meshwork of capillaries within the tissues, where the oxygen exchange actually takes place. The red blood cells are larger than the diameter of the capillaries, so they actually deform themselves as they snake their way through these tiny vessels. It's kind of like forcing a water balloon through a paper towel tube. The only way to get more of them through faster is to increase the diameter of the blood vessel and/or increase the deformability of the red blood cells so that more of them can work their way through more quickly. The good (series one) eicosanoids induced by our nutritional plan both dilate the blood vessels and increase the suppleness and deformability of the red blood cells, getting more of them to the working muscle faster.

8. Don't start your exercise program until at least a week after you start your new carbohydrate-restricted diet. We know you're fired up and ready to start pumping growth hormone today, but take our word for it and wait a week. When you change your diet from one of high carbohydrates to one of many fewer carbohydrates you are going to experience a few days of easy fatigability. You may even become a little short-winded just performing your normal daily tasks. After a few days, or maybe even a week, this breathlessness goes away and you will actually have more endurance. Why this phenomenon? Because of the enzymatic changing of the guard, as explained in the question-and-answer section at the end of Chapter 5.

What Will I Look Like?

You may be wondering what you'll end up looking like if you diligently follow all these instructions. For one thing, if you have a lot of weight to lose, you'll look great, not scrawny and wasted once you've come all the way down. And we can guarantee you'll feel better, look better, and enhance your performance in golf, tennis, squash, skiing, or whatever your activity of choice. If you don't have a sport you enjoy, find one. Athletics at any level improve your performance in life in general. No matter what you take up, you will find your coordination improved, your agility enhanced, your reflexes sharpened, and your outlook on life improved.

As the old saying goes, a picture is worth a thousand words, so take a look at the four photos in Figure 7.1. Amazingly, they are all of the same person, a 53-year-old printing supply salesman named Stan Kuter who lives in Little Rock. Let us give you a chronology of these truly astounding pictures. The first one (A) is Stan (with his daughter) when he was 43 years old and heavily into running and low-fat dieting. He appears kind of wasted and emaciated because . . . well, he was. The constant running—50 miles per week—was breaking down his muscles, and the inadequate protein component of his low-fat diet wasn't rebuilding them. To top things off, his carbo loading before his workouts ensured that he released no growth hormone to aid in the maintenance of his lean body mass. Because of his long-standing protein deficiency, he was immunosuppressed—a fate common to many distance runners—and was chronically afflicted with colds, sore throats, and a host of other minor illnesses.

Stan finally had all the fun he could stand and decided

FIGURE 7.1

A
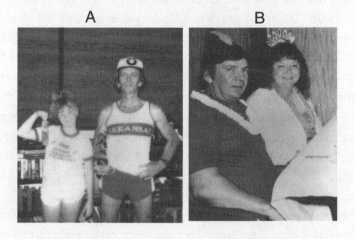

B

C
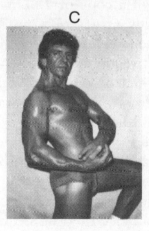

D
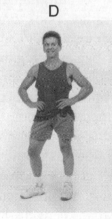

to take a break from it all for a while, only to find himself in picture B (with his wife) a short two years later. The protein malnutrition Stan suffered while running and dieting reduced his muscle mass significantly and consequently reduced his metabolic rate as well. He had compensated for the decreased-lean-body-mass-induced metabolic burn by expending large amounts of energy running. When he quit running, however, the combination of reduced metabolic rate and no exercise opened the floodgates of body fat accumulation. This situation is one familiar to many who try to maintain their weight by running or other endurance exercises. They often find themselves in a trap. They can maintain their weight only as long as they continue to run. When they quit or even slow down, they find their weight increasing at a frightening rate.

Photo C shows Stan in his body-building phase. After tiring of being fat, Stan decided to take a different approach to conditioning. He got a copy of *Thin So Fast*, Mike's earlier book on the advantages of a restricted-carbohydrate nutritional program, followed it to the letter, and began a regimen of weight training. Only six months of adequate protein intake combined with the growth-hormone-inducing effects of resistance training transformed him from photo B to photo C.

Stan doesn't work out regularly anymore and doesn't always follow his restricted-carbohydrate regimen, but he still looks great—photo D. The reason: the large mass of lean tissue he built when he did work out is a fat-burning furnace that keeps his metabolic rate fired up, so he can have much more leeway on his diet without suffering the consequences. When he does gain a little fat, he simply cuts back on his carbohydrates slightly, and in just a few days the excess is gone. He works out with the weights occasionally, which keeps him from losing the muscle mass he has built. He isn't trying for new gains; he's simply maintaining what he already has.

The take-home lesson is that Ted Williams had it only half right: adequate dietary protein in combination with resistance training is the key.

The Bottom Line

Regular exercise plays an important role in helping you reclaim your health and vitality, not only in weight loss and maintenance but also in lowered blood pressure and improved lipid values. More important even than that, dedication to regular physical exercise helps you milk all the pleasure you can from a long and healthy life. The goals of exercise are simple: increased muscle strength and endurance. Stronger, better-conditioned muscles lead to improved physical performance—not just in sporting endeavors but in everyday activities. And best of all, exercise keeps you young! Although that may seem impossible, it's true: the right kind of exercise, coupled with the proper nutritional structure, will increase your release of growth hormone, that magic elixir of youth.

Our *Protein Power* program provides the proper nutritional framework to enhance release of growth hormone—the miraculous substance of youth that allows adolescents to escape the consequences of profound dietary abuse and sloth and still appear thin and fit. Or to withstand hours of exhausting physical activity and bounce up the next morning rested, raring to go, and none the worse for wear.

Growth hormone encourages growth and repair of body tissues, helps build lean body mass, mobilizes your fat stores, and shifts your metabolism into fat burning as a fuel source. Adults have more than adequate amounts of growth hormone locked away in the brain—we just have trouble getting to it, whereas teens release it easily. The chief time of release is about an hour or so after you fall deeply asleep. A number of factors help stimulate growth hormone release: stable low blood sugar, increased protein intake, a diet low in carbohydrate, fasting, deep sleep, a "good" eicosanoid balance, and exercise. Our nutritional regimen brings about all these positives except exercise—and we're adding that now. Other factors reduce growth hormone release: elevated blood sugar levels, obesity, and pregnancy. Again, our regimen comes up a winner (except for pregnancy, of course).

Although aerobic or endurance exercise is great for improving cardiovascular fitness, the best exercise to encourage release of growth hormone is the resistance kind—working your muscles against a resistance (a weight) to the point of near exhaustion. Weight training builds muscle (every pound of which burns calories and keeps you thin), strengthens joints, and increases bone strength. And done properly, it helps reduce elevated insulin levels and promote the release of growth hormone—both essential to your physical and metabolic rehabilitation.

Although good books detailing weight training exercise abound, they're usually filled with nutritional misinformation and constant reminders to load up on pasta and power bars and the like for their "explosive high-carbo energy." You must ignore their nutritional advice, because that high-carbo explosion will ensure you release little or no growth hormone. It's essential to your physical rehabilitation that you eat no carbohydrate foods before bedtime or your exercise regimen and drink only water to hydrate yourself while you exercise. One book we can recommend is *Dr. Bob Arnot's Guide to Turning Back the Clock* (Little, Brown and Company) by Robert Arnot, M.D.

Your exercise guidelines should be:

1. Start with light weights first and work up slowly.

2. Work your biggest muscles first—thighs, shoulders, buttocks, and chest—because you get bigger lean mass gains quicker.

3. Use perfect form during the exercise—if you have to twist and arch your back to lift a weight, it's too heavy. Lighten it.

4. As you increase the frequency or intensity of your workouts, don't forget to recalculate your protein requirements.

5. Always work out on an empty stomach.

6. Perform all exercises slowly and perfectly, then

build speed—don't increase weight until you can smoothly, quickly, and perfectly perform the exercise at the current weight. This builds power and density of the muscle, not just strength.

7. Work aerobically during your weight training by moving quickly from one set to the next without long rest periods between.

8. Don't begin to exercise until you've been on your new nutritional regimen for at least a week. First set the stage and get stable nutritionally, then take off with your workouts.

If you bypassed the main body of the chapter in favor of this summary, you might want to back up for a moment to read the diet and exercise story of our patient Stan Kuter (page 200). As he has done for many of our other patients, Stan will amaze and inspire you. He's living proof that the right nutrition and resistance training are indeed the key to reclaiming your youth.

Chapter 8

Motivation: Plan Your Work and Work Your Plan

I'll purge, and leave sack, and live cleanly, as a nobleman should do.

Falstaff, in *Henry IV, Part One,*
WILLIAM SHAKESPEARE

If only it were that simple, Falstaff's name might never have become eponymous for gluttony, hedonism, and corpulence. Unfortunately, as anyone who has tried it knows, changing your eating behavior is tough, hard work. An enormous reality gap exists between the ease of dieting as presented in most books and magazine articles on the subject and the actual day-to-day grind of a particular diet. What's advertised as a fast, easy, painless, you-won't-believe-how-quickly-your-fat-melts-away approach to weight loss and other benefits all too often becomes monotonous, restrictive, and ultimately abandoned. If it weren't so, the notorious 95 percent of people who always regain all their lost weight would still be thin.

So, how is this program different? In many ways it

isn't—although unlike most other programs this one has a positive health approach that actually *will* heal you metabolically and make it easier to work your plan. Much as we'd like to tell you otherwise, the program we have outlined still requires discipline, self-denial, and just plain old hard work. But the reward for this' effort is spectacular. In the course of our work with thousands of patients we have developed many techniques to make life easier for them, but it still isn't magic. Although it "fixes" your health problems quickly, it's not just a quick fix. We feel it's important to inform you in advance of the discipline required because the approach you take and the outlook you have at the beginning are of paramount importance.

The first decision you need to make is not that you need to lose weight or lower your cholesterol or reduce your high blood pressure or any or all of these. Your first decision must be to make these changes a *permanent* part of your life. That sounds simple, but in reality making that decision means that you are willing to abandon life (and all its dangerous goodies) as you know it today. It will be one of the best decisions you've ever made, but we want you to understand it for what it is—a major life-altering decision. Assuming you've made that decision, you've got to realize and accept the fact that the responsibility for this change is yours and yours alone. You have to do the work. We have provided all the information you need to be successful, but we can't do it for you. What we can do is give you some tips and tricks that have helped us and our patients achieve our goals.

The Worst Will Be Over Soon

In Phase I and Phase II, when it's so critical to follow the program to the letter, it helps to adopt a boot-camp attitude. Recruits go to boot camp knowing it's going to be strict, grueling, difficult, and probably not particularly pleasant. They also know it's going to be over. You need to think the same way. Compared to maintenance, these intervention phases are much more rigorous, but they will be over soon. Look upon it as a finite period of time you're spending to turn your health around and get on with it. When it's over, you can rejoice. As long as you stay on maintenance and don't eat unconsciously, you'll never have to go back to boot camp again.

Don't Get Hungry

Never let yourself get hungry. If you're not hungry, you will be much better able to avoid the temptation to eat those foods you know you shouldn't. The best approach is to stay ahead of the hunger curve. In other words, always try to eat before you get ravenously hungry—not after. Never skip breakfast. Keep a quantity of allowable snacks at the ready. You need to prepare these yourself and keep them handy because virtually all of the commercially manufactured snacks you'll find will be crawling with carbohydrates and despite their *no-fat* or *low-fat* labeling will sabotage you in a hurry.

Visualize Your Goals

A question we're often asked by weight-loss patients is: Since I have 220 pounds to lose, how can I stay motivated to stick to any diet long enough to lose all that weight? The answer is that you are *not* going on a diet of a predetermined length; you are adopting a new way of eating for the rest of your life, so it doesn't really matter how long it takes. Several years ago, when a twenty-two-year-old patient of ours, Michael, began our program weighing 420 pounds, he wondered if he would ever lose the 200-plus pounds that stood between him and his ideal body weight. When we told him to expect to lose at least 2 to 3 pounds a week, he grumbled that at that rate he would be twenty-five before he reached normal weight. Well, of course, in two years he was going to be twenty-five whether he lost the weight or not, so we said he might as well reach twenty-five thin instead of overweight. He started our program on August 13, 1993, and by June 17, 1994, four months short of his twenty-fourth birthday, he had lost 169 pounds. As Michael lost his excess body fat and developed a more positive self-image, he developed a social life for the first time in his life and sought and found a better job that required his moving out of the area. He has since become engaged and continues to do well. The results of the diet *became* the motivation. So take heart: no matter how much you have to lose, every pound lost takes you closer to your ultimate goal—becoming a leaner, fitter, healthier person. You've got the rest of your life to live healthy and fit—don't get caught up in the trap of deadlines.

Learn to set reasonable goals and use the power of visualization to achieve them. We're not New Age fans, but we can tell you that visualization works. Visualize clearly and vividly the changes you wish to take place and visualize them as if they had already taken place. You will set in motion all kinds of subconscious activity that will work behind the scenes to make your visual pictures a reality.[1] An excellent book on this subject that we find indispensable and can't recommend highly enough is *Maximum Achievement* by Brian Tracy (Simon & Schuster, 1993). As with all books we recommend, ignore any nutritional advice—we can never understand why authors of books on nonnutritional subjects feel compelled to parrot the high-carbohydrate party line, but they do.

You're the Boss

It's astonishing that so many people fail at dieting. People who successfully overcome the uncontrollable vagaries of careers, higher education, marriage, and life in general succumb to the one, and maybe only, event over which they have total control—feeding themselves. We all seem to be about six years old when it comes to eating. But you need to realize that unless you are unconscious in a hospital bed undergoing tube feeding, *you, and only you, are in complete control over what you put in your mouth*. You may not be able to control the weather, the behavior of your children or your spouse, the intraoffice machinations at

---

[1] If it just seems completely unimaginable, you can send a current photo to Sound Feelings (see appendix), and they'll send you back a slimmed-down photo, carefully to scale so you can see how you'll actually look at the end of all this—but of course you'll have better muscles in real life. Phone: (818) 757-0600. E-mail: info@soundfeelings.com.

your workplace, the busybodies in your neighborhood, or the outcome of the Super Bowl, but you can take charge of the food you eat. We've all heard the excuse innumerable times from those who have been tempted from their diets by junk food of one sort or another: "I just couldn't resist it." As we say to our patients, "Yes, you *could* resist it; you just *chose* not to."

Temptation vs. You

It would be simplistic for us to act as though temptation doesn't exist or resisting it requires only a small effort of will. We love to eat, too (which is why we've built in occasional dietary vacations for maintenance). If it were easy, no one would be overweight. Although you can't make temptation go away, there are steps you can take to minimize its hold on you. In looking at these steps you'll get a better picture of how temptation actually works its wily magic on you and how you can turn the tables on it.

There are four components of any behavior—the physiological, the feeling, the thinking, and, finally, the doing. All behavior comprises some variation of these components in series. For example, let's say you suddenly find yourself in a threatening situation. The thinking component of behavior kicks in immediately with thoughts of all the potential harm you may be facing. Your adrenal glands begin pumping adrenaline—the physiological component. As a result you begin to feel the adrenaline rush we call *fear*. Finally, the doing component kicks in, and you remove yourself from the situation rapidly. These four behavioral components don't necessarily always proceed in this succession, but they are always there—some to a greater extent than others—driving all but unconscious activity. Although at first blush, especially in the situation we described, it appears that these progressions are beyond your control, in actuality by knowing what you're doing you can control them. How?

Of these four components you have total control over just one, the actual doing component, and partial control over one other, the thinking component. Over the other two, unfortunately, you have no direct control whatsoever, a fact not lost on your old adversary temptation, because these last two are its portals of entry into your behavior. If temptation can gain a foothold in your physiology and/or your feelings, it can often bend the other components to its will, resulting in self-destructive behavior. However, by controlling the doing portion of behavior you have the last say and can by force of your will drive the behavior the opposite way. You walk into the office break room to get your low-carb snack from the refrigerator and are overwhelmed by the fresh-baked aroma of still-warm doughnuts. There they are—at least a dozen fluffy, moist glazed ones in an open box with an attached note that says *help yourself!* Assuming you love doughnuts, what happens to you? You smell and see the doughnuts, which starts your physiology working. Your GI tract starts preparing for the incoming doughnuts, your pancreas actually releases a little squirt of insulin in preparation, and your whole being prepares for the consumption of the doughnuts—and all these changes are beyond your direct control. These physiological changes immediately cause you to feel consciously hungry and to crave the doughnuts. You begin thinking about how good the doughnuts would taste and how hungry you really are and how just one wouldn't hurt anything and how you could really buckle down to your diet tomorrow and . . . You break down and eat the doughnut, then another, then you say, "Oh, well, I've blown my diet. There's no sense in staying on it for the rest of the day. I'll start in earnest tomorrow. Now I think I'll have another doughnut." If someone who knows you're dieting walks in and discovers you in mid-debauch, you say, "I just couldn't resist." And temptation has played you like a violin. (If this happens in real life, jump right back into Phase I at the next meal.)

So you allowed the physiological and feeling components over which you have no control to run roughshod over your thinking and doing components. But you can drive the equation the other way. You walk into the break room, see and smell the doughnuts, and your physiology and feelings spring into action. Instead of allowing first your thinking and then your doing components to fall into line, reverse the order. Grab your low-carb snack and walk out. Get involved in some other activity. Think about something else. Make a phone call. Control the controllable components, and as you do your physiology will return to normal and your hunger will evaporate. By controlling the components you *can* control you end up indirectly controlling those you really have no direct control over. Take charge of your actions, and everything else will fall into line.

It sounds great in theory, you say, but it's difficult in real life. Sure it is, but so is getting up each morning when the alarm goes off, which you do day after day. Why? Because you have a job you have to get to and you enjoy the house you live in, the car you drive, and the clothes you wear—all courtesy of the money you make from the job you have to get to. Your physiological component and your feeling component and especially your thinking component all want to stay in bed, but your doing component rousts them all up and into the shower, and your day begins. Muster the same force of will with your eating behavior, revel in your domination of temptation, and watch with delight as you begin to make a reality of your visualized image of a lean, strong, healthy you. Good luck!

Chapter 9

Sample Menus

Once you've outlined your own unique requirements for protein (from pages 92–96 in Chapter 5) and determined whether you need to undertake a Phase I Intervention at about 30 grams of total effective carbohydrate a day or a Phase II Intervention at about a total of 55 grams of effective carbohydrate a day, you're ready to plan meals. The process is simple: each meal should contain a serving of lean protein adequate for you (refer to the Protein Equivalency Charts on pages 154–157 for the correct amounts) along with no more than the maximum amount of carbohydrate per meal recommended for that intervention level. Whether you cook the meals yourself, dine out, or catch a meal on the run at a fast-food restaurant, those rules apply.

To help you get started—or in case you're confused about how to put a meal together the *Protein Power* way— we've put together a week of menus with breakfast, lunch, dinner, and snack suggestions. You'll notice on these meal plans that we have not given you amounts of protein (meat, fish, chicken, eggs, dairy) since protein requirement varies with lean body weight and activity level. You already should have calculated your daily protein requirement and know whether Protein Equivalency Chart A, B, C, or D fits your needs. Use these portion sizes as your guide for the number of eggs or the amount of grilled chicken, lean beef, tuna salad, or other protein source you need. Each of these meals contains less than 10 grams of carbohydrate, so three meals plus snack will keep you at about 40 grams of effective carbohydrate per day. If you're following a Phase I Intervention, eat only the protein portion of a snack to keep your daily carbohydrate at 30 grams. At Phase II you can have two snacks, if you wish, and still be under the 55-gram level.

All meals interchange from a carbohydrate standpoint, so if you don't like or can't eat the foods listed for breakfast on a certain day, substitute another day's suggestion. The same is true for lunch, dinner, and snacks.

Vegetarians should substitute firm tofu (again refer to the Protein Equivalency Charts) for meat, fish, or poultry.

Meal Plans

BREAKFAST 1

Smoked salmon and cream cheese omelet
$^1/_2$ cup fresh strawberries
1 slice light bread toast with butter
Coffee, tea, or mineral water

LUNCH 1

$^1/_2$ avocado filled with tuna, chicken, or crab salad (made with mayonnaise, Dijon mustard, chopped hard-cooked egg, minced scallion, and minced dill pickle), served on a bed of fresh salad greens, drizzled with herbed olive oil vinaigrette, and garnished with black olives, pickle spears, and $^1/_2$ tomato in wedges
Coffee, tea, or mineral water

SNACK 1 (IF DESIRED AND ALLOWED)

1 oz. macadamia nuts, about $1/4$ cup
1 peach or $1/2$ apple with skin
Mineral water with lemon or lime

DINNER 1

Beef tenderloin (or other lean cut)
10 steamed fresh asparagus spears, dressed with hollandaise sauce if desired
1 or 2 cups mixed seasonal greens, dressed with herbed olive oil vinaigrette and garnished with carrot curls, olives, and radishes
$1/2$ tomato, sliced
$1/2$ cup dry red wine if desired
Coffee, tea, or mineral water

BREAKFAST 2

Cottage cheese
$1/2$ cup fresh strawberries
Coffee, tea, or mineral water

LUNCH 2

Sliced grilled chicken, served on a bed of fresh salad greens, black olives, and scallion, dressed with herbed olive oil vinaigrette
1 peach or $1/2$ apple with skin
Coffee, tea, or mineral water

SNACK 2 (IF DESIRED AND ALLOWED)

Cold leftover beef tenderloin with mustard for dipping
2 cups broccoli and cauliflower florets
Coffee, tea, or mineral water

DINNER 2

Grilled or sautéed jumbo shrimp, brushed or sautéed in olive oil and garlic

Sliced fresh tomato and mozzarella salad: 1 medium tomato, 2 ounces mozzarella, fresh basil, olive oil vinaigrette

1 cup sautéed broccoli florets

$^1/_2$ cup dry white wine if desired

Coffee, tea, or mineral water

BREAKFAST 3

Poached eggs on 1 slice light bread toast with butter

Grilled breakfast sausages

$^1/_2$ cup fresh or frozen berries

Coffee, tea, or mineral water

LUNCH 3

$^1/_2$ small pita filled with tuna, chicken, or crab salad (made with mayonnaise, Dijon mustard, chopped hard-cooked egg, minced scallion, and minced dill pickle), served with sliced tomato, lettuce, sprouts, and sunflower seeds and garnished with black olives and pickle spears

Coffee, tea, or mineral water

SNACK 3 (IF DESIRED AND ALLOWED)

1 or 2 ounces hard cheese (Gouda, Edam, cheddar, Swiss)

1 peach or $^1/_2$ Valencia orange

Mineral water with lemon or lime

DINNER 3

Grilled or boiled fish (salmon, swordfish, shark, tuna),
dressed with garlic or lemon dill butter
1 small zucchini, grilled or sautéed
1 or 2 cups mixed seasonal greens, dressed with herbed
olive oil vinaigrette and garnished with carrot curls,
olives, and radishes
1/2 medium tomato, sliced
1/2 cup dry white wine if desired
Coffee, tea, or mineral water

BREAKFAST 4

Strawberry Breakfast Fruit Smoothie, page 231
Coffee, tea, or mineral water

LUNCH 4

Quiche Lorraine (eat filling but not crust)
1 or 2 cups mixed seasonal greens, dressed with herbed
olive oil vinaigrette and garnished with black olives
and 3 or 4 tomato wedges
1/2 cup fresh or frozen strawberries, peaches, or raspberries
Coffee, tea, or mineral water

SNACK 4 (IF DESIRED AND ALLOWED)

1/2 cup cottage cheese with 1 peach or 1/2 apple with
skin
Mineral water with lemon or lime

DINNER 4

Grilled or roasted chicken

$^1/_2$ cup steamed spaghetti squash, dressed with butter and Parmesan cheese if desired

1 or 2 cups mixed seasonal greens, dressed with herbed olive oil vinaigrette and garnished with carrot curls, olives, and radishes

$^1/_2$ cup dry white wine if desired

Coffee, tea, or mineral water

BREAKFAST 5

1 serving Fluffy Pancakes, page 229, with butter

Crisp bacon

Coffee, tea, or mineral water

LUNCH 5

Double-patty burger, both buns removed, dressed with bacon, cheese, onion, tomato, lettuce, and avocado

1 or 2 cups mixed seasonal greens dressed with herbed olive oil vinaigrette

1 fresh peach

Coffee, tea, or mineral water

SNACK 5 (IF DESIRED AND ALLOWED)

Cold grilled chicken with mustard for dipping (leftovers work well)

1 ounce hard cheese

Mineral water with lemon or lime

DINNER 5

Garlic Shrimp with Salsa, page 239
1 or 2 cups mixed seasonal greens, dressed with herbed
   olive oil vinaigrette and garnished with $1/2$ sliced avocado and diced tomato
$1/2$ cup fresh or frozen strawberries, garnished with 1
   tablespoon whipped heavy cream if desired
$1/2$ cup white wine if desired
Coffee, tea, or mineral water

BREAKFAST 6

Omelet filled with mushrooms, cheddar, and onion
Crisp bacon
Coffee, tea, or mineral water

LUNCH 6

Grilled chicken or fish sandwich, both buns removed,
   dressed with bacon, cheese, onion, tomato, lettuce,
   and avocado if desired
$1/2$ cup cabbage coleslaw or fresh green salad
1 fresh peach
Coffee, tea, or mineral water

SNACK 6 (IF DESIRED AND ALLOWED)

Leftover cold grilled or sautéed shrimp
Low-carbohydrate cocktail sauce: dietetic ketchup, 1 ta-
   blespoon lemon juice, and 1 tablespoon horseradish
$1/2$ Valencia orange
Mineral water with lemon or lime

DINNER 6

Cabbage Lasagne, page 279

1 or 2 cups mixed seasonal greens, dressed with herbed olive oil vinaigrette

$1/2$ cup dry red wine, for Phase II only (will increase carb content of this meal too much for Phase I)

Coffee, tea, or mineral water

BREAKFAST 7

Raspberry Breakfast Fruit Smoothie, page 231

Coffee, tea, or mineral water

LUNCH 7

Smoked turkey and cheese sandwich (meat piled high on 1 slice light bread, dressed as desired with mayonnaise, mustard, lettuce, tomato slice, onion, sprouts, and sunflower seeds)

$1/2$ cup fresh or frozen strawberries or raspberries

Coffee, tea, or mineral water

SNACK 7 (IF DESIRED AND ALLOWED)

Hard cheese and salami with Dijon mustard

1 peach or $1/2$ apple with skin

Mineral water with lemon or lime

DINNER 7

Grilled Lamb Burgers with Roasted Eggplant Puree, page 283

1 or 2 cups mixed seasonal greens, topped with crumbled feta cheese, black olives, and 3 or 4 fresh tomato wedges and dressed with herbed olive oil vinaigrette

Strawberry sorbet: puree 4 whole frozen strawberries with 2 tablespoons heavy cream per serving until smooth, refreeze briefly to set, and spoon into cups

Coffee, tea, or mineral water

Chapter 10

Recipes

Protein is just as important as [carbohydrates in meal]
planning. Our protein calculations, unless otherwise
specified, are based on a 3-ounce portion in the
recipes. You can adjust to your protein needs for an
average of 7 grams protein per ounce of lean meat,
fish, or fowl.

What's for Breakfast?

The fastest answer is cottage cheese, our Breakfast Fruit
Smoothie, or hard-boiled eggs. But here are some more
interesting ideas. To pack in enough protein, breakfast
should include eggs, cheese or cottage cheese, meat,
chicken, or fish (well, maybe). On the carb front, don't
forget that milk contains 6 carbohydrate grams per half
cup, so in your coffee count .75 carbohydrate grams per
tablespoon—half-and-half is .6. If you'd like fruit, choose
a 5-carbohydrate-gram portion from pages 158–160 and
be sure to add it into your total meal count. When you
have time to sit down and really enjoy breakfast, try one
of the breakfast dishes in the main recipe section.

ON TOAST

...y salad mixture with finely chopped hard-
..., using 1 yolk to 2 whites, (2 ounces) slivered
...ed scallions, salt, and pepper and just enough
...r sour cream to bind it. Mound the mixture on
...r crackers (maximum count 6 grams).

SERVING: 8 GRAMS CARBOHYDRATE, 16 GRAMS PROTEIN

FRIZZLED ORANGE BEEF WITH POACHED EGG

Sauté 2 ounces slivered dried beef (still sold in jars in the canned-meat section) in a little butter along with several wire-thin strands of orange zest, a generous sprinkle of chives, and some freshly ground black pepper. Poach an egg in the microwave (40 seconds on medium). Stir a rounded tablespoon of crème fraîche (or cream cheese) into the beef and let it melt but not boil. Pour the beef over a Jaret toast and top with the poached egg.

PER SERVING: 7 GRAMS CARBOHYDRATE, 22 GRAMS PROTEIN

SMOKED SALMON AND FRUIT

Spread cream cheese and smoked salmon on 4 grams of bread or crackers (page 160) and enjoy with ¹/₂ cup of melon balls—these come frozen.

PER SERVING: 11.5 GRAMS CARBOHYDRATE, 10 GRAMS PROTEIN

ORANGE FRENCH TOAST WITH STRAWBERRIES

Soak a slice of Pepperidge Farm sandwich bread in 1 egg whisked with 1 tablespoon heavy cream. Sauté in a non-stick pan 1/2 pat of butter and a little grated orange zest until golden on both sides. Put 1/4 cup sliced berries in the microwave with NutraSweet or Equal to sweeten and cook for a few seconds until you have a chunky sauce. Pour over the hot French toast.

PER SERVING: 12 GRAMS CARBOHYDRATE, 8 GRAMS PROTEIN

BREAD PUDDING WITH HAM AND CHEESE

Soak 2 Jaret toasts in 1 egg beaten with 2 tablespoons heavy cream until almost all the egg is absorbed. Lift one toast into a flat-rimmed soup plate with a spatula, fold over a slice of Black Forest ham (or Canadian bacon) on top, cover it with 2 tablespoons grated cheddar, and sand-wich it with the second toast. Pour any remaining egg mixture over the top and sprinkle with a little more cheese. Microwave on high for 1 1/2 minutes.

PER SERVING: 13 GRAMS CARBOHYDRATE, 23 GRAMS PRO-TEIN

NOTE: Make this recipe open-faced with 1 Jaret toast and save 6 grams of carbs.

BLUEBERRIES AND CHEESE WITH COCONUT-CINNAMON TOAST

Mix $1/4$ cup fresh blueberries with $1/2$ cup cottage cheese and sweeten it to taste with NutraSweet or Equal. Toast 1 slice Pepperidge Farm Very Thin bread on one side only. Spread the other side with soft butter mixed $1/2$ teaspoon brown sugar, a sprinkle of cinnamon, and 1 heaped teaspoon of unsweetened grated coconut (at the health food store or the freezer case of some supermarkets). Broil until bubbly and golden brown. Serve toast with the cottage cheese and berries.

PER SERVING: 11 GRAMS CARBOHYDRATE, 16 GRAMS PROTEIN

STEAK AND EGGS WITH MANGO

Sauté a $1/2$-inch-thick beef tenderloin (or ham) steak in butter, with or without a minced fresh jalapeño chili, top with a boiled egg, and surround with $1/3$ cup diced ripe mango. Add salt and freshly ground pepper.

PER SERVING: 11 GRAMS CARBOHYDRATE, 27 GRAMS PROTEIN

BREAKFAST BURRITO

Moisten 1 small flour tortilla on both sides with lightly dampened hands and soften it by holding it briefly over a gas flame or brushing it across a medium-high electric burner. Spread the center of the tortilla with 1 tablespoon drained and rinsed canned beans mashed to a paste with a little sour cream. Sprinkle it with a tablespoon of Mexican salsa verde and $1/2$ cup (not packed) of grated Monterey Jack or cheddar cheese. Very lightly scramble 2 eggs and spoon them across the center of the tortilla. Roll up the burrito like an egg roll, tucking in the ends. Heat it in the microwave for about 20 seconds, just long enough to melt the cheese.

PER SERVING: 15 GRAMS CARBOHYDRATE, 21 GRAMS PROTEIN

Fluffy Pancakes

SERVES 2

>   2 extra-large eggs
> $1/4$ cup cottage cheese
>   2 tablespoons cream cheese
>   pinch of NutraSweet or Equal or to taste
>   3 tablespoons wheat germ
>   1 tablespoon rice flour or Wondra
>   1 teaspoon baking powder
>   pinch of baking soda

Whip the eggs in a food processor or by hand until frothy. Add the cheeses and beat until smooth. Add a little artificial sweetener. Add the rest of the ingredients and pulse to blend. Gently scrape the batter into a small bowl. Heat a nonstick skillet or griddle with a little butter as needed and when it's hot spoon the batter onto the griddle—about 10 pancakes. Cook over medium heat until the edges of the cakes are set and large bubbles appear across the surface, about 1 minute. Carefully flip them and cook for half as long as on the first side or until golden. Serve on heated plates, with a drizzle of dietetic maple

Berry Syrups

• In lieu of syrup, make up a little fresh berry puree by pulsing $1/2$ cup chopped fresh strawberries with 2 tablespoons orange juice and a pinch of artificial sweetener. Microwave the mixture to a simmer and then let it cool down to warm before using. Leftover puree will keep in the refrigerator for several days. Rhubarb is delicious in this mix too. Microwave it in a little water and add the sweetener after it's cooked.

Fresh raspberry puree is also wonderful with these pancakes. Use Raspberry Crystal Light to liquefy the berries in the food processor. If the Crystal Light doesn't sweeten them enough, add a little Equal or NutraSweet. After microwaving the berries, push them through a strainer with the back of a spoon to remove the seeds.

PER 2-TABLESPOON SERVING: 2 GRAMS CARBOHYDRATE

syrup or berry syrup (above) and a couple of breakfast link sausages or crisp bacon (about 2 grams protein each).

PER SERVING: 10 GRAMS CARBOHYDRATE, 13 GRAMS PROTEIN

• Rice flour is available at most health food stores and Asian markets. It's recommended for these pancakes because it results in a lighter texture.
• These pancakes don't keep particularly well, so just

cut the recipe in half if you're cooking them for yourself.

- Because this batter is very delicate, it's important that
the baking powder be fresh, not more than 2 months
old, so it will puff up properly.

Rain Forest Pancakes:

Add 1½ tablespoons finely chopped unsalted
macadamia nuts, 1 tablespoon toasted unsweetened coconut, and a few drops of coconut extract to the batter.

PER SERVING: AN EXTRA 3 GRAMS CARBOHYDRATE, 2 GRAMS
PROTEIN

If you're on maintenance, serve these little delectables
with alternating *thin* slices of banana and kiwifruit between the pancakes, adding 5 carbohydrate grams to each
portion.

Pecan Maple Pancakes:

Add 2 tablespoons finely chopped toasted pecans and a
few drops of maple extract to the batter. Use dietetic
maple syrup as a topping.

PER SERVING: AN EXTRA 2 GRAMS CARBOHYDRATE, 1 GRAM
PROTEIN

Breakfast Fruit Smoothie

SERVES 1

   ½ cup sliced strawberries, raspberries, or
        peaches, fresh or frozen
   ½ cup cottage cheese

¹/₄ cup plain yogurt
Sugar-free Tang or Crystal Light to taste
(enough to cover everything else in the
blender jar)

Mix in the blender. You can add ice if you're using fresh
fruit.

PER SERVING: 17 GRAMS PROTEIN, 9 GRAMS CARBOHYDRATE
(ALL STRAWBERRIES), 11 GRAMS CARBOHYDRATE (ALL RASP-
BERRIES), 14 GRAMS CARBOHYDRATE (ALL PEACHES)

Strawberry Jam

MAKES 2 8-OUNCE JARS, 32 TABLESPOONS

1 pint fresh ripe strawberries
  juice of ¹/₂ lemon
¹/₄ cup water
1 ¹/₄-ounce envelope of unflavored gelatin
5 teaspoons NutraSweet or 5 packets of Equal
  or less to taste

Wash, stem, and quarter the berries. In a medium
saucepan, heat the berries with the lemon juice, covered,
and simmer until the berries soften and give up their juice,
about 3 minutes.

In a mixing bowl, pour the water over the gelatin and
allow to soften for 1 minute. Add this to the berries and
remove from the heat.

Mix in the NutraSweet and store covered in the refrigerator. Keeps for several weeks.

PER 1-TABLESPOON SERVING: 1 GRAM CARBOHYDRATE

Blender Hollandaise Sauce

SERVES 6

Great over cooked vegetables—especially asparagus and broccoli—or for eggs Benedict.

1 **stick of butter**
3 **egg yolks (reserve whites for another use)**
2 **tablespoons fresh lemon juice**
  dash of cayenne pepper

Melt the butter in a saucepan over low heat or in the microwave. In a blender or food processor, mix the egg yolks, lemon juice, and cayenne. With the motor running, add the melted butter in a slow stream. Blend for 30 seconds or until thick.

PER SERVING: 0.5 GRAM CARBOHYDRATE, 1.2 GRAMS PROTEIN

Light and Speedy Meals

Here are some ideas for lunches and dinners to put together when you're too rushed to focus on real recipes. Some are familiar dishes, and you may have your own favorite way of preparing them, in which case these notes will serve as reminders that they're permissible on this diet. Where quantities are necessary, they're for one serving, but everything is easily multiplied.

QUICK SALADS

Egg Salad

Chopped hard-boiled eggs with minced celery, scallions, and fresh dill, salt and pepper, and mayonnaise seasoned with Dijon mustard and lightened with yogurt two to one.

PER SERVING: LESS THAN 1 GRAM CARBOHYDRATE, 6 GRAMS PROTEIN PER EGG USED.

Stuff a medium tomato with it for another 4.1 grams carbohydrate.

Greek Salad

Cut up $^1/_2$ medium ripe seeded tomato, $^1/_2$ medium green pepper, and $^1/_2$ peeled and seeded cucumber and toss into a salad bowl. Add a slice of sweet onion separated into rings, a minced garlic clove, some chopped fresh dill, and lots of chopped parsley. Drizzle olive oil and red wine vinegar over the salad and top it with an ounce of crumbled feta cheese.

PER SERVING: 8 GRAMS CARBOHYDRATE, 8 GRAMS PROTEIN

Ham and Cheese Salad

Sliver a $^1/_4$-inch-thick slice of deli baked (or Black Forest) ham along with an ounce of Jarlsberg or Gruyère cheese. Mix with $^1/_2$ cup sliced raw mushrooms, a little chopped celery, minced parsley, and a couple of tablespoons of freshly grated Parmesan cheese. Shake up the dressing in

a screw-top jar: 1 tab
white wine vinegar, ^{1}/
mustard, salt, and a t

PER SERVING: 3 GRAMS

Chicken Salad

Pull the meat from a
with minced scallior
chopped stuffed gree
half and half with sou

PER SERVING: 3 GRAMS CARBOHYDRATE, 21 GRAMS PROTEIN

Or mix the chicken with curried mayonnaise, grated orange zest, and yogurt. Add slivered jícama or water chestnuts for crunch and minced cilantro for sparkle. Serve
with a couple slices of fresh ripe mango or papaya and ^{1}/2
diced avocado.

PER SERVING: AN ADDITIONAL 10 GRAMS CARBOHYDRATE, 2
GRAMS PROTEIN

Tuna Salad

Flake the tuna and mix with minced scallions, parsley, and
grated lemon zest. Press a clove of garlic into mayonnaise,
add a squeeze of fresh lemon juice, and fold into the tuna
mixture.

PER SERVING: 2 GRAMS CARBOHYDRATE, 24 GRAMS PROTEIN

Cottage Cheese and To

Mix ^{1}/3 cup cottage
a minced clove of
over a big mix

PER SERVIN
TEIN

mato

neese with lots of minced parsley and
garlic. Stuff a medium tomato and serve
d green salad.

G: 6.5 GRAMS CARBOHYDRATE, 14 GRAMS PRO-

Parsley Salad

This salad tastes wonderful with grilled lamb or roast
chicken. Pull the leaves off a bunch of parsley and measure out 1 cup. Dress the parsley leaves with fresh lemon
juice and freshly grated Parmesan cheese, salt, and pepper. You don't really need oil, but you can add a little
olive oil if you like. Sliver 1 sun-dried tomato and toss
it in.

PER SERVING: 6.5 GRAMS CARBOHYDRATE

Melon and Prosciutto

Slice $1/4$ 5-inch cantaloupe and wrap each slice in thin prosciutto slices. Arrange the wrapped melon slices on a plate
and add a couple of wedges of lime to squeeze over them.
Pass the peppermill.

PER SERVING: 10 GRAMS CARBOHYDRATE, 4 GRAMS PROTEIN

CREAMED CHIPPED BEEF WITH MUSHROOMS

Stouffer's creamed chipped beef has 5 grams carbohydrate per 1/2 cup. Add 1/4 cup sautéed mushrooms, 1 table-spoon minced scallions, and a dash of Tabasco. (Serve it over 10 steamed spears of fresh asparagus for an extra 5 grams carbohydrate.)

PER SERVING: 7 GRAMS CARBOHYDRATE, 9 GRAMS PROTEIN

SAUSAGE AND PEPPERS WITH ZUCCHINI

Sauté 3 ounces of your favorite sausage, links or patties, with 1/2 cup chopped red or green bell pepper, 1/4 cup chopped onion, and 1/2 cup chopped zucchini.

PER SERVING: 7.5 GRAMS CARBOHYDRATE, 21 GRAMS PROTEIN

DILLED PANCAKES WITH SMOKED SALMON

Make the pancakes described on page 229, adding minced fresh dill and minced scallions to the batter and leaving out the sweetener. Stack 5 of the pancakes with a teaspoon of sour cream and a thin slice of smoked salmon on top of each one.

PER SERVING: 13 GRAMS CARBOHYDRATE, 28 GRAMS PROTEIN

Barbecue Sauce

Commercial BBQ sauces run between 5 and 14 grams carbohydrate per *tablespoon*. This one has only 2 grams per tablespoon (8.25 per $^1/_4$ cup). Mix together 2 tablespoons Heinz Light ketchup, 1 tablespoon Worcestershire sauce, 1 tablespoon Dijon honey mustard, 1 tablespoon minced shallot, 2 pressed garlic cloves, Tabasco sauce to taste, $^1/_4$ cup full-bodied red wine, a dash of liquid mesquite smoke, and a small pinch of NutraSweet or Equal.

HAM STEAK WITH BEET SALAD

Roast 2 medium beets at 375° for about 40 minutes or until a knife tip easily pierces the beet. Cool the beets and slip off the skins. Sliver the beets and dress them with 2 tablespoons minced scallion and $^1/_4$ cup heavy cream mixed with a scant teaspoon horseradish mustard (or mix your own), salt and pepper, and a few drops of fresh lemon juice. Serve with a grilled 3-ounce ham steak.

PER SERVING: 13 GRAMS CARBOHYDRATE, 22 GRAMS PROTEIN

STIR-FRY DISHES

Simple vegetable stir-fries with the addition of thinly sliced beef, chicken, pork, tofu, or whole shrimp are perfect hurry-up, low-carb meals. Look up in Chapter 5 the carbohydrate gram counts of the vegetables you want to use.

Choose from mushrooms, green beans, eggplant, red pepper, bok choy, asparagus, scallions, baby corn, carrots, spinach, snow peas or sugar snaps, celery, bamboo shoots, and water chestnuts. Heat the wok until it's hot and add peanut oil, minced garlic, a slivered coin of ginger, and a dried hot chili or two if you like your stir-fries spicy. Briefly cook the meat first, remove it (and chilies) to a side bowl, and then briefly toss and cook the vegetables. Add the meat back in and season with soy sauce, tamari, oyster sauce, or one of the many good liquid stir-fry seasonings available at gourmet stores. Check labels; some of these are loaded with carbs.

PER SERVING: Carbohydrate gram counts will vary according to the vegetables chosen. Watch the quantities!

GARLIC SHRIMP WITH SALSA

Sauté jumbo shrimp in garlic oil and add a tablespoon of hot Mexican salsa to each serving. Serve with a mixed green salad with 1/2 sliced avocado and 4 or 5 strips of jícama.

PER SERVING: 5 GRAMS CARBOHYDRATE, 21 GRAMS PROTEIN

SALMON OLIVADA

Smear olivada paste over a thick salmon fillet or steak and broil it. A 6-ounce salmon steak provides 42 grams protein.

Snacks: 5 Carbohydrate Grams or Less

Remember: subtract your snack carbohydrates from your meal allowance.

- $^1/_4$ cup Planter's mixed salted nuts with peanuts (3 grams)
- 1 Swedish ginger snap with a thin slice of natural cheddar (4 grams)
- 2 celery ribs filled with 1 tablespoon of chunky natural peanut butter or cream cheese with scallions (5 grams)
- 4 slices of hard salami (or cervelat with garlic and peppercorns) spread lightly with cream cheese and rolled around a thin scallion or half of a larger one (2 grams)
- 2 thin slices of boiled or baked ham spread with cream cheese and chives, rolled (1 gram)
- 2 thin slices of ham spread with spicy mustard and rolled up with thin slices of Gruyère (1 gram)
- 1 Wasa sesame cracker with 1 tablespoon of any cheese spread of your choice (3 grams)
- 2 slices of rare deli roast beef spread lightly with 1 tablespoon cream-style horseradish, rolled (1 gram)
- 5 pieces Talk o' Texas Okra Pickles—hot or mild (5 grams)
- $^1/_4$ cup roasted and salted sunflower seeds (4 grams)

- 5 Wheat Thins (5 grams)
- 2 ounces string cheese or mozzarella with 2 cherry tomatoes (3 grams)
- 1 deviled egg (1 gram)

CHEESE TOAST WITH TOMATO, BACON, AND AVOCADO

Melt 1 ounce grated cheese on 1 Jaret toast with a thin slice of tomato on the bottom. Top with 2 slices of crisp bacon and a slice of avocado.

PER SERVING: 7 GRAMS CARBOHYDRATE, 11 GRAMS PROTEIN

COD WITH TOMATO SHRIMP SAUCE

Mix 2 tablespoons crème fraîche or sour cream with minced chives, a squeeze of sun-dried tomato paste from a tube, a pinch of cayenne, and a squeeze of lemon. Fold in 1 ounce chopped cooked shrimp and serve the sauce over a *thick* 4-ounce fillet of cod steamed in the microwave.

PER SERVING: 3 GRAMS CARBOHYDRATE, 36 GRAMS PROTEIN

HUEVOS CARACAS

Frizzle some dried beef in butter with a little chili powder. Add 1/2 seeded and chopped tomato and a dash of hot sauce. Cook for about 2 minutes. Add a tablespoon of grated Parmesan cheese and then fold in 2 beaten eggs. Lift and turn until the eggs are firm.

PER SERVING: 2.5 GRAMS CARBOHYDRATE, 21 GRAMS PROTEIN

GRUYÈRE AND ZUCCHINI FRITTATA WITH SAUSAGE

In a nonstick omelet pan, melt butter and sauté ¹/₂ cup matchstick-cut zucchini with salt and pepper until it's tender. Pour in 3 beaten eggs and a handful of grated Gruyère cheese. Cook over low heat, continually lifting this flat omelet to let the uncooked portion flow to the bottom of the pan. Serve with a couple of small grilled sausages.

PER SERVING: 3.1 GRAMS CARBOHYDRATE, 31 GRAMS PROTEIN

Soups

Spicy Tomato and Celeriac Soup

MAKES 1 QUART; 4 SERVINGS

> 2 cups canned Italian plum tomatoes, drained
> 2 cups beef broth
> ³/₄ cup grated celery root
> 2 garlic cloves, minced
> 1 tablespoon minced flat-leaf parsley
> 1 teaspoon fresh thyme leaves or ¹/₄ teaspoon dried
> ¹/₄ teaspoon Tabasco sauce or to taste
> pinch of NutraSweet or Equal
> salt to taste

Put everything but the NutraSweet and salt in a saucepan and cook over low heat until the celeriac and garlic are soft. Add a small pinch of sweetener and some salt. Puree the soup in a food processor or blender.

PER 1-CUP SERVING: 7 GRAMS CARBOHYDRATE

• To serve this soup for a full meal, mix $^1/_2$ pound ground chicken with 6 minced scallions, $^1/_4$ teaspoon dried oregano, salt and pepper, and an egg yolk mixed with a bit of heavy cream. Form into little meatballs and sauté them quickly in olive oil. Put a few of them in the bottom of the soup bowls and freeze the rest for another use. Slices of cooked sausage would also be good. Additional protein grams: 16.

• Try replacing the beef broth with $1^1/_2$ cups clam broth and simmer chunks of sea bass or cod in the soup. Additional protein grams: 16.

Kind-of-Mexican Chicken and Vegetable Soup

MAKES 2 QUARTS; 5 SERVINGS

   2 tablespoons olive oil
$^1/_2$ cup chopped scallion
   1 garlic clove, minced
   1 tablespoon minced canned chipotle chili or
      canned green chili plus a shake of liquid
      smoke and hot sauce
   1 quart chicken broth
   2 celery ribs, chopped
   1 carrot, sliced
$^1/_2$ cup cut green beans
$^1/_2$ cup diced zucchini
   1 cup diced Muir Glen organic canned tomatoes

$^1/_2$ cup canned hominy, rinsed
1 cup shredded cooked chicken
  salt and pepper to taste
$^1/_4$ avocado, diced, per serving
1 thin slice of lime per serving

Heat the oil in a soup pot, then sauté the scallion, garlic, and chili in the hot oil over medium heat until the garlic is soft, about 2 minutes. Add the broth and all of the vegetables and simmer uncovered until the vegetables are soft. Add the hominy, chicken, salt, and pepper and heat for 2 minutes. Add more chipotle or some Tabasco sauce if you like the soup spicier. Garnish each portion with avocado and lime.

PER $1^1/_2$-CUP SERVING: 10 GRAMS CARBOHYDRATE, 12 GRAMS PROTEIN

Spinach, Leek, and Bacon Soup with Scallops

SERVES 2

4 strips of smoked bacon
3 leeks, trimmed, cleaned, and minced
  salt and pepper to taste
1 cup cooked frozen whole-leaf spinach, chopped
3 cups chicken broth
2 egg yolks mixed with $^1/_4$ cup heavy cream
  pinch of cayenne pepper
10 ounces bay scallops
2 lemon wedges for garnish

Crisp-cook the bacon and crumble it for garnish; set aside. Reserve 2 tablespoons of the bacon fat and sauté the minced leeks in it over medium heat until soft. Add salt and pepper. Add the spinach and broth and puree in a food processor or blender. Return to the stove over medium-low heat. Ladle a little hot broth into the yolk mixture and whisk, then whisk the mixture into the rest of the broth, stirring until the soup is thickened. Taste for salt and add the cayenne. Add the scallops and cook for a minute or two to heat through. Serve with the bacon bits on top and garnish with a lemon wedge.

PER SERVING: 9 GRAMS CARBOHYDRATE, 25 GRAMS PROTEIN

Double-Mushroom Soup

MAKES 1 QUART; 4 SERVINGS

- 4 tablespoons (1/2 stick) butter
- 2 cups chopped mixed mushrooms
- 1/2 cup minced scallion
- 2 garlic cloves, minced
  salt and cayenne pepper to taste
- 1 teaspoon dry mustard
- 2 teaspoons wild mushroom powder (grind dried wild mushrooms in a food processor)
- 3 cups chicken broth
- 2 tablespoons dry sherry
- 2 egg yolks mixed 1/4 cup heavy cream

Melt the butter in a large skillet over medium-low heat. Sauté the mushrooms, scallion, and garlic in the butter for about 30 minutes, until the mixture is thick. Add the salt and cayenne, dry mustard, and mushroom powder, mix well, and cook for 5 minutes. Pour in the chicken broth and sherry and bring the soup to a simmer. Whisk a little of the hot liquid into the yolk mixture and then whisk that mixture back into the soup, stirring until it thickens.

PER 1-CUP SERVING: 3 GRAMS CARBOHYDRATE, 5 GRAMS PROTEIN

• Serve before a roast chicken or a broiled fish fillet and add a big mixed green salad with lemon vinaigrette.

Gazpacho

SERVES 2

    1 16-ounce can Muir Glen organic stewed
       tomatoes
    2 garlic cloves, pressed
    1 tablespoon mayonnaise
       pinch of cayenne pepper
    1 teaspoon red wine vinegar
       salt and pepper to taste
  1/4 cup minced scallion
  1/2 medium cucumber, peeled if waxed, seeded and
       diced
  1/4 cup diced green bell pepper

Puree half of the stewed tomatoes in a food processor or blender with the pressed garlic, mayonnaise, cayenne, and vinegar. Add salt and pepper. Add the rest of the tomatoes and pulse on and off to blend, preserving some texture. Mix the remaining vegetables together and refrigerate separately from the soup base until both are well chilled. Serve the soup very cold with the chopped vegetables stirred in.

PER SERVING: 10.5 GRAMS CARBOHYDRATE

Chilled Red Pepper Soup with Cilantro

SERVES 2

- $3/4$ cup drained canned roasted red peppers
- 1 cup chicken broth
  salt to taste
- 1 garlic clove, pressed or minced
  pinch of cayenne pepper
- 2 tablespoons minced cilantro
- 3 tablespoons sour cream
- 1 tablespoon yogurt
- 1 tablespoon water

Puree the red peppers with the chicken broth in a food processor or blender. Add the salt, garlic, and cayenne and pulse to blend. Chill for at least an hour. Whisk the cilantro into the sour cream and yogurt. Serve the soup with the herbed cream feathered into it with a fork.

PER SERVING: 6 GRAMS CARBOHYDRATE, 3.5 GRAMS PROTEIN

- Serve this soup with a couple of broiled or grilled lamb chops and a mixed green salad, including some spinach.

Chilled Almond Avocado Soup

SERVES 2

- 1 ripe Hass avocado, chopped
- $1/2$ cup blanched almonds, toasted
- 1 cup chicken broth
- $1/4$ teaspoon fresh lime juice
  salt and pepper to taste
  pinch of nutmeg, preferably freshly ground

¹/₂ **cup light cream**
1 **tablespoon slivered almonds, toasted**

Puree the avocado and blanched almonds in a food processor or blender until smooth. Pour the mixture into a small saucepan and add the chicken broth, lime juice, salt and pepper, and nutmeg. Bring to a boil, then lower the heat, and simmer uncovered for 5 minutes. Stir in the cream. Chill the soup for at least an hour. Serve with the slivered almonds sprinkled on top.

PER SERVING: 15 GRAMS CARBOHYDRATE, 15 GRAMS PROTEIN

• Serve with jumbo shrimp sautéed in garlic oil and red pepper flakes over spinach salad. (12 cooked shrimp have about 21 grams protein.)

Gingered Egg Drop Soup with Chicken

SERVES 2

2 **chicken breast halves, skinned and boned**
1 **coin of fresh ginger**
3 **cups chicken broth, preferably homemade
   salt and Szechuan pepper to taste**
4 **scallions—the bulb, and 1 inch of the green
   parts, slivered**
8 **snow peas, trimmed and cut on the diagonal
   into thin strips**
1 **egg, beaten**

Cut the chicken breasts lengthwise into 3 sections and then into diagonal strips. Simmer the chicken strips with the ginger coin in the chicken broth in a small saucepan until the chicken is opaque, about 6 minutes. When the chicken is cooked, remove and discard the ginger. Salt the broth and grind in some Szechuan pepper. Add the scallions and snow peas. Whisk the egg and drizzle it into the broth. Serve the soup immediately.

PER SERVING: 4 GRAMS CARBOHYDRATE, 36 GRAMS PROTEIN

• Serve with 3 Japanese sesame rice crackers for an extra 4.5 carbohydrate grams.

Salads

Indonesian Vegetable Salad with Peanut Sauce

SERVES 2

- $1/2$ cup bean sprouts
- 1 cup very thinly sliced red cabbage
- $1/2$ cup sliced young green beans
- $1/2$ cup chopped zucchini
- $1/4$ large red bell pepper, cut into thin strips
- 2 tablespoons creamy natural peanut butter
- $1/4$ cup Thai unsweetened coconut milk
- 1 garlic clove, pressed
- $1/2$ teaspoon Thai hot chili sauce or to taste
- 1 tablespoon tamari or soy sauce
  pinch of NutraSweet or Equal

$^1/_6$ lime in a wedge
    water as needed
  8 scallions, trimmed and quartered
  2 tablespoons grated carrot
$^1/_2$ cucumber, peeled if waxed, sliced
  3 cups spinach, washed and dried
  2 hard-cooked eggs, sliced

Pour boiling water over the bean sprouts and let them sit for only a second. Strain and reserve. Steam the cabbage, beans, zucchini, and red pepper in the microwave together until crisp-tender, about 5 minutes. In a small bowl, mix the peanut butter, coconut milk, garlic, chili sauce, tamari, and NutraSweet into a sauce using the back of a spoon. Squeeze the lime wedge into the sauce. Add water to the sauce to bring it to the consistency of heavy cream. Adjust the seasoning. Arrange the cooked and raw vegetables around a bed of spinach, keeping each variety separate. Overlap the egg slices in the center and serve the salad with the peanut sauce on the side.

PER SERVING: 15 GRAMS CARBOHYDRATE, 8.5 GRAMS PROTEIN

• Serve with broiled or charcoal-grilled pork baby back ribs rubbed with salt and cayenne pepper.

Caesar Salad with Shrimp

SERVES 2

    4 hearts of romaine, broken into bite-size pieces

Dressing:

    6 tablespoons olive oil
    2 tablespoons fresh lemon juice
       salt and pepper to taste
       pinch of dry mustard
       dash of Worcestershire sauce
$^1/_2$ inch squeeze of anchovy paste from a tube (optional)
    1 egg yolk

Topping:

    2 tablespoons freshly grated Parmesan cheese
  12 large shrimp, cooked and peeled
  12 garlic croutons

Put the romaine into a salad bowl. Put the dressing ingredients in a screw-top jar and shake vigorously. Taste for seasoning and adjust—the dressing should be lemony and piquant. Toss the greens with enough dressing to coat the leaves, reserving a little. Sprinkle the leaves with the grated Parmesan. Dip the shrimp into the reserved dressing and place them on top of the salad along with the garlic croutons. (Make the croutons from diced rustic bread. Coat them with garlic olive oil and toast on a baking sheet in a 375° oven until golden and crisp.)

PER SERVING: 9 GRAMS CARBOHYDRATE, 13 GRAMS PROTEIN

Barbecued Pork, Zucchini, and Roasted Red Pepper Salad

SERVES 2

Dressing:

- 1/4 cup olive oil or avocado oil
- 2 tablespoons sherry vinegar
- 1 garlic clove, pressed
- 1/4 teaspoon ground cumin
  salt and pepper to taste

Salad:

- any amount of mixed salad greens
- 1 cup sliced mixed green and yellow summer squash
- 1/4 cup diced jícama
- 1 canned roasted red pepper, torn into strips
  any amount of barbecued pork tenderloin, sliced*

Shake the dressing in a screw-top jar. Toss the salad vegetables with the dressing and arrange the cold pork slices around the edge of the salad.

PER SERVING: 8 GRAMS CARBOHYDRATE, 21 GRAMS PROTEIN

---

*To barbecue the pork, rub a pork tenderloin all over with 1 tablespoon olive oil mixed with a minced garlic clove, 1/4 teaspoon oregano, 1/8 teaspoon ground cumin, and a jolt of liquid smoke and Tabasco. Massage the seasonings into the meat. Broil the pork 4 inches from the heat for 6 minutes on each side.

GOING FOR THE CRUNCH

You'll quickly notice that the low-carb kitchen is short on crunch—no rice cakes, no pretzels, no buckets of popcorn. But here are some ideas for snacks that offer a little crunch for very few carbs.

- unlimited pork rinds—zero carbohydrate
- 2 Wasa Sesame Rye crackers—4 grams carbohydrate
- 5 Wheat Thins—5 grams
- 1 cup Cape Cod cheddar cheese popcorn—5 grams
- 2 breadsticks—5 grams (check labels)
- 1/2 cup Planter's mixed salted nuts with peanuts—6 grams
- 1 Jaret (melba) toast—6 grams

Spinach, Avocado, Bacon, and Goat Cheese Salad

SERVES 2

Salad:

    any amount of spinach leaves
3   celery ribs, cut into 2-inch sticks lengthwise
6   scallions, trimmed and quartered
2   ounces goat Gouda or any firm goat cheese, cut into thin strips
1   medium Hass avocado, sliced

Dressing:

> 1/4 cup sunflower or light olive oil
> 2 tablespoons fresh lemon juice
> 1 teaspoon Dijon honey mustard
> 2 teaspoons minced fresh dill
> salt and pepper to taste

Toppings:

> 4 strips of smoked bacon, cooked and crumbled
> 2 tablespoons roasted sunflower seeds

Toss the salad ingredients with the blended salad dressing and add the toppings.

PER SERVING: 9 GRAMS CARBOHYDRATE, 12 GRAMS PROTEIN

Main Dishes

Antipasto Supper

SERVES 2

This long list of ingredients shouldn't intimidate you since there's no cooking involved. A great antipasto can be put together in minutes.

> arugula or other flat salad greens
> 3 tablespoons Hellmann's Light mayonnaise
> 2 large garlic cloves, pressed
> 1 tablespoon fresh lemon juice
> 1 6 1/2-ounce can white tuna, packed in oil

1 teaspoon tiny capers or minced large capers
1/2 cup Progresso or Giovanni's eggplant
     caponata
1/4 cup oil-packed artichoke hearts
     red wine vinegar
     salt and pepper to taste
4 slices of imported prosciutto
1 tablespoon whipped cream cheese with minced
   onion
8 slices of Italian hard salami
4 scallions, split lengthwise
2 red hot cherry peppers or pickled okra
8 mushrooms, thinly sliced
   oil and vinegar
   fresh thyme leaves
8 cherry tomatoes
8 Italian or Greek black olives
2 ounces ricotta salata or fresh mozzarella, cut
   into strips

Line a round serving platter with arugula leaves. Mix
the mayonnaise, garlic, and lemon juice in a small dish.
Turn out the tuna onto paper towels to drain, keeping the
fish in the round compressed shape. Blot the top and sides
and set the round of tuna in the center of the platter.
Spread with the garlic mayonnaise and dot with capers.
Set all the other components around the tuna like the
spokes of a wheel: First the canned caponata. Drain the artichoke hearts and drizzle some red wine vinegar over
them. Add salt and pepper. Next, ruffle the prosciutto.
Then place a dot of the cream cheese in the center of each
slice of salami. Place the white end of a scallion half on the
dot and gather the salami up around it, using the cream

cheese as the "glue." Next lay out the cherry peppers or okra. Dress the sliced mushrooms with oil and vinegar and the leaves from a couple of stems of fresh thyme. Arrange the tomatoes, the olives, and finally some fingers of cheese.

PER SERVING: 12 GRAMS CARBOHYDRATE, 31.5 GRAMS PROTEIN

Tex-Mex Cheese Flan with Chunky Salsa

SERVES 2

These puffy little flans are not only versatile and ready in a flash but are perfect for company, as either an accompaniment or a first course.

       vegetable or olive oil spray
   1   jumbo egg
 $^1/_4$ cup nonfat ricotta or large-curd cottage cheese
 $^1/_4$ cup grated Monterey Jack cheese, lightly packed
   2   tablespoons light sour cream
   1   tablespoon minced cilantro (optional)
       salt and pepper to taste
   2   tablespoons chunky Mexican salsa
   2   cilantro sprigs for garnish

Preheat the oven to 350°. Lightly spray $^1/_2$-cup soufflé ramekins or custard cups. Put all the ingredients except the salsa and cilantro sprigs in a blender or food processor. Blend or process until very smooth and creamy. Divide the mixture between the ramekins—they should be about two-thirds full. Bake for 20 minutes or until nicely domed and puffed. Run a sharp knife around the edge of the

ramekins and turn the flans out onto serving plates. Top
with a tablespoon of salsa, garnish with cilantro, and serve
immediately.

PER SERVING: 4 GRAMS CARBOHYDRATE, 12 GRAMS PROTEIN

• Serve the flan with chicken sausage and a large mixed
green salad with ¹/₂ avocado, sliced.

PER SERVING: AN ADDITIONAL 7 GRAMS CARBOHYDRATE, 24
GRAMS PROTEIN

Italian Flan:

Use grated fontina cheese or half fontina and half fresh
mozzarella—try smoked mozzarella. Arrange a couple of
basil leaves or one large one on the bottom of the ramekin
before filling it. Top the finished flan with a tablespoon of
hot marinara sauce (additional 1 gram carbohydrate).

Feta-Dill Flan with Shrimp:

Use cottage cheese, crumbled feta, minced dill, and 2
minced scallions in the flans. Serve with 6 large shrimp,
tails on, sautéed in olive oil with minced garlic and a sprinkle of hot red pepper flakes. Just before serving, toss a
large handful of baby spinach leaves into the shrimp and
toss until the spinach wilts but remains bright green.

PER SERVING: AN ADDITIONAL 5.5 GRAMS CARBOHYDRATE,
11 GRAMS PROTEIN

Nutty Chicken Thighs

SERVES 2

These crunchy baked chicken thighs are close cousins to southern fried chicken.

  4 tablespoons (¹/₂ stick) butter, melted
¹/₄ cup peanut oil
  1 egg, lightly beaten with 3 tablespoons butter-
      milk
¹/₄ cup ground raw peanuts
  1 tablespoon sesame seeds
  2 tablespoons flour
      salt and pepper to taste
  4 chicken thighs

Preheat the oven to 350°. Mix the melted butter with the oil and pour it into a shallow ovenproof pan. Slide the pan into the oven while you dip the chicken. Whisk the buttermilk and egg together in a flat soup bowl and mix the ground peanuts, seeds, flour, and seasoning in another. Dip the chicken pieces into the buttermilk/egg and then coat completely with the dry mixture. Place the chicken in the hot pan, spooning up the butter and oil to completely moisten the coating. Bake for 30 to 40 minutes or until the chicken is well browned and crisp.

PER SERVING: 10 GRAMS CARBOHYDRATE, 40 GRAMS PRO-
TEIN

• Serve the chicken with a large green salad, including some spinach, a few thinly sliced red onion rings, and 4 halved cherry tomatoes. Dress the salad with olive oil, red wine vinegar, and a dash of balsamic vinegar.

PER SERVING: AN EXTRA 3 GRAMS CARBOHYDRATE

Maintenance Additions:

Serve each portion of chicken with ¹/₂ cup steamed whole skinny green beans and coleslaw. To make the coleslaw, mix ¹/₂ cup shredded raw cabbage with 2 tablespoons grated carrot, ¹/₄ minced sweet red pepper, and a scant tablespoon of Hellmann's Light mayonnaise with a splash of apple cider vinegar.

PER SERVING: AN EXTRA 9 GRAMS CARBOHYDRATE, 2 GRAMS PROTEIN

Chicken with Chèvre, Smoked Bacon, and Pepper Salsa

SERVES 2

  4 single chicken breasts, pounded thin
¹/₄ cup soft goat cheese
  2 thick slices of smoked bacon, diced
  2 garlic cloves, minced
¹/₂ cup chopped onion
¹/₂ cup chopped mixed peppers (red, green, yellow, and jalapeño)
  2 tablespoons minced cilantro

Spread 2 of the pounded chicken breasts with the cheese. Cover them with the remaining chicken breasts and sandwich them together, securing them with toothpicks. Fry the diced bacon in a skillet large enough to hold the chicken breasts. Remove the crisp bacon and set aside. Pour off all but 2 tablespoons of the bacon fat. Sauté the chicken on both sides over medium heat until lightly golden. Remove them to a microwave-safe dish and cover with plastic wrap. Sauté the garlic, onion, and mixed pepper salsa until limp but not soft. Toss in the cilantro. When you're ready to serve, cook the chicken in the microwave for about 5–6 minutes. Top the chicken with the salsa and bacon.

PER SERVING: 6 GRAMS CARBOHYDRATE, 35 GRAMS PROTEIN

• Serve with a mixed green salad with slices of $1/2$ avocado, 3 to 4 cherry tomatoes, and a lime vinaigrette.

PER SERVING: AN EXTRA 8 GRAMS CARBOHYDRATE, 2 GRAMS PROTEIN

Turkey Burgers with Red Wine Sauce

SERVES 2

 3 tablespoons olive oil or butter
 2 tablespoons chopped shallot
 2 garlic cloves, minced
   pinch of dried thyme
   pinch of dried rosemary
   pinch of dried oregano
 1 teaspoon mustard with green peppercorns
 1 cup Zinfandel or other fruity red wine
 $3/4$ pound ground turkey or mixed chicken and
   turkey

Heat the oil in a small skillet and sauté the shallot and garlic over medium heat until wilted but not brown, about 2 minutes. Add the dried herbs and mustard and mix well. Add the red wine and reduce by half over high heat. Loosely form the meat into 2 patties and fry them over medium heat in another small skillet. Cook the burgers about 6 minutes on each side. Pour the sauce over the burgers.

PER SERVING: 8 GRAMS CARBOHYDRATE, 36 GRAMS PROTEIN

• Serve with $^1/_2$ cup chopped mushrooms sautéed with $^1/_2$ cup chopped green and yellow summer squash.

PER SERVING: AN EXTRA 3 GRAMS CARBOHYDRATE

Lemon Chicken with Choron Sauce

SERVES 2

This sauce is a French classic, named after the chef who invented it.

    1 roasting chicken or carryout rotisserie chicken
       salt and pepper to taste
    3 lemons
    6 garlic cloves, peeled
 $^1/_2$ medium onion
       olive oil

Choron Sauce:

    3 egg yolks
    2 tablespoons fresh lemon juice
 $^1/_2$ teaspoon salt
       pinch of cayenne pepper
 $3^1/_2$ tablespoons butter
 $^1/_2$ cup tomato puree

If you're roasting your own chicken, preheat the oven to 375°. Rinse the chicken inside and out and pat dry. Salt and pepper the cavity. Pierce the lemons all over with a fork and stuff them into the chicken along with the garlic and the half onion cut in two. Skewer the cavity closed (using meat skewers or wooden kebab sticks) and tie the legs together. Rub the chicken with olive oil and roast for 1 to 1½ hours, depending on its size. Remove the chicken from the oven, discard the stuffing, and let the bird sit while you make the sauce.

Beat the yolks in a blender until thick and yellow. Add the lemon juice, ½ teaspoon salt, and the cayenne. Melt the butter in the microwave and, while still hot, drizzle it slowly into the yolks with the blender running. The sauce will thicken quickly. Add the tomato puree and pour the warm sauce over the carved chicken.

PER SERVING: 4 GRAMS CARBOHYDRATE, 45 GRAMS PROTEIN (PER 6-OUNCE PORTION)

• Serve with 1 cup buttered steamed broccoli with toasted pine nuts.

PER SERVING: AN EXTRA 3 GRAMS CARBOHYDRATE, 2 GRAMS PROTEIN

Chicken Breasts Stuffed with Prosciutto and Mozzarella

SERVES 2

  2 whole chicken breasts, boned and split
  4 paper-thin slices of prosciutto

4 **thin slices of mozzarella**
1 **tablespoon Pillsbury Shake & Blend flour**
3 **tablespoons olive oil**
²/₃ **cup dry white wine**
¹/₂ **cup tomato sauce**
¹/₄ **teaspoon dried oregano**
    salt and pepper to taste
    minced parsley for garnish

Pound the chicken breasts between 2 pieces of wax paper until very thin. Put a slice of prosciutto and a slice of cheese on top of each. Roll the breasts up, tucking in the sides and securing the ends with toothpicks. Sprinkle each breast very lightly with the instant flour. Brown the rolls in the olive oil in a sauté pan over medium-high heat and transfer them to a microwave-safe covered dish. Pour the wine into the sauté pan and simmer vigorously, scraping up any browned bits and reducing the wine by half. Add the remaining ingredients and simmer for another minute or two. Pour over the chicken rolls and microwave on high for 3 to 4 minutes. Garnish with minced parsley.

PER SERVING: 10 GRAMS CARBOHYDRATE, 42 GRAMS PROTEIN

• Serve with a mixed green salad with arugula and bitter greens or spinach. Add ¹/₄ cup canned marinated artichoke hearts to each serving.

PER SERVING: AN EXTRA 3.5 GRAMS CARBOHYDRATE, 1 GRAM PROTEIN

Chicken Chile Verde with Pepitas

SERVES 4

    3   tablespoons peanut oil
    4   chicken thighs and 4 breasts, boned
    4   garlic cloves, minced
 1/2   cup chopped onion
        salt and pepper to taste
    2   teaspoons ground cumin
    4   tomatillos, husked and finely chopped
    1   cup chopped canned mild green chilies
    2   to 3 canned jalapeños to taste, minced
 1/2   cup chicken broth
 1/4   cup minced cilantro
    1   tablespoon per serving roasted, shelled pump-
        kin seeds
    2   tablespoons sour cream

Heat the oil in a large skillet over medium heat. Sauté
the chicken in the oil until golden, about 4 minutes on
each side. Add the garlic and onion, reduce the heat, and
cook until the garlic is soft, about 3 minutes. Add salt and
pepper and sprinkle in the cumin. Add the tomatillos,
chilies, and broth. Cover and simmer until the chicken is
tender and the sauce thickened, about 30 minutes. Add
the cilantro and serve the chicken sprinkled with the
pumpkin seeds and a dollop of sour cream.

PER SERVING: 7.5 GRAMS CARBOHYDRATE, 46 GRAMS PROTEIN

   • Serve with 1/2 sliced avocado on Caesar salad (page
251).

PER SERVING: AN EXTRA 3.7 GRAMS CARBOHYDRATE, 2
GRAMS PROTEIN

Barbecued Chicken Wings

SERVES 10

Our friend Bill Parker developed this wonderful recipe, which has become a family favorite. The secret is to cook the wings long and slowly, then dunk them in the sauce just before serving. Be careful not to burn the wings—if you don't have a cover on your grill, just use a big piece of foil.

The sauce:

1 cup water
$1/2$ cup olive oil
$1/2$ cup vinegar, white or apple cider
2 tablespoons chili powder
$1/2$ teaspoon cayenne pepper

Mix the sauce ingredients together in a saucepan and bring to a boil over high heat. Boil 5 minutes, then set aside.

The wings:

5 pounds chicken wings
salt and pepper

Prepare a grill for barbecuing. Snip the wing tips off and sprinkle the wings with salt and pepper. Arrange the wings on the grill when the coals are glowing red and covered with white ash or set the grill for medium-hot. Cook the wings covered for 1 to $1^1/2$ hours, turning frequently, until the wings seem a bit dry.

Remove the wings from the grill and immediately dunk them in the sauce. Arrange on a platter and serve.

PER SERVING: 1.4 GRAMS CARBOHYDRATE, 38 GRAMS PROTEIN

Baked Grouper with Parsley and Lemon

SERVES 2

³/₄ to 1 pound grouper, flounder, or any firm white fish fillet
1 egg beaten with 1 tablespoon milk
3 tablespoons wheat germ
2 tablespoons freshly grated Parmesan cheese
1 tablespoon almond or olive oil
1 tablespoon butter
2 tablespoons minced parsley
1 teaspoon grated lemon zest

Soak the fish in the egg wash for 30 minutes. Mix the wheat germ with the Parmesan and dip the fish into it on both sides to form a light coating—no more than needed. Preheat the oven to 375°. Heat the oil and butter together in a nonstick skillet with an ovenproof handle and lightly brown the fillet on both sides over medium heat. Remove the skillet to the oven and bake for 15 minutes or until the fish is firm. Garnish with parsley and lemon zest.

PER SERVING: 4.5 GRAMS CARBOHYDRATE, 47 GRAMS PROTEIN

• Serve with ¹/₂ cup peeled, seeded, and chopped cucumber sautéed in butter with 1 tablespoon grated carrot.

PER SERVING: AN EXTRA 4 GRAMS CARBOHYDRATE

Coconut Salmon

SERVES 2

> ¹/₄ cup peanut oil
> 2 large shallots, thinly sliced
> 1 tablespoon turmeric
>   pinch of cayenne pepper
>   pinch of ground mace
> ³/₄ pound salmon fillet, cut into 2 servings
> ¹/₂ cup Thai unsweetened coconut milk
>   cilantro sprigs for garnish

In a small skillet, heat the peanut oil over medium-high heat. When it's very hot, add the shallots and fry until deep brown, about 5 minutes. Strain them out onto a folded paper towel to crisp—set aside. Mix the spices in a small saucer and dip the salmon into them, rubbing the fillets all over to coat them lightly. Put the salmon into a covered microwave-safe dish and pour in the coconut milk. Microwave on high for about 3 minutes or until the salmon is opaque and just firm to the touch. Serve with the crispy shallots on top and a sprig of cilantro.

PER SERVING: 3 GRAMS CARBOHYDRATE, 36 GRAMS PROTEIN

• Serve with 1 cup sautéed fresh or cooked frozen spinach. Sauté the fresh spinach in a tablespoon or more of olive oil and a minced garlic clove or lightly butter the cooked frozen spinach. Add salt and pepper.

PER SERVING: AN EXTRA 3 GRAMS CARBOHYDRATE, 5.4 GRAMS PROTEIN

Portobello Mushrooms Stuffed with Salmon and Spinach

SERVES 2

> 2 large portobello mushrooms, stemmed
> 3 teaspoons sunflower oil or light olive oil
> salt and pepper to taste
> 2 tablespoons minced scallion
> 1/2 pound salmon fillet, skinned and chopped
> 1 10-ounce package frozen whole-leaf spinach, thawed
> 3 tablespoons cream cheese

Brush the mushrooms with the oil, and salt and pepper them. Broil them upside down for 3 minutes. Preheat the oven to 375°. Sprinkle a tablespoon of minced scallion on each mushroom and divide the chopped salmon between them. Cook the spinach according to the microwave instructions and drain well. Blot out most of the water and chop it coarsely. Put 1 cup of the spinach back in the microwave with the cream cheese just to melt the cheese. Mix it well with a fork. Add salt and pepper. Pile the spinach over the salmon and bake the stuffed mushrooms for 20 minutes.

PER SERVING: 4 GRAMS CARBOHYDRATE, 29 GRAMS PROTEIN

- Serve with a lettuce and tomato salad.

PER SERVING: AN EXTRA 4 GRAMS CARBOHYDRATE

Grilled Tuna Steak with Gingered Slaw

SERVES 2

  2   tablespoons avocado or light olive oil
1/4   teaspoon Sriracha Thai chili sauce or other hot
      sauce
  2   tuna steaks, 1 inch thick

Gingered Slaw:

  2   cups very thinly sliced red cabbage
  2   cups very thinly sliced Napa cabbage
  6   scallions, trimmed and slivered lengthwise
1/2   cup skinny green beans, slivered lengthwise
1/4   large yellow bell pepper, cut into thin strips
      salt and pepper to taste

Dressing:

1/2   teaspoon toasted sesame oil (Asian)
  3   additional tablespoons avocado or sunflower
      oil
  1   tablespoon rice wine vinegar
  1   teaspoon soy sauce
  1   tablespoon sesame seeds
  2   teaspoons minced pickled ginger
      small pinch of NutraSweet or Equal or a cou-
      ple of drops of Sweet 10

Mix the oil and chili sauce and rub it into the tuna
steaks on both sides. Combine all of the prepared vegetables in a large bowl. Lightly salt and pepper them. Whisk
together the dressing ingredients. Grill the steaks over

white ash-coated coals, or sauté them for about 1 minute on each side. Toss the salad and serve.

PER SERVING: 10 GRAMS CARBOHYDRATE, 29 GRAMS PROTEIN

• Tuna cooks particularly fast because of its oil content, so be sure not to overcook it or it will be very dry. As soon as the steak hits the heat you can actually monitor the cooking process by watching the edge of the meat. The opaque gray color will rise like a thermometer. Turn the steak before the color line reaches the center and remove it from the heat while the center is still red.

Crab Cakes

SERVES 2

1/2 pound lump or backfin crabmeat
2 tablespoons Hellmann's mayonnaise
1 tablespoon sour cream
   Tabasco sauce to taste
3 scallions, both white and green parts, minced
2 tablespoons minced parsley
1 teaspoon capers, chopped, or 1/4 teaspoon lemon zest
6 Sunshine oyster crackers, finely crushed
2 teaspoons Wondra flour
2 tablespoons butter

Pick over the crabmeat to remove any cartilage without breaking up the lumps. Mix together the next 6 ingredients and fold carefully into the crabmeat. Add the crushed oyster crackers and lightly form the meat into 4 round cakes without compressing it. Refrigerate the cakes for 1 hour. Lightly dust both sides with presifted flour. Melt the butter in a skillet large enough to hold the crab cakes. Sauté them in the melted butter over medium-low heat until golden brown and heated through, about 4 minutes on each side.

PER SERVING: 5 GRAMS CARBOHYDRATE, 28 GRAMS PROTEIN

• Serve with ¹/₂ avocado stuffed with radish salad: mix finely slivered red and white radishes with salt and pepper, then drizzle with a little balsamic vinegar.

PER SERVING: AN EXTRA 4 GRAMS CARBOHYDRATE, 2 GRAMS PROTEIN

Scallops and Ham with Honey Mustard Sauce

SERVES 2

2 scallions, minced
3 thin slices of domestic prosciutto or Black Forest ham
1 tablespoon safflower or light olive oil
12 large sea scallops
2 tablespoons Dijon honey mustard
1 teaspoon grated fresh ginger with juice
2 teaspoons Chinese oyster sauce

In a nonstick pan, sauté the scallions and ham in the oil over medium heat until the ham is lightly frizzled and the scallions soft, about 3 minutes. Blot the scallops dry on paper towels. Push the ham and scallions to the side of the pan and sauté the scallops over medium-high heat, turning them frequently. When the scallops have patches of golden brown, reduce the heat and add the mustard, ginger, and oyster sauce. Toss all the ingredients together and simmer until the scallops are cooked through.

PER SERVING: 4 GRAMS CARBOHYDRATE, 12 GRAMS PROTEIN

• Serve the scallops with $1/2$ cup sugar snap peas or snow peas stir-fried with 2 sliced water chestnuts and mushrooms.

PER SERVING: AN EXTRA 6.5 GRAMS CARBOHYDRATE, 1 GRAM PROTEIN

Greek Shrimp with Feta Cheese

SERVES 2

    3 tablespoons olive oil
    2 garlic cloves, minced
       hot red pepper flakes to taste
 $1/2$ teaspoon crushed dried oregano
 $1/2$ cup strips of drained canned Italian plum
       tomatoes
    3 tablespoons bottled clam juice
    2 tablespoons chopped fresh dill
    1 tablespoon drained capers
       salt and pepper to taste
$1^{1}/2$ tablespoons butter
   12 to 16 large shrimp, peeled but tails left on
    3 tablespoons crumbled feta cheese

In a small skillet over medium heat, sauté the garlic, pepper flakes, and oregano in the olive oil until the garlic is soft and golden, about 2 minutes. Add the tomatoes and clam juice and simmer until most of the liquid evaporates, about 3 minutes. Add the dill, capers, and salt and pepper. Preheat the oven to 400°. Pour the sauce into a bowl and wipe out the skillet. Heat the butter over medium-high heat until it starts to brown. Toss and sauté the shrimp very briefly—just sealing and glazing the exterior and not cooking them through. Divide the shrimp between 2 ovenproof gratin dishes, arranging the tails up. Spoon the sauce over the shrimp and sprinkle the cheese on top. Bake for 15 minutes.

PER SERVING: 4.5 GRAMS CARBOHYDRATE, 15 GRAMS PROTEIN

• Serve with a big green salad.

Beef Provençal

SERVES 4

Make this dish the day before you plan to serve it to give the flavors a chance to develop fully.

1/4 pound sliced slab bacon
2 pounds boneless chuck or rump roast, cut into 2-inch cubes
2 medium onions, quartered
  salt and pepper to taste
1 small fennel bulb, trimmed and thinly sliced
1 head of garlic, separated into cloves and peeled
6 large strips of orange zest
1 bay leaf
  pinch of dried thyme

>   1 cup full-bodied, fruity red wine
>   1 cup canned beef broth
> 12 Mediterranean black olives, pitted

Use a 12-inch sauté pan with a tight lid. Sauté the bacon over medium heat until crisp and set it aside. Leave the bacon fat in the pan. Brown the meat and glaze the onions in the bacon fat. When they're golden, salt and pepper the meat and onions and add the rest of the ingredients except the olives, barely covering them with the liquid. Cover the pan and simmer the stew over very low heat for a couple of hours. Let it cool with the cover on, then refrigerate. Before reheating the next day, skim off any solidified fat that's risen to the surface. Serve the stew garnished with the crumbled bacon and the black olives along with a large green salad vinaigrette sprinkled with grated Parmesan.

PER SERVING: 8 GRAMS CARBOHYDRATE, 60 GRAMS PROTEIN

Zesty Beef Sangria

SERVES 4

Since leftovers of this dish are delicious, this recipe makes enough for 2 meals for 2 people.

>   2 pounds rump roast, chuck, or brisket
>   2 tablespoons chili powder
>   salt to taste
> 1/4 pound smoked slab bacon, diced
> 1/4 cup chopped onion
>   4 garlic cloves, minced
>   2 canned chipotle chilies, minced (optional)

1 cup Zinfandel or Spanish Rioja
2 tablespoons Triple Sec
   zest of $^1/_2$ medium orange

Rub the meat well with the chili powder and salt. Let it sit until it comes to room temperature. Cut it into $1^1/_2$-inch cubes. In a large skillet with a tight cover, sauté the diced bacon over medium-high heat until most of the fat is rendered. Pour off all but about 3 tablespoons of bacon fat. Sauté the beef in the skillet with the bacon until it's well browned on all sides. Add the onion, garlic, and minced chipotle. Stir and toss until the onion and garlic softens and browns lightly. Add the wine, Triple Sec, and orange zest, cover the pan, and simmer over very low heat until the meat is fork-tender, about 1 hour, or longer, depending on the cut of beef selected.

PER SERVING: 4 GRAMS CARBOHYDRATE, 56 GRAMS PROTEIN

• Serve with $^3/_4$ cup baked acorn squash, buttered and sprinkled with a little cinnamon. Or serve it over $^3/_4$ cup spaghetti squash.

PER SERVING: AN EXTRA 8 GRAMS CARBOHYDRATE, 1 GRAM PROTEIN

Bulgogi

SERVES 2

This is an indoor version of the classic Korean beef barbecue. Actually you'll end up eating less than the 5 grams of carbohydrate listed here, since most of the marinade stays behind.

    1   pound flank steak, rib-eye, or tenderloin
    3   tablespoons peanut oil

Marinade:

  ¹/₄ cup chopped scallion
    2 garlic cloves, minced
  ¹/₂ teaspoon grated fresh ginger
    2 tablespoons soy sauce
    1 tablespoon toasted sesame seeds, crushed
       pinch of NutraSweet or Equal
    2 teaspoons freshly ground black pepper
1¹/₂ tablespoons sake or dry sherry
    6 scallions, sliced diagonally, for garnish
    1 teaspoon toasted sesame seeds for garnish

Slice the meat across the grain into very thin slices about ³/₈ inch thick. Combine the marinade ingredients and rub into the beef with your hands. Place in a covered dish or plastic bag and leave it to develop flavor for 2 hours in the refrigerator.

Drain the meat and sear in the hot peanut oil in a non-stick skillet or a wok over high heat for 1 minute. Do not overcook. Serve garnished with the sliced scallions and a sprinkling of sesame seeds.

PER SERVING: 5 GRAMS CARBOHYDRATE, 57 GRAMS PROTEIN

• Serve with 1 cup steamed broccoli pieces tossed with 2 sliced water chestnuts for an extra 4 grams carbohydrate and 2 grams protein.

• You can also omit the peanut oil and simply add the meat, marinade and all, to the hot skillet.

Chili-Stuffed Peppers

SERVES 2

- 2 large red or green bell peppers
- 3/4 pound ground chuck
- 2 garlic cloves, minced
- 1 small red onion, minced
- 1 canned chipotle chili in adobo or 1 canned jalapeño plus a dash of liquid smoke
  salt and pepper to taste
- 1 teaspoon ground cumin
- 1 teaspoon dried oregano
- 1/2 cup grated cheddar or Monterey Jack cheese

Grill the peppers over an open flame or directly under the broiler, turning often, until the skin is totally charred. Watch them closely so the peppers don't collapse. As soon as they are blackened, put them into a plastic bag and let them sit for a few minutes until they're just cool enough to handle. (Don't let them sit too long, or the steam in the bag will soften the peppers too much.) Rub off all the skin. Carefully cut around the stem and pull it out. Carefully scoop out the seeds with a teaspoon. If you mistakenly tear a pepper, don't despair; they'll taste good anyway. Preheat the oven to 350°.

Mix the meat well with the remaining ingredients except the cheese. Stuff the peppers and stand them up or sit them down on a pie plate or shallow oven pan. Bake them for about 20 minutes and then remove them from the oven to mound the cheese on top. Return the peppers to the oven to melt the cheese and ensure that the meat is cooked.

PER SERVING: 8.5 GRAMS CARBOHYDRATE, 32 GRAMS PROTEIN

• Serve with an avocado salsa made with $1/2$ cubed avocado tossed with a couple of slivered cherry tomatoes, minced scallion, and cilantro. Add salt and pepper to taste.

PER SERVING: AN EXTRA 6 GRAMS CARBOHYDRATE, 2 GRAMS PROTEIN

Microwaved Stuffed Peppers:

Slice the stem end from the peppers at the point where the edge is straight. Shake and pull out the seeds and stand the peppers up in a small microwave-safe dish. Stuff them with the meat mixture and $1/2$ inch beef broth in the bottom of the dish. Cover the dish with plastic wrap and microwave for 6 to 8 minutes on high. Remove the plastic wrap, pile the cheese on top, and put them back in the microwave for 20 seconds.

Italian Stuffed Peppers:

Using green bell peppers and the same procedure, stuff them with $3/4$ pound of ground veal or mixed ground chicken and turkey. Season the meat with 3 slivered slices of prosciutto, 2 pressed garlic cloves, 3 tablespoons minced parsley, 1 teaspoon lemon zest, and salt and pepper to taste. Mix in 1 egg whisked with 2 tablespoons of crème fraîche or sour cream, a pinch of freshly grated nutmeg, and $1/4$ cup of grated Parmesan cheese. Top off each cooked pepper with a little dollop of crème fraîche or sour cream.

Cabbage Lasagne

SERVES 8

The "noodles" here are cabbage leaves. You can use Swiss chard the same way.

- 1 medium to large head of cabbage
- 1 tablespoon olive oil
- 2 garlic cloves, minced or pressed
- 1 medium onion, chopped
- 1 green bell pepper, chopped
- 3/4 pound ground beef
- 1 6-ounce can Hunt's tomato paste
- 1 8-ounce can Hunt's tomato sauce
- 1 teaspoon dried oregano
- 2 teaspoons salt
- 1 teaspoon black pepper
- 1 cup grated mozzarella cheese
- 1/2 cup ricotta or cottage cheese
- 1/2 cup freshly grated Parmesan cheese

Preheat the oven to 350°. Wash the cabbage and remove the tough outer leaves. Cut the head in half. Carefully peel back the leaves, trying to keep them intact; these will serve as the lasagne noodles. Arrange the individual leaves on a steamer basket or tray and steam until nearly tender, about 3 to 5 minutes. (You can also do this in the microwave.) Set aside.

Put the olive oil in a large skillet over medium-high heat. Sauté the garlic, onion, and green pepper until the onion is translucent. Add the ground beef and brown thoroughly. Drain or skim the accumulated fat and water.

Add the tomato paste, tomato sauce, and seasonings to the mixture and combine well.

Coat a 9- by 13- by 2-inch baking pan with a little olive oil. Line the bottom with a layer of cabbage leaves. Top with half of the meat mixture. Add a third of the mozzarella and half of the ricotta cheese. Add another layer of cabbage leaves, the remaining half of the meat mixture, another third of the mozzarella, and the remaining half of the ricotta. Top with the remaining mozzarella and finish by scattering the Parmesan on top.

Bake, covered, for about 20 minutes. Uncover and bake for 5 minutes more.

PER SERVING: 9 GRAMS CARBOHYDRATE, 20 GRAMS PROTEIN

• This dish freezes well. Cool, then cut into 8 servings. Wrap individually in freezer wrap. To reheat, thaw and heat in the microwave for approximately 4 minutes on high.

• Serve the lasagne with a big green salad tossed with a red wine vinegar and olive oil dressing.

Finnish Meat Loaf

SERVES 6

This typical Finnish meat loaf is traditionally wrapped with sour cream pastry and taken along on cross-country skiing picnics. It's delicious either hot or cold and should be served with a big dollop of sour cream.

    1 cup chopped mushrooms
    $^1/_2$ cup chopped onion

4 tablespoons (¹/₂ stick) butter
3 pounds ground meat: 1¹/₂ pounds beef and ¹/₂
   pound each pork, ham, and veal
¹/₄ cup minced parsley
   freshly ground pepper to taste
1 cup grated Gruyère cheese
¹/₂ cup heavy cream

Preheat the oven to 350°. Sauté the chopped mushrooms and onion in the butter over medium heat until the
onion is soft, about 5 minutes. Add the cooked mixture to
the ground meat and remaining ingredients, reserving ¹/₄
cup of the cheese for the top. Mix it all together with your
fingers and press the mixture into a loaf pan. Sprinkle the
top with cheese and bake the meat loaf for an hour.

• If you don't use the ham, add a teaspoon of salt to
the mixture.

PER SERVING: 2.5 GRAMS CARBOHYDRATE, 66 GRAMS PRO-
TEIN, PLUS SOUR CREAM GARNISH AT .5 GRAM CARBOHY-
DRATE AND 1 GRAM PROTEIN PER TABLESPOON

• Serve with ¹/₂ cup sliced roasted beets seasoned with
olive oil, salt and pepper, and a splash of balsamic vinegar.
(Roast whole unpeeled beets in a 375° oven for about 1
hour or until the tip of a knife pierces them easily. When
cool enough to handle, slip the skins off with your fingers.
These beets reheat well in the microwave.) Add a spinach
salad with slivered scallions.

PER SERVING: AN EXTRA 6 GRAMS CARBOHYDRATE, 38 GRAMS
PROTEIN

Veal Scaloppine with Ricotta and Swiss Chard

SERVES 2

$^3/_4$ pound veal scaloppine
2 eggs, beaten with a pinch of salt and pepper
1 bunch of Swiss chard, stemmed
2 garlic cloves, minced
2 tablespoons butter
$^1/_2$ cup ricotta cheese
3 tablespoons sour cream
    nutmeg, preferably freshly grated
    salt and pepper to taste
1 tablespoon freshly grated Parmesan cheese

Soak the veal in the beaten egg for 30 minutes. Meanwhile, stack and roll up the Swiss chard leaves, then slice across the roll into 1-inch ribbons. Sauté the chard with the garlic in the butter over medium-high heat for 10 minutes. Remove and reserve 1 cup.

Preheat the oven to 375°. In the same skillet, over low heat, add half the veal slices one at a time and cook just long enough to set the egg coating on both sides. Remove the slices as they're cooked to an ovenproof gratin dish. Put the ricotta and sour cream in the processor or blender with a pinch of nutmeg, salt and pepper, and the grated Parmesan. Blend until smooth. Spread half the cheese mixture over the veal with the back of a spoon. Layer $^1/_2$ cup Swiss chard on top. Cook the rest of the scaloppine and cover the first batch. Layer on the other $^1/_2$ cup Swiss chard and then spread the rest of the cheese on top. Bake for about 30 minutes or until the cheese topping is set.

PER SERVING: 9.5 GRAMS CARBOHYDRATE, 46 GRAMS PRO-
TEIN

- Serve with a mixed green salad vinaigrette.

Grilled Lamb Burgers with Roasted Eggplant Puree

SERVES 2

The spicy eggplant puree transforms simple ground lamb patties into something special. The leftover puree will keep for several days in the refrigerator and is equally good as a vegetable dip or an accompaniment to a cold roast chicken.

  1 medium eggplant
  2 tablespoons roasted garlic paste, Consorzio
     brand or homemade
 1/2 teaspoon harissa (Moroccan hot sauce), avail-
     able at specialty food stores and some super-
     markets, or other hot sauce
 1/4 cup minced cilantro
  3 tablespoons minced scallion
  1 tablespoon fresh lemon juice
  3 tablespoons olive oil
     salt to taste
     grilled lamb burgers

Pierce the eggplant skin in a few places and roast it in a 400° oven until it's soft all the way through, about 30 minutes. Slit it lengthwise and let it cool. Meanwhile, mix together everything else but the olive oil, salt, and lamb into a thick paste, then slowly whisk in the olive oil. Spoon out the eggplant flesh into a food processor and add the seasoning paste. Blend until smooth but not soupy. Add salt to taste. Add more harissa if you like things spicier. Add more oil if necessary. Grill the lamb burgers and top with a spoonful of eggplant.

PER SERVING: 3 TO 5 GRAMS CARBOHYDRATE, DEPENDING ON HOW MUCH EGGPLANT YOU DEVOUR, 28 GRAMS PROTEIN

• Serve with ¹/₂ cup baby carrots, blanched in the microwave and then sautéed in butter until lightly brown.

PER SERVING: AN EXTRA 3 GRAMS CARBOHYDRATE

Cold Lamb with Raw Vegetable Salad

SERVES 2

This is not only a great way to make a meal from leftover roast lamb or any roast meat or poultry, but it's delicious enough not to seem like leftovers at all.

      sliced roast lamb, turkey, chicken, or ham,
         about 6 ounces
 ¹/₄ pound cream cheese, softened in the microwave
 ¹/₄ teaspoon paprika
 ¹/₄ teaspoon salt
   2 tablespoons fresh lemon juice
   2 tablespoons minced parsley
   2 tablespoons minced fresh dill
 ¹/₄ cup olive oil
 ¹/₂ cup sliced firm white mushrooms
 ¹/₂ cup red bell pepper strips

1 cup thin slices of zucchini
8 cherry tomatoes, cut in half
6 scallions, both white and green parts, minced
   pepper to taste

Use a food processor to blend the cream cheese with the next 5 ingredients. When it's smooth, drizzle in the olive oil a little at a time until the seasoned cheese absorbs it all and the sauce is thick but pourable. Taste for salt, pour over the mixed vegetables, and give the salad a few grinds of fresh pepper. Serve alongside the cold sliced meat.

PER SERVING: 11 GRAMS CARBOHYDRATE, 26 GRAMS PROTEIN

Butterflied Pork Chops with Bourbon Mustard Sauce

SERVES 2

       salt and pepper to taste
   2 butterflied pork chops, ³/₄ inch thick
   3 tablespoons butter, preferably clarified
   1 tablespoon olive oil
   3 tablespoons bourbon
   2 tablespoons minced shallot
   1 cup thinly sliced mushrooms
 ¹/₈ teaspoon dried thyme
   1 tablespoon Dijon mustard
 ¹/₄ cup heavy cream
   1 tablespoon minced parsley

Salt and pepper the chops. In a skillet large enough to hold the chops, sauté them in 2 tablespoons of the butter and the olive oil over medium-high heat until nicely browned on both sides. Pour in the bourbon and swirl it around in the pan over medium-high heat until it reduces to a thin syrupy glaze. Add the shallot and mushrooms, cover the pan, and cook for 5 minutes. Crush the thyme between your fingers and sprinkle over the chops. Add the mustard and cream, cover the pan, and simmer for 25 minutes. Remove the chops to serving plates, add the remaining butter to the pan, and swirl it into the mustard sauce. Pour the sauce and mushrooms over the chops and sprinkle with the parsley.

PER SERVING: 3 GRAMS CARBOHYDRATE, 21 GRAMS PROTEIN

- Serve with 1 cup steamed spinach.

PER SERVING: AN EXTRA 3.1 GRAMS CARBOHYDRATE, 5.4 GRAMS PROTEIN

Ranch Chili with Cheese

SERVES 2

   3 tablespoons peanut oil
   1 pound beef chuck, minced or ground once
  1/2 cup chopped onion
   2 garlic cloves, minced
   2 tablespoons chili powder
  1/2 teaspoon crushed dried oregano
  1/2 teaspoon paprika
  1/2 teaspoon ground cumin
  1/4 teaspoon cayenne pepper
  1/2 cup Contadina tomato puree
  1/2 cup strong leftover black coffee or canned beef
      broth

1   tablespoon masa harina or cornmeal, optional
3   tablespoons grated cheddar cheese

Heat the oil in a large skillet over medium-high heat. Add the beef and brown it, then add the onion, garlic, and all the seasonings. Stir and cook until well mixed and the onions are limp. Transfer to a covered saucepan and add the tomato puree and coffee. Cover and simmer the chili for an hour, adding a little water if it becomes dry. The chili should be thick and soupy. Add the masa and simmer for 10 more minutes. Serve in bowls, sprinkled with cheddar.

PER SERVING: 10 GRAMS CARBOHYDRATE, 56 GRAMS PROTEIN

• You can add chopped green bell peppers to this chili—1 medium pepper, added along with the onions, will contribute a little less than 2 additional grams carbohydrate. You may want to delete the cornmeal in that case to keep the dish under 10 grams.

Desserts

Chocolate Chip Cheesecakes

SERVES 12

You don't have to use ersatz sugar for these little tarts, but each cheesecake is only 2 grams carbohydrate if you use NutraSweet instead.

12 1³/₄-inch fluted paper cups
    12-cup mini-muffin tin

1 large graham cracker, finely crushed
1 extra-large egg
$^1/_4$ cup sugar or NutraSweet Spoonful
$^1/_4$ teaspoon vanilla extract
1 8-ounce package Philadelphia cream cheese, softened
2 tablespoons semisweet mini chocolate chips

Preheat the oven to 350°. Place the paper cups in the muffin tin and distribute the crushed graham cracker among the cups. Put all the ingredients except the chocolate chips into a food processor and blend thoroughly—or beat the egg, sugar, and vanilla together well with a whisk and then incorporate the cheese. Fold in the chocolate chips and then spoon the blended mixture into the cups. Bake for 15 minutes or until the edges are set and the center is still moist. Remove the cheesecakes from the muffin tin and let them cool. Refrigerate for at least an hour before serving.

PER SERVING: 5 GRAMS CARBOHYDRATE (MADE WITH SUGAR), 2 GRAMS CARBOHYDRATE (NUTRASWEET), 3 GRAMS PROTEIN

• Use different flavorings to change these little treats. Substitute a couple of teaspoons of instant espresso coffee powder for the chocolate chips or leave in the chips for a mocha cheesecake. Use lemon extract or a tablespoon of fresh lemon juice instead of the vanilla and add some grated lemon or lime zest. Sprinkle the tops of the cheese-cakes with toasted unsweetened coconut for a little crunch-or bury a single whole toasted almond in each cake and flavor with almond extract. Remove the paper and serve two on a plate with a drizzle of fresh raspberry puree (page 230) for an extra 1 gram carbohydrate.

Sweets If You Must

Unfortunately, one sweet treat usually begs another, and the unhealthy devotion to sugar can last a lifetime. The good part is that the craving quickly disappears if the temptation is just ignored. Try it— wait ten minutes and reconsider. Once you're into the dynamic phase of weight loss, your cravings will virtually disappear. But we recognize that this is a particularly tough habit to break, so here are a few mini-desserts for when your chin starts to wobble. Since the insulin rush of sugar is lessened if it's consumed or digested with protein, having a sweet with your after-dinner coffee is the best time to sin. If you must indulge between meals, precede it with $1/2$ cup of cottage cheese or other available protein. The suggested candy on this list is individually wrapped to make it easier not to exceed the calculated portions.

Grams	Candy
5	1 Hershey's Nugget with Almonds
6	1 Milky Way Miniature
5.5	1 Chocolate Parfait Nips
4.2	1 tablespoon (12) Nestlé's Goobers (chocolate-covered peanuts)
5	8 Starbucks chocolate-covered espresso beans
5	2 Andes chocolate crème de menthe thins
2	1 Life Savers sugar-free popsicle
4.5	2 Hershey's Kisses with Almonds
4	1 Irish Lace Cookie (page 292)

Meringue Tart Shells
___

SERVES 6

These elegant little company dessert jewels can be filled with berries and whipped cream. It may take you a few trial runs to get them crispy. Don't open the oven door too soon.

     3 egg whites
  1/4 teaspoon salt
     3 teaspoons NutraSweet Spoonful or 3 packets
         of Equal
     1 teaspoon almond extract
  1/2 cup grated almonds
  1/2 cup shredded unsweetened coconut (optional)

Preheat the oven to 250°.

In a bowl, combine the egg whites, salt, NutraSweet, and almond extract. Beat until stiff. Add the almonds and coconut.

Drop by large spoonfuls onto a buttered cookie sheet. Create a depression in each mound with the bottom of a glass. Bake for 30 minutes. Then turn off heat—*don't* open the oven door. Leave the meringues in the oven for another 30 minutes.

PER SERVING: 3.5 GRAMS CARBOHYDRATE, 5.5 GRAMS PROTEIN

Coconut Flan

SERVES 6

> 1 cup unsweetened coconut milk
> 1 cup light cream
> 1/4 cup sugar or NutraSweet Spoonful
> 4 extra-large eggs
> 1 teaspoon vanilla or coconut extract
> nutmeg, preferably freshly grated

Preheat the oven to 325°. Heat the coconut milk, cream, and sugar in a glass pitcher in the microwave for 5 minutes on high or in a saucepan over medium heat until a skin begins to form on the surface. In a heatproof bowl, whisk together the eggs and extract and, continuing to whisk, add the hot cream in a thin stream. Divide the mixture evenly among six 1/2-cup custard or soufflé cups. Dust the tops with nutmeg. Space the cups apart in a shallow pan—or a glass or ceramic casserole for the microwave—and pour water into the pan about a third of the way up to the top of the cups. Bake for 30 minutes or cook on high for about 6 minutes. Do not overcook; the centers should wiggle slightly. After cooling them completely, refrigerate for at least 4 hours before serving.

PER SERVING: 9.5 GRAMS CARBOHYDRATE (NUTRASWEET), 16.5 GRAMS CARBOHYDRATE (SUGAR), 6 GRAMS PROTEIN

- Try adding a little rum extract or Myers's dark rum. Decorate with a slice or two of kiwifruit or a strip of ripe mango.
- If you're not fond of coconut, leave the coconut milk out and make this flan with 2 cups light cream.

Irish Lace Cookies

MAKES 2 DOZEN COOKIES

- $1/2$ cup boiling water
- 2 cups rolled oats
- 1 tablespoon unsalted butter
- 4 teaspoons NutraSweet or 4 packets of Equal
- 2 extra-large eggs
- 1 teaspoon vanilla extract
- 2 teaspoons baking powder
- $1/2$ teaspoon salt

Preheat the oven to 375°.

Pour boiling water over the oats, mix, cover, and set aside to soak. Meanwhile, beat the butter, NutraSweet, eggs, and vanilla together until fluffy and smooth. Add the baking powder and salt to the oats, then pour the oats into the creamed mixture and combine well.

Drop teaspoonsful 2 to 3 inches apart on a lightly greased cookie sheet. Bake for 12 to 15 minutes. Cool completely on a rack. Store in an airtight container in layers separated with wax paper or paper towels.

PER COOKIE: ABOUT 4 GRAMS CARBOHYDRATE, LESS THAN 1 GRAM PROTEIN

Warm Brie with Chutney and Almonds

SERVES 4

This makes an unusual dessert served with the apple slices—or an interesting hors d'oeuvre, for that matter.

- 1¼-pound wedge of Brie cheese or a mini Brie wheel with the rind
- 2 tablespoons Major Grey chutney, finely chopped
- 1 to 2 tablespoons sliced blanched almonds to taste

Preheat the oven to 350°. Put the cheese on a piece of aluminum foil on a baking sheet. Spread the chutney over the top of the cheese. Sprinkle with sliced almonds and bake for 5 to 7 minutes or until the cheese is slightly runny. Using a wide spatula, transfer the cheese to a serving plate. Serve with crackers or thinly sliced apples dipped in lemon juice for an additional 1–2 grams of carbohydrate per cracker or apple slice.

PER SERVING: 6 GRAMS CARBOHYDRATE, 7 GRAMS PROTEIN

Espresso Ice Cream with Cinnamon

SERVES 5

- ⅓ cup Italian espresso powder
- 1 quart light cream or 2 cups heavy cream plus 2 cups milk or half-and-half
- ½ teaspoon ground cinnamon
- ½ cup NutraSweet Spoonful to taste

Put the coffee powder, cinnamon, and cream in a microwave-safe bowl and bring it to the brink of a boil in the microwave. Or heat the mixture in a saucepan on top of the stove. Remove from the heat, stir well, and let the coffee and cream steep for at least 30 minutes. Strain it if there are any lumps. Add NutraSweet. Freeze in an ice cream maker according to the manufacturer's directions.

PER SERVING: 9 GRAMS CARBOHYDRATE, 8 GRAMS PROTEIN

Part III

Why This Plan Will Leave You Healthy and Thin

Chapter II

The Deadly Diseases of Civilization

Hydra. A monster with many heads slain by Hercules: whence any multiplicity of evils is termed a hydra.

SAMUEL JOHNSON'S DICTIONARY

In Greco-Roman mythology it fell to Heracles (Hercules) as one of his twelve labors to slay the Hydra, an enormous beast with a doglike body and a writhing cluster of snaky heads. Heracles drove the beast from its lair and began to bash at its many heads with his club, but no sooner had he destroyed one head than two or three replacements sprang from its bleeding stump. Heracles doubled his efforts and summoned his nephew Iolus into the fray, and together, with Heracles slashing and bashing the heads and Iolus cauterizing the stumps before new heads could sprout, they reduced the Hydra to its last and supposedly immortal head. Heracles took it off with one mighty swipe, and the deadly Hydra was gone forever.

The myth of the Hydra is a perfect metaphor for the

diseases of civilization. Conventional medical wisdom has unfortunately approached the treatment of these interconnected diseases in much the same way that Heracles first attacked the Hydra—one head at a time—usually with the same results: other heads springing up to confound and frustrate doctor and patient. Just as Heracles finally discovered, however, it is only by going for the immortal head—insulin resistance and hyperinsulinemia—that medical science can hope to complete the Herculean task of ridding the patient of the diseases of civilization. Treating one disease at a time will at best merely hold them at bay; at worst it will actually contribute to the formation of other diseases. How? By worsening the underlying insulin problem, which in turn aggravates high blood pressure, diabetes, heart disease, and all the rest. Before we examine this phenomenon in detail, let's look at how several other medical researchers define this common problem.

Norman Kaplan, M.D., head of the Hypertension Division at the University of Texas Southwestern Medical Center at Dallas, published an article in the July 1989 *Archives of Internal Medicine* entitled "The Deadly Quartet" describing his version of the Hydra. Dr. Kaplan first presents the traditional view that glucose intolerance (a precursor of diabetes), hypertension, and high triglycerides (excess fat in the blood) are usually found in conjunction with upper-body obesity.[1] This view holds that as a person develops upper-body obesity the hypertension, glucose intolerance, and excess triglycerides start to become evident, leading to the conclusion that upper-body

---

[1] The distinction between upper-body and lower-body obesity is significant; it's addressed in Chapter 4.

obesity *causes* these disorders. It makes sense: first you get fat, then you develop all these other problems; therefore the excess fat must be causing them, right?

When Dr. Kaplan examined the data closely, he found that upper-body obesity is not necessarily the cause of the other three *but is simply found in conjunction with them most of the time.* He goes on to demonstrate that hyperinsulinemia, which has been found to coexist with each of these conditions, can be more realistically represented as the root cause of upper-body obesity, glucose intolerance, hypertension, and excess triglycerides—the deadly quartet of his article's title. Excess body fat—the first thing most people notice—doesn't come first; it comes *after* and as a result of the hyperinsulinemia.

The inevitability of this health progression—first hyperinsulinemia, followed by any or all of the related disorders: obesity, hypertension, diabetes, and heart disease—may not be pleasant to contemplate, but you can take comfort in the fact that if all have one root cause and we can effectively deal with that single troublemaker, we can solve them all at once.

Here's another way to look at it. Imagine hyperinsulinemia as a huge iceberg floating along with only its tips exposed. Ralph DeFronzo, M.D., professor of medicine and head of the Diabetes Division of the University of Texas Health Science Center at San Antonio, a pioneering researcher on hyperinsulinemia and insulin resistance, uses this metaphor to explain the disorder. At meetings he draws a picture of a huge iceberg with peaks labeled *hypertension, heart disease, high cholesterol, diabetes,* and *obesity* protruding above the water. The great mass of the iceberg extending deep into the water, the part hidden from view, he labels hyperinsulinemia—as doctors and patients chip away at the tips, the great dangerous mass remains hidden from view.

The Hydra, Dr. Kaplan's deadly quartet, Dr. De-Fronzo's iceberg—all are simplistic descriptions of the somewhat complex medical problem of hyperinsulinemia, which until recently hasn't even had a name. Gerald Reaven, M.D., professor of medicine at Stanford University and a longtime researcher into the metabolic effects of insulin, finally remedied that shortcoming. In a 1988 article in the journal *Diabetes* on the cluster of metabolic disorders typically found in association with insulin resistance and hyperinsulinemia, he dubbed it *Syndrome X*. Syndrome X includes the following disorders:

- elevated VLDL (a type of blood fat)
- low level of HDL (the so-called "good" cholesterol)
- insulin resistance
- hyperinsulinemia
- hyperglycemia (elevated blood sugar)
- hypertension

Says Dr. Reaven: "The common feature of the proposed syndrome is insulin resistance. All other changes are likely to be secondary to this basic abnormality."

Although the name *Syndrome X* has gained fairly wide usage in the medical literature, we prefer the more descriptive representation of the Hydra's many heads or the iceberg chunking along beneath the surface en route to a metabolic catastrophe. However you choose to think of it, the important thing is to realize that *these diseases of civilization are in reality only different manifestations of one complex disorder.* As we begin our discussion of the individual manifestations, always keep in mind that they are interrelated through hyperinsulinemia and that any one always lurks around the corner from any other. Let's start by considering what is without doubt the most common insulin-driven disorder-obesity.

The O Word: Obesity

For some of us are out of breath, and all of us are fat.

LEWIS CARROLL

How much of a problem is obesity? According to the government, obesity is an enormous problem. The most recent figures, reported in 1995, place the segment of Americans who are "significantly overweight" at 33 percent—nearly a 30 percent *jump* in one decade while the population has *cut* fat consumption. Although the Centers for Disease Control had set goals for a reduction in obesity from the nation's lower-fat efforts, Americans went off in the opposite direction and got even fatter. If you believe your eyes, obesity is virtually epidemic—as anyone who's ever been to a shopping mall knows.

Despite the manifold health problems associated with obesity, people continue to gain weight; despite the many disadvantages obesity inflicts on its victims on the job, the cultural stigma against them, the plethora of weight-loss centers, books, and products available, more people than ever are overweight. Why?

HOW WE GET FAT

Obesity is defined simply as the accumulation of excess fat on the body; obesity has nothing to do with excess weight. Based on the standard height-weight tables, Arnold Schwarzenegger would be considered overweight, but he obviously isn't overfat or obese.

Although it's almost always attributed to excess calories, obesity is more related to the multifaceted actions of insulin and glucagon on the storage of fat. As any juvenile-onset diabetic can readily attest, in the absence of insulin one can eat and eat and eat while continuing to lose weight; it's not just a matter of how much is consumed but the result of a complicated interplay among insulin, glucagon, and what and how much is consumed. These two hormones exert a profound influence on all the metabolic pathways, but especially on those involved in the burning and storing of fat and the development of obesity.

When you eat food, your body either breaks it down and burns it for energy or stores it away as body fat in the fat cells (or as glycogen, the storage form of glucose, in the muscles) for later use. Both functions occur simultaneously, and although both the storing and burning pathways are active to some degree all the time, one pathway usually predominates. What is important is the net direction of fat flow over time—i.e., are you mainly storing fat or mainly burning it for energy? Which pathway predominates most of the time? If you mainly store it, you develop obesity; if you mainly burn it, you lose weight.

The flow of fat is composed of the fat you eat, the fat released from storage in your fat cells, and the fat you make from excess protein and carbohydrate. Yes, the body can make fat from carbohydrate and plenty of it. That's why you can't eat fat-free cookies and ice cream and potato chips and expect to lose fat!

Obviously if the direction of fat flow is from our mouths to our fat cells for storage, we are going to gain fat; if this pathway predominates, in time we will become obese. Conversely, if the fat flows in the opposite direction, from the fat tissue to the muscle cells and other tissues to be burned for energy, we won't; in fact we will lose weight. If our goal is to remain—or become—slender and fit, obviously this second pathway is preferable. Is it possible to change the flow of fat and redirect it from the fat tissue to muscle cells? The exciting answer is yes, and here's how.

Directing the Flow of Fat Through Food Selection

Insulin and glucagon, the hormone twins, are the primary regulators of these metabolic pathways and actually direct the flow of fat down one pathway or the other. By altering the ratio of insulin to glucagon—*which we can do through our selection of foods*—we can determine which pathway predominates. Instead of allowing our biochemistry to control us, we can control it.

Taking as our starting point the fat in the blood, let's walk through the fat metabolism pathways and follow the flow of the fat molecules. Fat travels through the blood in a form called *triglyceride,* a molecule composed of three fatty acids. At the surface of the cells enzymes break down the triglyceride molecule, and the fatty acids can enter the cells.

Once inside the cells, fat reaches its first hormonal regulation point—the mitochondria. These tiny sausage-shaped power plants within the cells burn the fat—but only if the fatty acids can actually get into the power plant. To do that they need carnitine, which operates a little shuttle system to bring the fat in for oxidation. Insulin inhibits this fat-carnitine shuttle system, saying, in effect, "Hey, we're full; we don't need any more energy. Send that extra fat to the fat cells." Which is precisely what happens when there's too much insulin: the fatty acids turn back into triglycerides and move back into the blood. Glucagon in contrary fashion *accelerates* the shuttle, rapidly moving fat into the mitochondria. Glucagon's signal: "We need energy; let's start breaking that fat down and getting it in here to the furnace."

Muscle, liver, kidney, lung, heart, and other cells break down fat and burn it for energy, but it's a different story with the fat cells. Fat cells merely store the fat molecules. Residing on the surface of the fat cells are two enzymes—both regulated by insulin and glucagon—responsible for herding fat into or out of the fat cells. The first, *lipoprotein lipase,* transports fatty acids into the fat cell and keeps them there. (Lipoprotein lipase, as we shall see shortly, also plays a major role in the rapid regaining of lost weight that plagues so many dieters.) The other, *hormone-sensitive lipase,* does just the opposite—it *releases* the fat from fat cells into the blood. As you might imagine, insulin stimulates the activity of lipoprotein lipase, the fat-storage enzyme, and glucagon inhibits it; glucagon stimulates the fat-releasing enzyme, and insulin inhibits it.

THE BUILT-IN NO-WIN SITUATION

It turns out that the biological activity of this enzyme increases prodigiously immediately *after* weight loss. That's right, *the very act of losing weight strengthens and makes more potent the enzyme that is in great measure responsible for the overweight state to begin with*. Although it no doubt has an evolutionary purpose, this is a sorry state of biological affairs: while working hard to lose weight, you reinforce the biochemical underpinnings of your obesity. Add to this the fact that insulin by itself *further* activates the already hyperactive lipoprotein lipase and you begin to understand why 95 percent of people who manage to lose weight will not be able to keep it off.

What standard treatment is brought to bear against this combined force? The only weapon in the arsenal, *the low-fat, high-complex-carbohydrate* diet, a diet that *stimulates* the release of insulin. Expecting a formerly obese person with a history of hyperinsulinemia not to gain fat on a carbohydrate-rich diet is like throwing gasoline on a fire, then wondering why it flares. In fact, it's amazing that even 5 percent of successful dieters manage to keep it off. But that may correlate with the percentage of overweight people who *don't* have hyperinsulinemia and insulin resistance.

What about our goal, to divert the flow of fat away from the fat cells? Although we can't control lipoprotein lipase directly, we can control it *indirectly* by controlling the metabolic hormones—insulin and glucagon—that modulate it. By keeping insulin levels low, we can remove any stimulation this hormone provides; by keeping glucagon *elevated*, we can continue to inhibit lipoprotein lipase and thus counteract the stimulatory effect brought on by the weight loss. The nutritional plan in this book lowers insulin and raises glucagon levels, the ideal combination both to achieve and to *maintain* a lower fat mass. We've seen it happen in thousands of our patients, and in our experience it's the *only* approach that works.

Amazingly, obesity remains much less treatable than the vast majority of cancers, a grim statistic in and of itself. Are 95 percent of the overweight doomed to live out their lives swaddled in layers of fat?

Most physicians, dietitians, and nutritionists have been locked in the notorious clean and well-lit prison of a single idea for decades. These experts have been treating obesity with low-calorie, low-fat, high-complex-carbohydrate diets, then standing around wringing their hands, watching 95 percent of their patients regain their weight. Perhaps inevitably they blame the patient for the failure. In a brilliant and controversial essay on intelligence published in the winter 1969 issue of *Harvard Educational Review*, Arthur R. Jensen, a professor of psychology at the University of California at Berkeley, wrote: "In other fields, when bridges do not stand, when aircraft do not fly, when machines do not work, when treatments do not cure, despite all conscientious efforts on the part of many persons to make them do so, one begins to question the basic assumptions, principles, theories, and hypotheses that guide one's efforts."

The evidence seems clear that the low-fat, high-carbohydrate diet—the standard obesity therapeutic agent—is flawed in principle, out of sync with biochemical reality. So why not try something different?

Diabetes

Diabetes. A morbid copiousness of urine; a fatal colliquation by the urinary passages.

SAMUEL JOHNSON'S DICTIONARY

Almost 2,000 years ago physicians first wrote of diabetes, describing it as a disease causing its sufferers to urinate frequently and in great quantity and to have a great thirst. These early physicians watched helplessly as their patients consumed enormous volumes of fluids that seemed to pour through them unstopped, became progressively more ill and emaciated, and finally died. The disease causing this wretched condition they named *diabetes,* which means "to run through like a siphon." It took 1,600 years before physicians realized that along with vast quantities of body fluids their diabetic patients were losing sugar in their urine. Thomas Willis, a professor at Oxford University in the seventeenth century, wrote of his experience with diabetic patients that their urine was "wonderfully sweet, as if imbued with honey or sugar." He added to the name the Latin term *mellitus,* meaning "sweetened with honey."[2]

Although *diabetes mellitus* is accurate in targeting a couple of the primary symptoms, it's a useless description of the underlying disease mechanisms. By naming diseases by their signs and symptoms, early physicians often created confusion, leading to misspent effort by those who fol-

---

[2] You may be wondering how Professor Willis knew his patients' urine was "wonderfully sweet" without actually tasting it. He did taste it. In fact, up until the middle of the 1800s physicians routinely tasted their patients' urine to check for diabetes mellitus.

lowed. Diabetes is a case in point. Today we subdivide diabetes mellitus into two separate and distinct diseases—type I and type II diabetes—with two different pathological causes but essentially the same symptoms. Sixty or seventy years ago, however, physicians believed that all diabetes was the same—there was just a difference in severity. Some people got it in childhood or early adulthood, suffered a progressively rapid course, were unresponsive to treatment, and died within a few years. Others developed it much later, had much less severe cases, and could be "cured" or at least treated fairly successfully by diet. Both groups of patients produced large amounts of sweet urine and so were diagnosed as having diabetes mellitus.

Physicians now recognize that although both disorders are called *diabetes* the circumstances and pathology leading to their development are entirely different. Type I diabetes, the more rapidly serious of the two, usually develops in childhood or adolescence when a virus or other toxic substance destroys the insulin-producing cells in the pancreas and requires aggressive treatment with insulin in shot form. It is a disease of insulin lack. In contrast, type II diabetes develops later in life, can usually be treated with diet and/or oral medicines, and is a disease of insulin *excess*. It seems strange that the same disease can be caused by both an excess *and* an insufficiency of insulin, but that is precisely the case.

Although our dietary plan is in most cases the ideal nutritional regimen for optimal health in those with type I diabetes, it is not the total treatment. Since their damaged pancreases can produce no, or at best very little, insulin, these patients require injections of insulin daily to meet their metabolic needs. Should they not receive their insulin, they face serious illness and even death in fairly short order. The treatment of this complex disease is beyond the scope of this book, but a brief discussion of the pathology involved illustrates well the indispensable role insulin plays as the overseer and regulator of metabolism. Our attention has so far focused so exclusively on the disorders of insulin excess that you may believe that insulin has no redeeming qualities or that glucagon is a metabolic panacea. A quick look at type I diabetes will dispel this notion in a hurry. Type I diabetes is a disorder of insufficient insulin and unrestrained glucagon excess, and as such it serves to clarify the importance of a regulated *balance* between insulin and glucagon.

TYPE I DIABETES: GLUCAGON RUN AMOK

In type I diabetics, with no insulin to hold it back and only glucagon to stimulate its release, fat pours out of the fat cells into the blood. For the same reason any incoming dietary fat can't get into the fat cells and so joins with the fat rushing from the fat cells and heads toward the tissues for disposal. As this blood, laden with fat, courses through the liver, the fatty acids enter the liver cells and then, without insulin to stop them, easily enter the mitochondria for breakdown. In contrast to other cells, liver mitochondria process fatty acids differently in that they don't burn the fatty acids for energy but instead partially break them down into molecules called *ketone bodies* and release them into the circulation. Normally the ketone bodies produced in the liver cells travel through the blood to the muscle and other tissues that burn them for energy. In type I diabetics, however, the enormous quantities of ketone bodies generated by the massive fat flux far exceed the needs of the tissues and outstrip the body's capacity to jettison them via the urine, the stool, and the breath. As the ketone bodies, which are acids, accumulate in the blood, the blood becomes more and more acidic until the victim is in the throes of a metabolic nightmare called *diabetic ketoacidosis,* which leads to coma, then death if not treated quickly.

This reverse flow of fat makes it impossible for a person without insulin to gain weight. Indeed the first symptom a person with undiagnosed type I diabetes usually experiences is an unexplained weight loss in the face of constant hunger and greater-than-normal food intake; *it's not unusual for such a person to lose 30 or 40 pounds in a month or two.*

TYPE II DIABETES: THE SLOW ROAD

Type II diabetes represents approximately 90 percent of all cases of diabetes, and although less immediately sinister than its type I counterpart, it is every bit as deadly over the long run. Like heart disease, high blood pressure, and obesity, type II diabetes doesn't develop overnight but requires years of underlying metabolic disturbance before the symptoms become apparent. As a result, since most cases of type II diabetes surface during middle age, the disorder is often referred to as *adult-onset diabetes.* The development and diagnosis of the type II variety usually follows a weight *gain,* a fact easily explained by the difference in insulin dynamics between the two disorders.

In both cases blood sugar is elevated but for different reasons. The blood sugar level rises in type I because there is no insulin present to hold it down by moving it into the cells; blood sugar goes up in type II because the cells have become so resistant to the effects of insulin that even large amounts can't adequately move the sugar out of the blood and into the cells. In type II diabetes there may exist the paradoxical situation in which both insulin and blood sugar are elevated—at least for a while. In the early stages insulin is always elevated, but as the disease progresses insulin levels often decrease as the pancreatic beta cells (the cells that produce the insulin) fatigue or "wear out" from constantly producing insulin at prodigious rates under the stimulation of the increasing blood sugar. During the early stages, which can last for years, the constantly elevated insulin levels give rise to high blood pressure, heart disease, elevated cholesterol, and obesity—all disorders that afflict type II diabetics with great frequency. During the later stages of the disease the elevated blood sugar damages the kidneys, eyes, blood vessels, and nerves in the same way it docs in type I diabetes.

Type II diabetes is without doubt of genetic origin; if your parents have or had it, then the odds are high that you will inherit the predisposition to the disease. If you follow the proper diet, you can ward off the onset of type II diabetes or even reverse its damaging effects. Conversely, in the susceptible person, dietary imprudence can certainly hasten the development and worsen the severity. Our diet is the optimal nutritional regimen for patients with type II diabetes because by correcting the underlying insulin resistance it lowers the abnormally elevated blood sugar levels, begins to repair any pancreatic damage, and can restore the tissues to normal.

From Insulin Resistance to Type II Diabetes

This vicious cycle begins slowly and develops over many years. Beginning with a genetically susceptible person, years of insulin bombardment brought on by teenage dietary and lifestyle abuse finally take their toll on the insulin sensors in the tissues and they begin to become resistant. To make the system work, the pancreas cranks out more insulin and thus begins the upward creep of chronically elevated insulin. Ultimately enormous levels of insulin may be required to keep the blood sugar within the normal range in the face of severe insulin resistance. In the majority of cases this is as far as the progression goes: insulin remains elevated, doing its damage through enhanced cholesterol synthesis, arterial thickening, increased fat storage, and all the rest but still managing to keep the blood sugar controlled. In genetically predisposed people, however, the condition progresses further, leading first to glucose intolerance, then ultimately to type II diabetes.

Consider a person with severe insulin resistance, who to keep blood sugar normal must produce huge amounts of insulin every day. At some time his overworked pancreas will reach the point at which it can no longer accommodate a bigger need—it's already making as much insulin as it possibly can. If his blood sugar level now rises he can no longer step up insulin production to overcome the increased resistance necessary to force his blood sugar back into line. At the limit of pancreatic insulin output type II diabetes is just around the corner.

Once the patient's blood sugar reaches diabetic levels, it begins to cause many but not all of the problems of type I diabetes: sugar spills into the urine, causing frequent urination and increased thirst, and the increased blood glu-

cose causes degenerative complica
kidneys, and blood vessels. *Glucose*
trations is toxic to many tissues, inclu
beta cells. Under constant overstimulatio
glucose the beta cells may finally give up a
ducing insulin altogether—a condition called
tigue or *beta cell burnout*. As long as the patient's
are producing some insulin, the patient avoids th
gerous ketoacidosis of type I diabetes because the ins
prevents the stored body fat from rushing out and con
verting to ketone bodies under the influence of unop-
posed glucagon. If, however, enough beta cells fatigue
and insulin production falls sufficiently, glucagon can predominate and all the problems of type I diabetes ensue.
Usually the beta cells continue to make more than enough
insulin to prevent ketoacidosis, indeed enough insulin to
cause all the symptoms of insulin excess, including hypertension, excess cholesterol production, obesity, and heart
disease, the disorders with which most type II diabetes
victims are afflicted. Typically most physicians focus on
these disorders—the tips of the iceberg—instead of the
cause of the problem, aberrant insulin metabolism.

Once again by aiming efforts at the underlying hyperinsulinemia people can reverse and often rid themselves of
another of the major diseases of civilization. Even those
with type I diabetes can markedly lower their insulin doses
and attain much better control over their blood sugars
with our plan—but *only under the supervision of a physician.*

Dr. Richard K. Bernstein, a diabetologist in Mamaro-
neck, New York, is the author of *Diabetes: Type II* (originally published by Prentice-Hall), an excellent primer on
the merits of carbohydrate restriction as applied specifi-

> ...believes that strict ad-
> ...is the cornerstone of
> ...ry importance in the
> ...control necessary to
> ...n to victims of both

...ions of the eyes, nerves,
at high blood concen-
...ding the pancreatic
...n by the excess
...nd cease pro-
...beta cell fa-
...beta cells
...dan-
...lin

> *...ment killer, and the first*
> *...symptom may be death.*

KENNETH COOPER, M.D.

Our patient Tom Edwards came in weighing about 315 pounds and was taking three different medications for his high blood pressure, which at 160/105 still wasn't particularly well controlled. We had just started treating weight-loss patients with the protein-sparing modified fast described in Mike's earlier book *Thin So Fast,* and we hadn't yet used it on anyone with a serious blood pressure problem. Back in our do-it-like-everyone-else days, we treated many overweight patients with blood pressure problems by putting them on low-calorie diets. As their weight came down slowly (which it usually did *if* they stayed on the diet; getting them to stay on it was the hard part), so did their blood pressure. On successive visits a month or so apart we'd gradually reduce their blood pressure medications, sometimes getting them completely medication free if they lost enough weight. There was no reason to assume Tom would be any different.

We didn't yet know about the dramatic insulin-lowering

properties of this new nutritional
point we didn't know that insulin
thing other than blood sugar control. W
off any of his medications but told him we
to as soon as he lost some of his weight. Tom
days into the program.

"Doc, I'm dizzy," he said. "When I get up out of a c
I almost pass out. When I stand on my feet for a while a
work I get so spacey-headed I feel like I'm going to faint."

We told him to come to the office right away. When he
arrived, the nurse found his blood pressure to be
100/60—an unduly low figure compared to the pressures
he had been running—and his weight had dropped to 309
pounds. Six pounds is a lot of weight to lose in only three
days for most people, but not for someone weighing in at
315. Most of his early weight loss was fluid loss, but we
couldn't square it with the dramatic fall in blood pressure.
Even using potent diuretic drugs, we hadn't gotten that
kind of response. Mike told him to quit taking one of his
medications, and his symptoms improved as his blood
pressure went up a little. He was back in a few days with
the same symptoms. Within the first two weeks of his diet
his blood pressure had fallen to the point that we took
him off all but one of his medicines and that one at reduced dosage. By this time he had lost only 13 pounds or
so, less than 5 percent of his body weight, and we couldn't
figure out what was going on.

Shortly after this experience we attended a scientific
meeting at which a researcher from Switzerland gave a paper on the effects of insulin on fluid retention. His data
showed that a rapid reduction in serum insulin levels
would bring about a rapid and substantial diuresis. And of
course that would mean a rapid and substantial decrease in

happened with Tom
some other strange
with patients on the
place way too soon af-
ated to the minuscule
s on our study of the
sulin resistance, and hy-

approach, in fact at that
was involved in any-
e didn't take him
would be able
alled three
hair

LOOD PRESSURE

Excess insulin causes high blood pressure in basically three
ways: it causes fluid retention, alters the mechanics of the
blood vessels, and increases nervous stimulation of the arterial system. Let's examine these processes in order, starting with insulin's propensity to raise blood pressure by
driving the body to retain excess fluid.

Along with transporting nutrients to the tissues and
hauling waste products away, the blood bathes the cells
with electrolytes in the proper mix and concentration.
These electrolytes—sodium, potassium, chloride, bicarbonate, and others—are critical for normal cell function
and are, like blood sugar, maintained within a narrow
range. The kidneys filter the blood that runs through
them, removing waste products and regulating the concentration of the electrolytes. Here's another of the
body's great balancing acts. If the blood contains too
much sodium, the kidneys pull it out, deposit it in the
urine, and send it to the bladder to be removed; if there is
too little, the kidneys assiduously conserve what there is
and remove just enough fluid to ensure the proper concentration of sodium in the blood.

Diuretics work by forcing the kidneys to get rid of more sodium than they normally would. As the kidneys eliminate this sodium they jettison fluid along with it to maintain the blood concentration of sodium within the proper range.

Insulin has exactly the opposite effect: it forces the kidneys to retain sodium—even when there's too much and the kidneys would rather get rid of it. To maintain the sodium concentration in the blood at the proper level, the kidneys must then retain excess fluid to dilute the excess sodium. More insulin means more sodium retention and therefore more fluid retention. As the body retains more fluid and the blood volume increases, the blood pressure begins to rise and can in due course reach dangerous levels, requiring treatment. The typical first-line therapy is the administration of diuretics to override the effects of insulin, forcing the kidneys to release excess sodium and fluid, returning the blood pressure to normal. Or the patient can use nutrition to reduce the elevated insulin levels and achieve the same results in a less costly fashion.

Insulin also increases blood pressure by altering the mechanics of the vascular walls, namely, by making the arteries less elastic. Recall from the last chapter that insulin acts as a growth hormone on the smooth muscle cells in the walls of the arteries and that as the insulin level increases the excess stimulation of these smooth muscle cells causes them to enlarge. As these smooth muscle cells grow, they increase the thickness of the arterial walls, making them stiffer and less supple while at the same time decreasing the volume within the arteries. The heart then has to exert more force to push the blood through these narrowed, more rigid arteries, resulting in elevated blood pressure.

The third way insulin causes elevated blood pressure is by stimulation of the nervous system, leading to the increased release of norepinephrine, an adrenalinelike substance, into the blood. Adrenaline is a neurotransmitter whose effects we've all experienced during times of stress, excitement, or after a bad scare. If you narrowly avoid an automobile accident, you typically feel flushed, notice your heart beating faster, and have a shaky, uncomfortable feeling—all brought on by the sudden outpouring of adrenaline. Not only does this rush of adrenaline cause these uneasy feelings; it drives up the blood pressure at the same time. Elevated insulin levels acting through unknown mechanisms engender an increase in blood norepinephrine that, although not of the magnitude of the rush occasioned by the near disaster, nevertheless raises blood pressure and causes an increased heart rate, placing the heart under continuous stimulation and keeping the blood vessels constricted.

The three ways insulin induces and sustains high blood pressure all complement one another. Insulin-spawned adrenaline acts to constrict insulin-thickened, less supple arterial walls, while at the same time the entire vascular system tries to cope with all the excess fluid retained by the insulin-stimulated kidneys. It's difficult to imagine how the blood pressure *wouldn't* rise under these conditions.

Heart Disease

More commonly the arterio-sclerosis results from the bad use of good vessels.

SIR WILLIAM OSLER, M.D.

Heart disease, the last head of the Hydra, is responsible for more death and disability than the rest of the heads combined. Hyperinsulinemia exerts its sinister influence on the heart in a number of ways: by increasing the blood cholesterol in ways we'll examine in Chapter 13 and by acting directly on the coronary arteries, making them more prone to occlusion, spasm, and clot formation. Before delving into the precise ways in which insulin acts, let's take a moment to review what medical science knows about the progression of coronary artery disease and heart attack first from a clinical and then from a cellular perspective.

WHAT IS A HEART ATTACK?

A heart attack occurs when, for whatever reason, the blood flow to an area of the heart is cut off or severely diminished. The heart is nothing but a large muscle that contracts rhythmically, pumping blood throughout the body. How hard does this muscle work? Imagine that you are holding a 5-pound weight in your hand and you begin to flex your arm at the elbow, bringing the weight to your shoulder. Your biceps, the muscle on the front of your upper arm, is doing most of the work during this exercise. The various arteries servicing your biceps carry oxygen- and nutrient-enriched blood to the working muscle as the veins bear away the waste products and deoxygenated blood. If you flex your arm repetitively faster and faster, you will ultimately reach the point at which the oxygen needs of the hardworking biceps exceed the capacity of the arteries to supply it. When your muscle begins to get inadequate amounts of oxygenated blood, it begins to hurt, more than likely prompting you to discontinue the exercise and allow your muscle to recover. Now, if your arm were hooked up to some kind of device that beeped electrical impulses into your biceps to make it contract involuntarily regardless of the pain involved, you can imagine the consequences. The pain would rapidly become excruciating. If the stimulation continued, some of the muscle fibers would begin to die, and ultimately the entire muscle would be damaged irreparably and fail. Your arm would dangle uselessly at your side, unable to contract despite the relentless beeping of the electrical stimulator.

Only in the nightmarish fiction of a Stephen King novel might this torture be inflicted on a human arm; in real life it is inflicted on human hearts daily. The heart has a built-in, mindless stimulator, the *sinoatrial node,* that beeps out an electric current across the body of the cardiac muscle about 72 times per minute. (Just try contracting your biceps a little faster than once per second and you will realize what an amazing muscle the heart is. It contracts at this rate—or even much faster if, for example, the body needs more oxygen due to exercise or fever—day in and day out, awake or asleep, never resting until the day you die.)

Due to the enormous demands for energy required to continuously contract 72 times per minute throughout life, nature has endowed the heart with an extensive circulatory system, the coronary arteries that wrap around

the heart carrying large quan
all segments of the muscle. If one
ies—as a result of blood clot, spasm, o
instance—fails to supply a portion of
enough blood to meet its demands, the hear
ble. But the sinoatrial node continues to stimu
heart muscle, including the segment that is now recei
inadequate oxygenated blood. And as with our biceps, the
heart muscle that can't quit beating to rest becomes
racked with agonizing pain—the pain of a heart attack. If
the blockage is severe enough and continues long enough,
the segment of heart served by the involved coronary
artery becomes irreversibly damaged and dies.

Along with the severe pain, the aftermath of coronary
arterial blockage typically includes shortness of breath,
weakness, nausea, drenching sweat, and the feeling of impending death. Medical science has defined and attached
names to all the different degrees and manifestations of
this phenomenon: angina pectoris, the pain associated
with the lack of heart muscle oxygenation; myocardial ischemia, the situation in which the heart muscle receives
inadequate oxygen, but before it is permanently damaged;
and myocardial infarction, death of a segment of heart
muscle. For our purposes we can lump all these together
under the rubric of heart disease.

As long as the coronary arteries provide adequate supplies of oxygen-rich blood to the heart, it will pump on forever. The problem arises when the flow of blood to an area
of the heart is cut off or reduced significantly. How does
this happen? Usually by occlusion of a coronary artery created by the buildup of plaque—cholesterol-filled fibrous
growths—on the inner linings of the arteries involved.
Plaque forms over a long period of time, progressing in a

LY DISEASES OF CIVILIZATION

tics of oxygen-rich blood to

of these coronary arter-

r plaque growth, for

the heart with

t is in trou-

late the

ing

321

...tion of cholesterol

...ding to the develop-

...zingly, insulin, once

...oints along the way.

IN?

several points along the

...on, starting with elevated

...he blood. Although arterial damag... ...n occur in the face of nor-mal—or even ...holesterol, elevated LDL levels usually hasten its o.... And insulin, by its action on the cholesterol synthesis pathway located within the cells, helps to create and sustain excess amounts of LDL in the blood.

Insulin also increases the proliferation of smooth muscle cells in the artery and their migration into the area of plaque formation. This not only accelerates the development of plaque but increases the thickness and rigidity of the arteries as well. Once these smooth muscle cells migrate into the developing fatty streak and plaque growth continues, insulin stimulates the increased synthesis of collagen and other connective tissue that make up a large part of the forming mass. At the same time insulin enhances cholesterol synthesis within the plaque lesion, the source of its greasy appearance.

As you can see, the only stage in this pathway that insulin *doesn't* affect (or at least hasn't yet been shown to affect) is that of LDL modification. Although insulin itself apparently doesn't play a direct role in the alteration of the LDL molecule, making it a target for the macrophages, the metabolic changes that go along with insulin resistance and hyperinsulinemia do. As blood sugar rises, increased amounts of glucose are irreversibly attached to LDL molecules, altering their structure and making them attractive to the macrophages; free radicals form and attack other LDL molecules—a process enhanced by an insulin-resistant environment—rendering them susceptible to the same fate.

Insulin and Plaque—A Direct Correlation

In the early 1960s a research team led by Dr. Anatolio Cruz in a now-classic experiment demonstrated the changes wrought by chronically elevated levels of insulin. His team injected insulin into the large arteries in the legs of dogs: each day each dog was injected with insulin in the artery of one leg and the same-size dose of sterile saline in the other. This procedure was followed daily for almost eight months. Upon examination the arteries injected with the insulin were found to have a pronounced accumulation of cholesterol and fatty acids along with a thickening of the inner arterial lining; the opposite arteries, injected with saline, remained normal. Dr. Cruz induced these profound changes with a relatively small dose of insulin given only once a day for a little over seven months. Picture the changes he might have found had he been able to keep the insulin level consistently elevated for several years! With this in mind it's not difficult to imagine the changes in our own coronary arteries after many years of chronic hyperinsulinemia.

Can You Undo This Damage?

Are we doomed to live with the current state of our coronary arteries barnacled with plaque, or can we reclaim them? We can reclaim them, but not overnight. The development of plaque takes time, and so does its regression; it's a process that takes years, not months. It can also be done only in the face of a *lowered insulin level.*

In the words of one researcher, a consistent finding in animal studies is that insulin "inhibits regression of diet-induced experimental atherosclerosis, and insulin deficiency inhibits development of arterial lesions." In other words, if you want to clean up your coronary arteries, you can't do it in the presence of hyperinsulinemia. Unfortunately, when plaque has reached the point of calcium deposition, hemorrhage, and excess fibrous tissue formation, it is irreversible despite insulin lowering; even at that point, however, dietary intervention can forestall further formation. And if plaque hasn't reached the final stage, our program, by removing the harmful stimulation of insulin in excess, allows the arteries to recover, slowly become more supple, and ultimately rid themselves of the dangerous cholesterol deposits beneath their inner linings. Another head of the Hydra severed.

When the Deadly Quartet Isn't a Foursome

If hyperinsulinemia indeed causes all these disorders we've been discussing, why doesn't everyone with hyperinsulinemia have high blood pressure, heart disease, diabetes, and obesity? How, for example, can a person have hyperinsulinemia, elevated cholesterol, and high blood pressure and not be overweight? We know that insulin causes the storage of fat, so a person with greatly elevated insulin levels is bound to be overweight, right? Not necessarily. Take the case of Linda Mot. Ms. Mot is a slender (5'8" tall, 110 pounds) 44-year-old woman with high cholesterol. She'd been to another physician who had recommended that she start medications to remedy the problem, but she wanted a second opinion. We began by asking her about her diet.

"What do you usually eat? What are your favorite foods?"

"Well, I don't eat a lot of fats," she assured us. "I try to eat a balanced diet with lots of different foods."

"What's your favorite food?"

"Anything with chocolate in it," she answered without hesitation.

"So, you eat a lot of sweets along with your balanced diet?"

"Oh, yes, I love sweets, especially chocolate," she answered, "and I've always considered myself fortunate in that I could eat them without worrying. All my friends have to watch their weight and either don't eat junk food or do and feel guilty about it. I can eat all the cake, pie, doughnuts, and especially chocolate candy and ice cream that I want and never gain a pound. I guess I'm really lucky."

"Do you have any other health problems besides the cholesterol?"

"I've had some problems with high blood pressure, but that's all okay now because my doctor gave me some pills for my fluid retention that keep the blood pressure down."

"Fluid retention?"

"Yeah, I don't ever gain any weight—you know what I mean; I don't get fat—but I do have a problem with holding on to fluids. My ankles swell a little, sometimes I can't get my rings on, my eyes get puffy, that sort of thing. But the water pills get rid of it and keep my blood pressure down to boot."

"Does your father have heart problems?"

"Yes . . . how did you know?"

Ms. Mot's blood pressure was moderately elevated, and her blood tests revealed a total cholesterol of over 300 and an insulin level that was 56 mU/ml, *almost twice the highest limit of normal by the lab's standards and over five times the limit of what we consider normal.* We set about revising Ms. Mot's diet, not an easy task since she was confronted with a major diet overhaul and had all her life eaten everything she wanted. People who have never had a problem with excess weight have the most difficult time sticking with any kind of diet because dieting has never been a part of their mind-set. Ms. Mot was no exception to this rule, but she has persevered—with an occasional chocolate debauch—and her insulin level has come down along with her blood pressure and cholesterol. Although her blood values haven't quite reached normal yet, she has completely eliminated her problem of fluid retention and hasn't had to take a "water" pill since she started our dietary plan.

Getting back to our original question, why does the slender Ms. Mot—who falls into a category we call *normal weight, metabolically obese*—have most of the problems associated with hyperinsulinemia yet no excess weight, while others who are overweight may not have high blood pressure or elevated cholesterol? Why do some have diabetes or high blood pressure only, while others have the whole full-blown syndrome of hyperinsulinemia?

The answers to these questions lie in the genetic basis of these diseases of civilization. It is well known that these diseases run in families, and when all the studies are in it will be apparent that hyperinsulinemia does too. Depending on our own unique genetic makeup, we each have different propensities to develop these disorders once our insulin levels begin to climb.

WHEN YOUR GENES CATCH UP WITH YOU

Some fortunate people are genetically programmed so that even in the face of a lifetime of reckless eating they don't develop much insulin resistance. Most of us, however, are not so lucky and do gradually develop some degree of insulin resistance and hyperinsulinemia. Our genetics then determine what happens after our insulin levels go up: some of us inherit genes that program us to develop high blood pressure; others will develop diabetes; most will gain weight; and an unfortunate group will develop the whole full-blown cluster of disorders. If your parents developed high blood pressure and diabetes as they began to age, chances are they had underlying hyperinsulinemia and your odds are greater of developing the same problems. Although you can't do anything to change your genes, you can at least be aware of the source of the problem and take steps to avoid or remedy it.

By attacking the individual diseases, we physicians and patients are at best playing a delaying game; only by focusing our energies and treatments on insulin resistance and hyperinsulinemia can we hope to kill the Hydra instead of merely replacing one of its heads with another. Unfortunately, we can't just take a pill and lower our insulin levels; the only way is by changing the foods we eat, by changing our diet to one that is closer to what nature designed us to eat in the first place. The good news is that once we do undertake the proper dietary treatment the proof that we're on the right track is usually dramatic and not long in coming. Thanks to the profound biochemical activity of the correct foods, hyperinsulinemia usually disappears in a hurry, taking with it most of its untoward side effects. Your body will simply heal itself if you give it the right fuel.

The Bottom Line

The major diseases of Western civilization—obesity, high blood pressure, heart disease, elevated blood fats, and diabetes—have a common bond. In truth these "diseases" that afflict, disable, and kill so many people in America today aren't diseases at all; they're symptoms of a more basic single disorder: hyperinsulinemia (excess insulin) and insulin resistance. Here's how the problems develop:

When you eat, your body breaks down the food into its basic components—protein, carbohydrate, and fat—and absorbs them into the bloodstream, causing a rise in blood sugar. This rise signals your pancreas to make and release insulin that attaches to sensors in the tissues, enabling the sugar to come out of the blood and move into the cells, where it can be either burned for energy or stored away for later use (as fat in the fat cells or as glycogen in the muscles). Years of dietary and lifestyle abuse in susceptible people can lead to malfunctioning of the insulin sensors and the progressive development of chronically elevated insulin levels. This sluggish system favors the storage signals for fat and sugar, leading to the development of excess body fat. Continued dietary abuse (with excess carbohydrate) can finally result in such severe resistance to insulin (insulin sensors so sluggish) that no matter how much insulin your pancreas can make, it's no longer enough to make the system work. The combined forces of the high insulin and the rising blood sugar damage the pancreas and limit its ability to produce insulin, which then sends the blood sugar level skyrocketing, and adult-onset diabetes (type II diabetes) results.

The excess insulin works in several ways to cause elevation of blood pressure: it prompts the kidneys to hold on to salt and fluid; it promotes growth in the muscular layer of the artery walls, making them thicker and less pliable; it increases the levels of norepinephrine, an adrenalinelike substance that raises the heart rate and constricts the blood vessels. Many cases of hypertension in this country can be laid at the door of hyperinsulinemia and insulin resistance.

Insulin also plays several key roles in causing the formation of hard plaque that blocks the arteries, obstructs blood flow through them, and leads to heart attack. Insulin increases the liver's production of LDL cholesterol, increases the thickness and rigidity of the artery walls, and favors the laying down of the cholesterol beneath the artery lining, where it can harden and create blockage.

The bad news is that all these disorders are related—if you suffer from one, another might be in your future. The good news is that by simply restructuring your diet to reduce excess insulin and restore the insulin sensors to their normal sensitivity, you can undo much of the damage. Blood pressure, blood cholesterol and triglycerides, and blood sugar respond very quickly to dietary correction. Thickening of the arteries and early plaque formation takes years of insulin control to correct; in the late stage, even with the best nutritional control, it's doubtful that you can dissolve a rock-hard obstructive plaque. Still, you'd be preventing further damage by using this program. But the beauty of this concept is in the awesome power of food to correct these disorders. If you simply give your body the proper nutritional tools, it will take them and heal itself.

Chapter 12

The Microhormone Messengers: Meet the Eicosanoids

You can view eicosanoids as the biological glue that holds together the human body. In that regard they are the most powerful agents known to man, yet they are totally controlled by the diet.

BARRY SEARS, PH.D., author of *The Zone*

You may never have heard of eicosanoids before, but understanding how they work in your body is as important to your health as understanding hyperinsulinemia.

Early in Goethe's *Faust* the devil appears to Dr. Faust, who inquires of him, "Who are you?" Mephistopheles replies, "Part of that force which would do evil evermore, and yet creates the good." This exchange could be applied to eicosanoids, a gang of at least 100 powerful hormonelike substances that control virtually all physiological actions in your body. The most important thing about eicosanoids is to keep them in balance. If you have too little of one, too much of another, eicosanoids can send your body hurtling down the slippery slope of biochemical evil toward arthritis, blood clots, and dozens of other dangerous conditions. In fact, they play a major role in *most* diseases, including heart disease and cancer. When they're balanced, the system hums along smoothly in perfect health. In fact, Dr. Barry Sears, a prominent researcher in the area of eicosanoids and diet, describes the maintenance of the dynamic balance between the various eicosanoids as the *definition* of optimal health. The most exciting thing about eicosanoids is that you can control these powerful agents simply by making the right food choices.

The bad news is that many things we *can't* exert much control over—aging, viral illnesses, and stress to name a few—drive our body's production of eicosanoids in the wrong direction, leading to arthritic aches and pains, blood clots, arterial constriction, heart disease, dry skin, and a host of other problems: in short, all the signs and symptoms of aging and stress. The good news is that our nutritional regimen reverses many of these changes, leading to dramatic health improvements difficult to correlate with a simple change in diet. As you progress on our program you should begin to notice many of these changes caused by the shift to more "good" eicosanoids: increased luster and body in your hair, increased skin moisture and suppleness, increased endurance, sounder sleep, to mention just a few. We began to notice these changes in our patients years ago and, in fact, were puzzled by them—before we fully understood the role diet plays in eicosanoid modulation.

Patients would start on the program and return for their follow-up visits reporting that rashes they'd had for ages had cleared up.

"Why did my rash go away?" they would ask.

"We don't really know, but we're glad it did," we would reply.

"How come my allergies are better?"

"Why don't my knees hurt as much anymore?"

"Why did my headaches go away?"

"Why did my nails stop splitting?"

"How come my asthma got better?"

"We don't know, we don't know, we don't know."

But after seeing these changes occur time and time again as patients reduced their insulin levels, we became confident enough to change the dialogue a little and make it more proactive.

"Well, Mrs. Smith, this little rash on your arms will more than likely disappear once you get going on your program and get your insulin down."

"Really? How come?"

"We don't really know; it's just a good side effect of the program."

Now that we understand eicosanoids and their effects, not only can we predict with a fair degree of confidence exactly what kinds of changes and improvements our patients are likely to experience; we can also tell them why. We draw them a simple diagram, point out the critical points along the eicosanoid synthesis pathway, tell them what specific foods to avoid, and explain why it's so important to get their insulin levels under control. As you progress through this chapter, you will learn about the power of diet to control eicosanoids, and you'll understand the good changes you'll begin to experience in your own body.

What Are Eicosanoids?

You're probably thinking, *If these eicosanoids are so potent, why have I never even heard of them?* Even your doctor may not be familiar with the term: this is cutting-edge research. But you've probably heard of at least one type, prostaglandins, first discovered in secretions of the prostate gland about sixty years ago. Prostaglandins, along with their cousins prostacyclins, thromboxanes, and leukotrienes, are known collectively as *eicosanoids* because they are all compounds composed of twenty carbon atoms (Greek *eikosi*, twenty). If you've ever taken an aspirin—or any other of a large number of drugs—you've done so specifically to interfere with the formation of prostaglandins and other eicosanoids. If you've ever had a headache, menstrual cramps, abdominal discomfort from ulcers, swelling or inflammation, or a rash, you have likely been the victim of too many of the wrong eicosanoids.

Although prostaglandins and the other eicosanoids act in many ways like hormones, there is one critical difference that explains why we've understood so little about them until recently. Hormones, which are produced in specific glands and travel through the blood, can readily be measured by blood tests. Eicosanoids, on the other hand, are produced inside the cells, act inside the cells, and vanish in fractions of seconds, much too quickly to be detected easily. Development of exceptionally sophisticated instrumentation has allowed scientists to identify more than 100 different eicosanoids—in fact, the 1982 Nobel Prize was awarded for research in eicosanoids.

What Do Eicosanoids Do?

Eicosanoids exert powerful physiological effects at extremely low concentrations. How powerful? Comparing the physiological effects of fiber (which has been touted widely for its many health benefits) to those of eicosanoids would be, to use a baseball analogy, about like comparing the home run power of, say, Woody Allen to that of Babe Ruth. Fiber isn't even in the same ballpark with eicosanoids. Fiber exerts a slight chemical and bulking effect in the colon, whereas eicosanoids control and direct the regulation of such diverse functions as blood pressure, blood clotting, the inflammatory response, the immune system, uterine contractions during birth, sexual potency in men, the pain and fever response, the sleep/wake cycle, the release of gastric acid (the potent new antiulcer drugs now under investigation are eicosanoid modulators), the constriction and dilation of airways in the lungs and blood vessels in the tissues, and many others. In short, eicosanoids exert major effects on just about everything that goes on in the body. As a result, numerous drugs work by increasing or decreasing the body's synthesis or response to eicosanoids. We mentioned aspirin earlier, so let's consider that as an illustration.

Doctors have recommended aspirin forever to relieve pain and reduce fever. More recently, however, they've begun prescribing it to reduce the risk of heart attack and, most recently, to reduce the risk of colon cancer. How can one inexpensive, simple drug do all this? Because aspirin is a potent inhibitor of eicosanoid synthesis. Certain eicosanoids are responsible for pain, fever, increased blood clotting and constriction of arteries, as well as increased cell growth and intestinal secretions, and by blocking the synthesis of these eicosanoids aspirin eliminates or reduces the problems they cause. The downside of aspirin, however, is that it doesn't block the production of *only* the offending eicosanoids; it blocks the production of many others as well. This generalized blockade results in the development of the unpleasant side effects we associate with aspirin: stomach pain, severe ulcer problems, and allergic reactions. Aspirin itself doesn't do any of these things; it simply causes the change in the eicosanoid balance that does the actual work—or damage.

Your Diet and the Eicosanoid Factory

Drugs are not the only modulators of eicosanoid production: food plays an even greater role. In fact of all the things you can do to alter your eicosanoid balance, regulating your insulin and glucagon levels with diet is the most potent. And with what you've already learned about insulin, it should come as no surprise that it is a major stimulant of the production of the wrong kinds of eicosanoids. Since the structure of the diet—particularly the carbohydrate content—determines the level of insulin, following our program allows you to regulate eicosanoid synthesis without using drugs. The fat content of the diet also plays a significant role in the production of eicosanoids. The essential fatty acids that are the building blocks of eicosanoids come from the diet—i.e., no essential fatty acids, no eicosanoids. An *essential fat* is one required to sustain life that can't be made by the body's own biochemistry and consequently must be obtained from the diet. Linoleic acid is the only truly essential fat; all the others can be made from other substances or made from linoleic acid. Fortunately linoleic acid is commonly found in many foods, so unless you starve or go on a *totally* fat-free diet you are likely to get all the linoleic acid you need.

A plentiful dietary source of fatty acids in combination with the appropriate ratio of insulin and glucagon provides the optimal circumstances for the production of beneficial eicosanoids. Basically, with a few modifications that we'll deal with later in the chapter, you can think of this system as a factory where linoleic acid is the raw material, insulin and glucagon the processors, and cicosanoids the finished products. Each of our billions of cells houses these little factories turning out the various eicosanoids that regulate the function of these cells and, consequently, the tissues and organs these cells compose.

Heroes and Rogues: Two Kinds of Eicosanoids

Eicosanoid end products fall into two basic groups that have opposing functions:

"The Good"	"The Bad"
Series one eicosanoids:	*Series two eicosanoids:*
act as vasodilators	act as vasoconstrictors
act as immune enhancers	act as immune suppressors
decrease inflammation	increase inflammation
decrease pain	increase pain
increase oxygen flow	decrease oxygen flow
increase endurance	decrease endurance
prevent platelet aggregation	cause platelet aggregation
dilate airways	constrict airways
decrease cellular proliferation	increase cellular proliferation

It should be pretty obvious that we want more of the series one eicosanoids. It should also be apparent that eicosanoids play a major role in most diseases—either a disease-enhancing role or a disease-suppressing role. Take heart disease, for example: when you combine the blood vessel narrowing (vasoconstriction), the decreased oxygen flow, and the increased platelet aggregation (clot formation) caused by the series two eicosanoids, you have the setup for a heart attack. Most cardiac drugs work to offset these effects of the series two eicosanoids. Cancer offers another example: cancer occurs when cells lose their ability to regulate their own division and replication, and the cells begin to proliferate madly in an uncontrolled fashion. Series one eicosanoids suppress this rogue cell growth and are being investigated extensively for use as cancer chemotherapeutic agents; series two eicosanoids *promote* tumor growth. Victims of asthma and bronchitis who suffer tightness of the small airways in their lungs need more series one eicosanoids to reverse this airway constriction; series two eicosanoids make it worse.

Strange as it may seem, you wouldn't want to have all good and no bad; you do, however, want to have more good than bad. The bad serve a useful purpose—blood clotting when we get cut, for instance—you just don't want to be overwhelmed with them. Your goal is to do whatever you have to do to make more good than bad eicosanoids so that the balance is shifted toward the good side most of the time. Of all the means available to accomplish this goal, we can say without hesitation that following our nutritional program is the most potent. It provides the necessary essential-fat building blocks to make plenty of eicosanoids while at the same time keeping insulin and glucagon—the most powerful forces in eicosanoid synthesis—in the appropriate range to maximize the output of good eicosanoids.

Controlling the Eicosanoid Production Line

There are three points along the eicosanoid synthesis pathway where we can exert dietary influence over the eicosanoid end products. The first control point is at the start of the process, where linoleic acid, the raw material for eicosanoid synthesis, enters the system. The second is by altering the synthesis process itself in a way that results in the production of predominantly good eicosanoids. The third is by restricting the dietary intake of arachidonic acid, a precursor of many of the bad eicosanoids. Figure 12.1, a schematic representation of the eicosanoid synthesis pathway, shows how our program affects these control points.

The first step in eicosanoid synthesis is getting the raw material—linoleic acid—into the production line. Linoleic acid is a ubiquitous fat found in practically all foods, so you should have plenty available unless you've been on a slash-and-burn, extreme-low-fat diet for a long time. The problem then is not the amount of available linoleic acid but getting it into the system. The key to getting sufficient linoleic acid into the pathway is the critical gatekeeper enzyme—*delta 6 desaturase.* If this enzyme is active and working properly, linoleic acid flows continuously into the system, providing the material for all the eicosanoids your body needs to make. Inhibiting the action of this enzyme denies entry to adequate amounts of linoleic acid, and deficient eicosanoid production results. The first step in modulating your eicosanoid balance is to ensure that you have plenty to work with, which you can do by keeping this gatekeeper enzyme happy and working efficiently. You can do this by catering to its wants while avoiding, as much as possible, those things that slow it down. The following chart lists the major factors affecting this enzyme.

FACTORS THAT INFLUENCE GATEKEEPER ENZYME ACTIVITY

SPEEDS UP GATEKEEPER	SLOWS DOWN GATEKEEPER
Dietary protein	Aging
	Stress
	Disease
	Trans fatty acids
	Alpha Linolenic Acid
	High-carbohydrate diet

A quick glance should alert you that the deck is not exactly stacked in your favor in terms of getting sufficient linoleic acid into the pathway. On the positive side the nutritional regimen we recommend will provide you with plenty of protein, so by following it you're doing all you can to activate the enzyme pumping linoleic acid into the system. The next step is to eliminate those things that slow down the gatekeeper enzyme's activity.

It's pretty obvious that you can't really do anything about aging. You can try to control your stress levels by meditating and using other relaxation techniques, removing yourself from stressful situations, and just kicking back and relaxing, but as a practical matter stress is something most of us must endure as part of the fast-paced American way of life. You can do everything possible to stay disease free, but you're still going to be laid low by the occasional cold or flu and sometimes by even more serious afflictions.

Since these three factors—aging, stress, and disease—are pretty much beyond your control, you're left with the remaining three factors, all dietary and over which you do have control, to effect the synthesis of eicosanoids.

ACCENTUATE THE POSITIVE; ELIMINATE THE NEGATIVE

Trans fatty acids: The Myth of Margarine

Trans fatty acids are made when polyunsaturated fats are partially hydrogenated. Polyunsaturated fats have multiple double-carbon bonds in their structure. The instability of these bonds makes polyunsaturated fats more liquid, whereas fats that contain single carbon bonds "saturated" with hydrogen atoms are more solid. The fat that you find around the edge of a steak, for instance, is solid at room temperature and is predominantly a saturated fat; butter, also a saturated fat, is solid at room temperature. Corn oil, a polyunsaturated fat of vegetable origin, is liquid at room temperature. To make corn oil solid so that with the addition of artificial flavoring it can be used as margarine, it must be partially hydrogenated, an operation that forces hydrogen into the oil molecules under high temperature and pressure and in effect artificially saturates it. That's why it remains solid on the dinner table. If that's all that happened, there wouldn't be much of a problem, but unfortunately artificially hydrogenating the fat permanently alters the structure of the double-carbon bonds to an unnatural configuration (called the *trans configuration* in chemical parlance). In the process, what was once a good-quality polyunsaturated oil is converted to a hybrid called

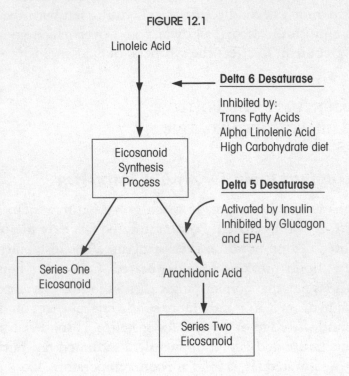

FIGURE 12.1

Linoleic Acid

Delta 6 Desaturase

Inhibited by:
Trans Fatty Acids
Alpha Linolenic Acid
High Carbohydrate diet

Eicosanoid
Synthesis
Process

Delta 5 Desaturase

Activated by Insulin
Inhibited by Glucagon
and EPA

Series One
Eicosanoid

Arachidonic Acid

Series Two
Eicosanoid

a *trans fatty acid*. The virtue of trans fatty acids from a food manufacturing and processing perspective is their stability and longer shelf life along with the fact that the fat molecules thus changed pack together better to make a more solid substance. (*Partially hydrogenated* is the villain here; fats labeled *hydrogenated* are not a problem.)

Trans fatty acids, found not only in margarine but in any of the thousands of commercial food products that have been partially hydrogenated, cause the health damage they do because they inhibit the formation of the good eicosanoids. For this reason margarine—that very substance Americans have been eating to save themselves from heart disease—can *increase* the risk for heart disease, cancer, and all the other problems caused by a relative abundance of bad eicosanoids.

Alpha Linolenic Acid (ALA): All Oils Are Not Created Equal

This omega-3 fatty acid found in the oils of various plants also slows down the gatekeeper. Canola oil (10 percent ALA), flaxseed or linseed oil (57 percent ALA), black currant oil (14 percent ALA), and soybean oil (7 percent ALA) are its primary sources. To avoid undermining your body's production of good eicosanoids, you need to minimize your consumption of the oils containing ALA, and that means limiting your intake of canola oil and soybean oil. Over the past few years there has been a boom in canola oil consumption because of reports that monounsaturated fats decrease the risk of heart disease. Indeed canola oil contains 60 percent monounsaturated fat, which is good, but it also contains 10 percent ALA, which is not so good. We have switched to olive oil; it has more flavor, contains more (82 percent) monounsaturated fat, and has no ALA. If you don't like the flavor of olive oil, try light olive oil. For recipes that won't work with the distinctive olive flavor, use sesame oil (the light one, not the dark toasted Asian sesame oil); it contains 46 percent monounsaturated fat, no ALA, and has a much more delicate taste. If you just can't bring yourself to abandon canola oil, you can offset the negative effects of the ALA by scrupulously avoiding trans fatty acids and carbohydrate excess and by keeping your protein intake up. In fact, of all the things you can do to enhance the production of good eicosanoids, eliminating canola oil is probably the least important.

Not so, however, with flaxseed oil, another oil many people consume for its supposed health benefits. Promoters of flaxseed oil—a reputed panacea for a variety of disorders—tout as one of its virtues its ability to help relieve the pain and inflammation of arthritis. You will recall that a bit earlier we discussed how aspirin, the archetypal drug for arthritis relief, works through an indiscriminate blocking of eicosanoid production, both good and bad, and that the shift away from so many bad ones eases the pain, but at the expense of potentially unpleasant side effects. By virtue of its high ALA content, flaxseed oil is a sort of biological version of aspirin: it blocks the synthesis of all eicosanoids, giving some relief to arthritis victims in the short run. You may be thinking at this point, *So what? If it gives relief, isn't flaxseed oil okay, at least for arthritis sufferers?* It would be if it were the only means available to afford relief, but it's like using a nine-pound hammer to kill a fly: it kills the fly, but it does a lot of other damage, too. With the techniques you learn in this chapter you'll be able to fine-tune your eicosanoid pathway to reduce inflammation, enhance immune function, and all the rest without having to resort to the blunt-instrument approach of flaxseed oil and other health food store remedies we've yet to deal with.

Another oil containing some ALA—soybean oil—is hard to avoid entirely since it's incorporated into most processed foods. Fortunately, it has a low percentage of ALA, so a little of it won't slow down your eicosanoid factory much. Just make sure that it isn't partially hydrogenated soybean oil, or you'll have trans fatty acids compounding the problem.

The following chart lists most commonly used oils and their composition. In general, select oils for cooking that contain a high percentage of monounsaturated fatty acids and little or no ALA.

FATTY ACID PERCENTAGES OF COMMONLY USED OILS

OIL	SATURATED	MONOUNSATURATED	LA	ALA
Almond	9	65	26	0
Canola	6	60	24	10
Corn	13	27	57	2
Flaxseed	9	16	18	57
Hazelnut	7	76	16	0
Olive	10	82	8	0
Peanut	18	49	29	0
Safflower	8	13	79	0
Sesame (light, not Asian)	13	46	41	0
Sunflower	12	19	69	0
Walnut	16	28	51	7

High-Carbohydrate, Low-Protein Diets: Trouble at the Gate

According to several studies, high-carbohydrate, low-protein diets inhibit the activity of the gatekeeper enzyme, leading to deficient eicosanoid production. High-carbohydrate diets compound the problem because they also stimulate the release of excess insulin, an even more serious problem for good eicosanoid synthesis, which we'll discuss in due course.

To ensure that you get the linoleic acid into the production pathway needed to synthesize all the eicosanoids necessary for optimal health, you must consume a diet of at least 30 percent protein, while avoiding trans fatty acids, ALA, and high-carbohydrate intake. But that's not the whole equation; it's only the first part. If you follow these steps, you will have all the raw material in the system that you need to make plenty of eicosanoids; the next step is to make certain these raw materials are converted to the *right* eicosanoids.

CONTROLLING INSULIN AND GLUCAGON

The most critical step in the entire eicosanoid synthesis process is the next one, the one over which we have the most nutritional control—directing the flow in either the good or bad direction. The direction of the flow is under the control of a second critical enzyme called, confusingly enough, *delta 5 desaturase*. This enzyme, when activated, shifts the synthesis process away from the good and toward the production of primarily bad eicosanoids; conversely, inhibiting this enzyme increases the production of good eicosanoids. As with all enzymes, this one has its own particular set of activators and inhibitors. And guess what? Insulin is a major activator. That's right, elevated levels of insulin send the production of bad eicosanoids soaring. What inhibits this enzyme? Glucagon, of course, which always works in opposition to insulin. In fact, short of drug therapy, of all the things that can modulate your eicosanoid balance insulin and glucagon are the most potent. Control them and you control your eicosanoids.

If we look at this from a dietary perspective, we can begin to make even more sense out of the current state of ill health gripping our society. The low-protein, high-carbohydrate diets most people try to follow first compromise the entry of adequate linoleic acid into their eicosanoid factories and then by increasing insulin and decreasing glucagon actually drive whatever gets in toward the production of the bad eicosanoids, causing aches, pains, vasoconstriction, platelet aggregation, and all the rest. The nutritional plan described in this book, however, does just the opposite. The increased protein content stimulates the entry of adequate raw material into the pathway, while the lowered insulin levels and the increased glucagon levels drive the production in the good direction, reversing the problems caused by an overabundance of bad eicosanoids. Knowing what you know so far, it's easy to understand the unexpected benefits our patients experienced when they began our program.

The Fish Oil Rescue

Eicosapentaenoic acid (EPA) is another substance that works like glucagon to divert the production of eicosanoids in the good direction; it just doesn't work nearly as well. EPA, an omega-3 fatty acid found in the oil of such cold-water fish as mackerel, herring, and salmon, adds another measure of dietary control over the eicosanoid balance. It also provides another example of how eicosanoids—and science—work in real life.

You have no doubt read that fish oil helps prevent heart disease. Somewhere along the way researchers stumbled onto this phenomenon—which we now know is eicosanoid related—and decided to study it. They gave subjects varying amounts of fish oil for varying lengths of time and checked them for platelet aggregation, vasoconstriction, all the other components of heart disease, and the development of heart disease itself. The results were frustratingly inconclusive: sometimes, in some subjects, fish oil worked like a charm; in others it showed no benefit. For anything to be scientifically valid it must be reproducible in the majority of cases; the case of fish oil was a hit-or-miss proposition at best. What happened?

Heart disease is a complicated, multifactorial problem, but for purposes of illustration let's confine our discussion to just a couple of the underlying actions contributing to the disorder. Platelets aggregate around a tiny injury on the lining of the coronary artery and form a clot. The artery may then constrict, further reducing the blood flow to the heart tissue beyond. As we have seen, both these actions are a consequence of bad eicosanoids, so if we can deliver an overwhelming force of good eicosanoids to the area, we should be able to reverse these changes, or so thought the researchers using fish oil rich in EPA for the purpose. But let's say that one group of subjects was following the standard low-fat, high-carbohydrate diet (which you now know means low protein as well). These people would be running their eicosanoid factories in the wrong direction because of their elevated insulin and lowered glucagon levels. Since EPA isn't nearly as potent as glucagon in driving the eicosanoid flow in the good direction, just about all the fish oil in the world would have trouble overcoming the forces driving eicosanoid production in the wrong direction. You would not expect these subjects to have a positive result. People who ate more protein or who had no insulin problems would likely show different results. These subjects would have a smaller insulin response to the diet and consequently would be making both good and bad eicosanoids in a fairly balanced fashion. The addition of fish oil to the diets of these subjects would then be enough to drive their eicosanoid production predominantly in the good direction, manifested in decreased platelet aggregation, diminished vasoconstriction, and all the rest—in short, positive results showing the benefit of fish oil as a therapeutic agent.

So, you have two groups of patients showing different results with the same amount of EPA. The reason: the metabolic hormonal effects of the difference in their underlying diets. This factor confounds many studies that are otherwise vigorously controlled. You can't get meaningful results unless you make sure to control for the extremely powerful druglike effects of food on insulin and glucagon—a step most researchers forget or don't understand.

Because of the relative weakness of fish oil as an agent to drive eicosanoid synthesis, we like to use it mainly as a fine-tuner. If our patients aren't getting the full benefit of the positive eicosanoids driven by the dietary reduction of insulin, we sometimes add fish oil to the regimen. We also use fish oil to counter the effects of dietary arachidonic acid, the third and final variable in the eicosanoid equation.

ARACHIDONIC ACID: NATURE THROWS US A CURVE

Arachidonic acid is one of those curves nature loves to throw at us just to keep us from being able to wrap everything up nicely and simply. Arachidonic acid (AA) is a fatty acid essential to life but also incredibly destructive in excessive amounts. Lab animals injected with large amounts of all other fatty acids go on about their business with no apparent ill effects—those injected with arachidonic acid are dead within moments. AA is made in the eicosanoid

Are You Sensitive to Arachidonic Acid?

The main symptoms associated with too much AA (or sensitivity to it) are:

- chronic fatigue
- poor or restless sleep
- difficulty awakening or grogginess upon awakening
- brittle hair
- thin, brittle nails
- constipation
- dry, flaking skin
- minor rashes

synthesis pathway and is the immediate precursor of the bad eicosanoids. If you keep your insulin down and your glucagon up, you should make very little arachidonic acid, but—and here's the curve—arachidonic acid doesn't come from just the eicosanoid pathway; it also comes in directly via the diet. Unfortunately, the dietary variety can also transform into bad eicosanoids. So, you may be asking, *I can do everything right, watch my carbohydrate intake, keep my insulin down, and still be sabotaged by dietary AA?* Yes, but *only* if you're particularly sensitive to arachidonic acid and eat a large amount of it.

AA is found in all meats, especially red meats and organ meats, and in egg yolks. It probably hasn't escaped your notice that these foods are the same ones that most people identify as being loaded with fat and cholesterol. Despite popular opinion, though, it's not the saturated fat and cholesterol that cause most of the problems associated with these foods: it's their arachidonic acid content—for those who are sensitive to it.

The AA in meat is located both in the muscle tissue and in the fat. The quantities are higher in red meat because red meat has more fat, which, at least in today's domestic feedlot animals, contains high levels of AA. Animals have the same eicosanoid synthesis cascade that we do, and when they are grain-fed and fattened, the high-carbohydrate grain stimulates their insulin just as it does ours. Fats are stored in fatty tissue in the same ratio that they occur in the blood, so cattle—and people—having large quantities of circulating AA will store large quantities as well. The good news is that range-fed cattle and wild game have much less fat to begin with, and what fat they have contains little AA. You can add wild game to your diet by following in the footsteps of your ancestors and bagging it in the field or by purchasing it from one of the purveyors listed in the appendix. But the easiest first step in avoiding dietary AA is to avoid as much visible fat as possible on your meat, especially red meat.

Does this mean you should avoid beef entirely if you're sensitive to arachidonic acid? Not at all. Here are a couple of techniques that will decrease the amount of AA you get in the beef you eat. First, after you trim as much of the visible fat as you can, *grill* your steaks. This method of cooking reduces the amount of AA in beef by about 35 percent. You can also follow our favorite way to marinate a steak that is not only healthful but actually makes the beef taste better—we've provided that method in the box on page 352. Most alterations you make in foods for health reasons really take a toll on taste, but not this technique for steak. The only drawback is that it takes a little advance preparation, so it doesn't work for spur-of-the-moment meals.

A Trick for Reducing Arachidonic Acid in Steaks and Roasts

Trim all the visible fat from the steak, then place it in a large resealable plastic bag along with a mixture of 1 cup of red wine and 1 cup of olive oil or light sesame oil (or any other oil you like as long as it contains no ALA). Allow the meat to marinate in this mixture in the refrigerator for a full 24 hours, flipping the bag and contents over a couple of times. Take the steak out, drain it for an hour or so, discard the marinade, rub the beef with some pepper or other spices to your taste, then grill it. You won't believe the taste. The wine acts as a solvent to leach out a fair amount of the saturated fat in the steak, which is replaced in part by the monounsaturated fat in the olive oil or other oil you use. These oils permeate the steak, giving it a juicy, succulent taste that you have to experience to believe—and make it more healthful to boot. You can use this technique with roasts as well. You won't get quite the same arachidonic acid decrease you will with the steak because you will be roasting the meat instead of grilling. Roasts taste even better if you make cuts all over the meat and insert slivers of garlic.

No advance work is necessary to decrease your arachidonic acid consumption from egg yolks. Make omelets using one or two whole eggs and the remainder egg whites. Or use one egg and add ricotta or tofu to scramble it. Try to remove yolks from egg recipes as much as you can because the yolks are very high in arachidonic acid. If you must eat a lot of eggs and you're AA sensitive, add some fish oil to your diet.

What about sautéing and frying? You now know how the trans fatty acids in margarine prevent the building blocks from getting into the eicosanoid production pipeline, so we want you to avoid margarine. Many polyunsaturated fats undergo a trans alteration during the high temperatures required for panfrying, so your health will also be best served by avoiding those. We need heat-stable fat that also imparts great taste, and the substance that fits the bill is butter.

I Can't Believe You Said Butter

That's right, the much-maligned butter is much better for you than almost anything else under these circumstances, because it is a naturally saturated fat—no trans fats to gum up your eicosanoid factory. But it can be made even more useful by clarifying it (so it won't burn) using the method described on page 355.

Remember that all of these precautions are necessary only if you have a problem with arachidonic acid. If you follow an insulin-lowering diet—the most important change you can make as far as modulating your eicosanoids is concerned—and you solve all your health problems to your satisfaction, eat all the red meat and eggs you want. If you do everything else right, keep your insulin levels low, and still have a problem (with hypertension, for instance), maybe you're exceptionally sensitive to dietary arachidonic acid (see page 350). You might want to try reducing your intake and see what happens.

The Case of Mr. Gorden

Mr. Gorden is forty-seven years old and extremely sensitive to dietary arachidonic acid. He came to see us initially for weight loss—he weighed over 350 pounds. On examination we found him to have high blood pressure, 180/115, and high cholesterol, over 300 mg/dl. We started him on an insulin-lowering weight-loss diet. When he returned in a week for follow-up, he had lost nine pounds, but his blood pressure was down only slightly. A few weeks later he had lost more than fifty pounds, and his cholesterol was much improved, but his blood pressure, though somewhat improved, was still elevated. His diet diaries showed that he ate several eggs and at least one serving of red meat every day. We instructed him to substitute fish and chicken for his steak, gave him the recipe for beef preparation described in the box on page 352, and recommended that he make his scrambled eggs using only one yolk. He did, and within two weeks his blood pressure was normal. He had been making enormous quantities of vasoconstricting eicosanoids from dietary AA, causing his elevated blood pressure.

Fine-Tuning Your Eicosanoids

You can fine-tune by paying attention to how you feel and what kind of symptoms you are experiencing. Do any of the symptoms listed in the box on page 350 apply to you?

If you've been on the plan for a while and you are still experiencing any of these symptoms, you probably need to reduce your AA consumption and/or increase your in-

Clarified Butter

Clarified butter, a mainstay in the culinary reper-
toire of great chefs everywhere, is also called *ghee* in
some recipes. You can purchase ghee already prepared in Indian markets. To make your own:

1. Place a pound of unsalted butter, cut into large
pieces, in a saucepan over medium heat.

2. As the butter melts and begins to bubble, reduce the heat to a level at which small bubbles continue to surface. These bubbles bring the
yellow-white milk solids to the top, where you can
skim them off and discard them.

3. After 10 to 15 minutes of bubbling and skim-
ming, you will have taken most of the milk solids off
the top or they will have congealed on the bottom.

4. At this point, strain the hot melted butter
through cheesecloth. *Voilà!* You have clarified butter.

5. Pour the clarified butter into an airtight container and store it in the refrigerator for up to 6
weeks.

6. Whenever you need to panfry or sauté, put a
few teaspoons of it into your skillet. You can also
mix clarified butter with a little olive oil, light
sesame oil, or other fairly heat-stable oil and have an
unmatched taste sensation.

take of EPA. Remember, EPA works in the same way as
glucagon to drive eicosanoid production in the good direction, so if you're following your insulin-lowering,

glucagon-enhancing diet and not getting quite the results you expect, you can boost glucagon's efforts with EPA. To increase your consumption of EPA you can eat mackerel, salmon, herring, or other cold-water ocean fish several times a week, or you can take fish oil capsules.[1] The standard dose of EPA in the typical fish oil capsule is 180 milligrams—not a lot. To get enough EPA to achieve results, you will need to take at least four to six capsules a day, more if you've strayed from your diet and don't have glucagon working for you at full capacity. Fish oil capsules may be purchased from most drugstores and all health food stores.

One easy way to monitor how you're doing is to notice your bowel movement frequency and composition. Good eicosanoids tend to increase the flow of water into the colon, whereas bad eicosanoids made from AA tend to reduce water flow into the colon. The more water in the colon, the looser the stools. If you're constipated, you probably need a little more EPA; if you develop diarrhea, you need less EPA. Another bowel sign that reveals your eicosanoid balance is whether your stools float or sink. Increased water flowing into the colon produces stools that are less dense and tend to float.

As you begin to get your eicosanoids in balance by controlling your insulin and by increasing your intake of essential fats, you should notice increased luster and body in

---

[1] When you purchase fish oil capsules, make sure they are labeled *cholesterol free*. Fish tend to concentrate many pollutants, including heavy metals and PCBs, in their fat, and this fat is where fish oil comes from. The refining process that removes all these pollutants also removes the cholesterol, so if the label says *cholesterol free,* you can be sure that the oil you are buying is pollutant free.

your hair, your skin should become more moist and supple, your endurance should improve, and you will probably sleep much better. We've noticed many of these changes in our patients as they have begun following our program, even before taking any extra essential fats at all.

The Bottom Line

Your body works as a balance of opposing forces. Control of these forces—whether your blood vessels dilate or constrict, you have pain and inflammation in a joint or none, you breathe freely or wheeze, you sleep well or poorly, you suffer allergies or don't react, to name a few—occurs through cell-to-cell messenger microhormones called *eicosanoids*. Your body manufactures two families of these messengers—those beneficial to your health and those detrimental to it—by making alterations to one essential dietary fat. Whether the fat becomes a "good" messenger or a "bad" one depends primarily on your diet.

Your first task is to eat a diet that provides you with plenty of linoleic acid—the essential fat from which all the eicosanoid messengers are made. The best dietary sources for ensuring you always get plenty of this raw material to build eicosanoids are naturally pressed oils. We recommend olive oil, but other good oils are almond, hazelnut, safflower, light sesame, sunflower, and walnut. Oils that have been altered by the manufacturer to make them more stable for sale (cheap cooking oils are altered to keep the polyunsaturated fats in them from spoiling, and this damages the oil irrevocably) or to change them from their natural form to something else (liquid vegetable oil is artificially saturated to make it become margarine or shortening) contain trans fats that interfere with normal eicosanoid production.

The next step in production is getting that raw material onto the assembly line, and a number of factors beyond your control influence this step: aging, stress, and disease (but also trans fats and a high-carbohydrate diet) all slow down entry of the linoleic acid into the eicosanoid production pathway. Dietary protein enhances entry of linoleic acid to the pathway. Following the guidelines of our program, you will be eating the proper balance of protein, carbohydrate, and fat to ensure that the raw material gets into the system.

Once it does, whether it becomes primarily a "good" messenger or a "bad" one depends again on diet. Excess insulin from a high-carbohydrate diet favors the formation of "bad" eicosanoids; so does the dietary fatty acid arachidonic acid (AA), found in red meat and egg yolk, which the body turns directly into the "bad" eicosanoids. Although you don't have to avoid these AA-containing foods unless you seem to be especially sensitive to AA (see page 350 for more information), you can reduce your consumption of this fatty acid by using a few tricks of food preparation we describe for you on pages 351–353.

Fish oil (omega-3 fatty acid) helps to offset the detrimental effects of AA by slowing down the production of bad eicosanoids coming off the assembly line. You can use fish oil capsules to supplement your intake of dietary fish oil found in cold-water ocean fish: mackerel, herring, salmon, tuna.

Eating a diet like the one we recommend maximizes your production of "good" messengers and favors a balance of eicosanoids to optimize your health.

The important points to remember are:

1. The most potent means to restore your eicosanoid balance and keep it there is to follow an insulin-lowering diet such as ours.

2. Next in importance is to avoid as much as you can partially hydrogenated fats and ALA to ensure adequate supplies of eicosanoid building blocks getting into the production line. Use olive oil instead.

3. Keep an eye on your dietary arachidonic acid, especially if some of your health problems such as hypertension don't completely disappear with steps 1 and 2.

4. Fine-tune your essential fat status by adding EPA (fish oil) as described.

Chapter 13

Cholesterol Madness

Thus we should beware of clinging to vulgar opinions, and judge things by reason's way, not by popular say.

MONTAIGNE (1533–1592)

If the sixteenth-century French essayist Montaigne were alive today, he might write about the various groups who are whipping the world into an anticholesterol frenzy in much the same way he did about certain philosophers of his time: "[they] have created in their feeble imaginations this absurd, gloomy, querulous, grim, threatening, and scowling image, and placed it on a rock apart, among brambles, as a bogey to terrify people." Cholesterol is indeed a bogey and one that terrifies people beyond reason. We are obsessed with it. Obsessed to the point that, like the Eskimos who have in their language twenty-seven different words for *snow*, we have come up with almost as many to describe cholesterol. We have HDL cholesterol (which can be further subdivided into HDL_2 and HDL_3 cholesterol), LDL cholesterol, VLDL cholesterol, IDL cholesterol, and a whole slew of others if you start differentiating by apoprotein type (apoproteins are protein structures found on the surface of the various cholesterol complexes).

Although the average American is not likely to be conversant with this arcane language of cholesterol research, he's certainly alert to the specter of high cholesterol and all its sinister ramifications. In fact most people recall the results of their last cholesterol test faster and with greater accuracy than their hat size. Cholesterol levels have become the ultimate measure of health and fitness—to be bragged about if low and confessed to if elevated.

And, of course, cholesterol has become big business. Whenever mass paranoia starts to brew, a legion rises up ready to exploit it. The food processing industry and its advertisers now emblazon the containers of edibles as diverse as soft drinks and cornflakes with the superfluous statement "contains no cholesterol." Cholesterol angst is not lost on the various governmental and private research funding bodies responsible for underwriting all kinds of medical research. These groups disburse hundreds of millions of dollars to eager research labs throughout the world, allowing them to pursue the secrets of cholesterol in ever-more-intricate studies. As a measure of this scientific interest, more than a dozen Nobel Prizes have been awarded for cholesterol's study.

Why all this fuss? What exactly is cholesterol? Should you be concerned about it? Where does it come from? How do you get rid of it, or how, at the very least, do you control it? You're about to learn everything you need to know to make an accurate assessment of your own health as it relates to cholesterol, and you'll learn how you can dramatically lower your cholesterol level—if it's elevated—without using drugs and without going on a bare-subsistence, low-fat diet. In fact, if you are a careful reader, by the time you finish this chapter you will know more about cholesterol than 95 percent of the physicians in practice today. You won't learn all the esoteric terms for all the minute components of the various cholesterol complexes, but you will gain an understanding of the actual workings of the cholesterol regulation system that will put you way ahead of many doctors.

Cholesterol: Essential for Life

Despite the mounting fervor against it, the average American doesn't know exactly what cholesterol is but is quite certain that it's dangerous. The consensus on cholesterol seems to be *the lower, the better,* but as we shall see, this is not always the case. Far from being a health destroyer, cholesterol is absolutely essential for life.

Although most people think of it as being a "fat in the blood," only 7 percent of the body's cholesterol is found there. In fact, cholesterol isn't really a fat at all; it's a pearly-colored, waxy, solid alcohol that is soapy to the touch. The bulk of the cholesterol in your body, the other 93 percent, is located in every cell of the body, where its unique waxy, soapy consistency provides the cell membranes with their structural integrity and regulates the flow of nutrients into and waste products out of the cells. In addition, among its other diverse and essential functions are these:

Cholesterol is the building block from which your body makes several important hormones: the adrenal hormones (aldosterone, which helps regulate blood pressure, and hydrocortisone, the body's natural steroid) and the sex hormones (estrogen and testosterone). If you don't have enough cholesterol, you won't make enough sex hormones.

Cholesterol is the main component of bile acids, which aid in the digestion of foods, particularly fatty foods. Without cholesterol we couldn't absorb the essential fat-soluble vitamins A, D, E, and K from the food we eat.

Cholesterol is necessary for normal growth and development of the brain and the nervous system. Cholesterol coats the nerves and makes the transmission of nerve impulses possible.

Cholesterol gives skin its ability to shed water.

Cholesterol is a precursor of vitamin D in the skin. When exposed to sunlight, this precursor molecule is converted to its active form for use in the body.

Cholesterol is important for normal growth and repair of tissues since every cell membrane and the organelles (the tiny structures inside the cells that carry out specific functions) within the cells are rich in cholesterol. For this reason newborn animals feed on milk or other cholesterol-rich foods, such as the yolks of eggs, which are there to provide food for the developing bird or chick embryos.

Cholesterol plays a major role in the transportation of triglycerides—blood fats—throughout the circulatory system.

A quick review of this list should give you a better idea of what cholesterol does and dispel any notion that it's a destroyer of health to be feared and avoided at all costs. Far from being a serial killer, cholesterol is absolutely essential for good health; without it you'd die. Without cholesterol we would lose the strength and stability of our cells, rendering them much less resistant to invasion by infection and malignancy. In fact, a grave sign of serious illness, such as cancer development or crippling arthritis, is a *falling* cholesterol level.

Where does cholesterol come from? Although some cholesterol indeed does come from food, the vast majority (80 percent) is produced by the body itself. In fact, every cell in the body is capable of making its own cholesterol. Most don't, however, and rely instead on that made in the liver, intestines, and skin, with the liver responsible for the lion's share of the production. Due to the body's need for large amounts of cholesterol, a feedback loop exists so that whenever dietary intake decreases the liver's synthesis increases. And, in opposite fashion, when the diet is rich in cholesterol, the liver synthesizes less. This self-regulation helps explain the baffling research finding that blood cholesterol levels vary only minimally in the face of enormous variations in dietary intake. As a matter of fact most people, contrary to what you read and hear daily, can consume almost unlimited amounts of cholesterol without significantly increasing their blood cholesterol levels. That being the case, people having excessive blood cholesterol levels—and many do—must have a problem with the ability of their bodies to regulate cholesterol levels internally. That is precisely the case. *The key to lowering elevated cholesterol levels is not in the restriction of dietary cholesterol or fat but in the dietary manipulation of the internal cholesterol regulatory system.* Unfortunately, there's a glitch in the works that causes all the problems.

THE FLY IN THE OINTMENT

Nature endowed—or afflicted—us with a minor design flaw that creates most of the problems we have with excessive cholesterol: *cholesterol levels are regulated only inside the cell.* Why is this a design flaw? Because problems

arise due to excess cholesterol in the blood, yet the cholesterol level in the blood isn't regulated—there is no
feedback loop to signal the need for the body to lower
cholesterol levels in the blood when they get too high.

The cells of the body require a steady supply of cholesterol to build and repair cell membranes and to carry out
all the other tasks required of them to make life possible.
Where does the cholesterol for all this construction come
from? Basically two sources: the cell either extracts cholesterol from the blood or makes its own or both. The important thing is that the interior of the cell needs plenty of
cholesterol, so the interior is where the cholesterol sensors
are located. Falling cholesterol levels within the cell trig-
ger these sensors to fire off messages to the production
machinery within the cell to increase the supply—make it
or get more from the blood. By these means the level of
cholesterol inside the cell is maintained tightly within a
narrow optimal range. The point to remember is that the
sensors that dictate cellular need for cholesterol are *inside*
the cells (primarily of the liver), not out in the bloodstream.

When cholesterol causes its artery-clogging mischief,
where does that occur? In the walls of the arteries supplying the heart and the major arteries supplying the body
and brain, *not* in the cells with cholesterol sensors. This
system glitch is analogous to having a big, powerful air
conditioner in a house and putting the thermostat that
controls it into a small, hot, airtight closet. The cooling
machinery could be cranking out enough cold air to form
icicles on the woodwork throughout the house, but the
thermostat in the closet would never know. As far as it
knows, the air is hot and needs cooling, so it calls for more

cold air, and in spite of the icicles forming on it, the air conditioner keeps huffing and struggling along to pump cold air out.

The cholesterol plaques choking the interiors of the arteries are like the icicles in the house. Deposits of cholesterol fill the arteries, but the sensors inside the cholesterol-producing cells never know it because they, like the thermostat in the closet, are concerned only with cholesterol levels within the cell, not what's going on outside in the arteries. What are these feedback controls, these cholesterol sensors that often work against us? And what can we do to escape or confound this apparent design glitch? There is a way.

HOW CHOLESTEROL GETS AROUND: INTRODUCING THE LIPOPROTEINS

A few years ago patients came into our office wanting to know their cholesterol levels; now that's not enough. Now most patients want to know their *total* cholesterol levels along with their LDL and HDL levels and the various ratios of all the above. At this stage of the cholesterol awareness game, most people know that LDL is the "bad" cholesterol and HDL is the "good" cholesterol but don't have an inkling of what HDL and LDL actually are. Although it's possible to live a long and prosperous life without ever knowing what LDL and HDL are, it's important to be familiar enough with them to see how they, along with cholesterol in general, fit into the insulin, glucagon, and insulin control equation—especially if elevated cholesterol or heart disease runs in your family or is a problem for you.

You can think of the various lipoproteins as envelopes

that enclose cholesterol and triglycerides, making them soluble in blood so that they can be transported to the tissues. Since neither cholesterol (a waxy, fatty solid) nor triglycerides (the storage form of fat) are soluble in blood, the only way they can get around is to be wrapped up in and carried by a substance that is soluble in the blood. The lipoproteins fit the bill.

LDL is the abbreviation for *low-density lipoprotein,* while *HDL* stands for *high-density lipoprotein.* The names of these complex molecular compounds tell us nothing about what they do but are instead reflective of their densities: how light or heavy they are. The lightest of all the blood fats are the triglycerides. In a slurry of blood fats they would float to the top, like cream. Next lightest are the very-low-density lipoprotein (VLDL) molecules. These are carriers of some triglyceride and a little cholesterol. Next heavier are low-density lipoprotein (LDL) molecules that carry mainly cholesterol. And finally are the densest, heaviest molecules of all, the high-density lipoprotein, or HDL.

A Day in the Life of a Lipoprotein

Your liver cells make and release VLDL (very-low-density lipoprotein) into the bloodstream as a molecule composed mainly of triglyceride but with a little cholesterol. As this young particle circulates through the blood, it matures by acquiring more cholesterol. The mature VLDL particle ferries triglycerides to the body tissues to be burned for energy or stored. The cholesterol-rich remnants left after most of the triglyceride has been released become a low-density lipoprotein (LDL) molecule that is practically all cholesterol. This cholesterol-rich LDL, the so-called "bad" cholesterol, circulates through the bloodstream and is the primary means the body has for transporting cholesterol to the outlying tissues. Three fates can befall these LDL particles: they can be removed from the circulation by the liver—as we shall see, a critical operation in the maintenance of normal cholesterol levels; they can be requisitioned by other tissues needing cholesterol; or, unfortunately, they can be deposited in the arteries. Figure 13.1 summarizes the sequence of events in the life of a lipoprotein.

LDL: The Heart Disease Heavy

Since LDL is the main culprit in the development of coronary artery disease, the secret of cholesterol control is in knowing how your body deals with LDL and how you can influence the cells to remove as much LDL from the blood as possible. How do the cells remove LDL from the circulation? With LDL receptors.

Remember, cholesterol is regulated from *within* the cell, and when the level inside the cell falls, the cell either makes more or procures more from the blood outside the cell. The cell gets the cholesterol from the blood by sending structures called *LDL receptors* to the surface of the cell to grab the cholesterol-filled LDL particles and pull them into the interior of the cell, where the cholesterol is removed and used for cellular functions. Remember those obscene winged monkeys in the movie *The Wizard of Oz*, the ones the Wicked Witch sent to get Dorothy and Toto? They swooped down, grabbed Dorothy and her dog, and carried them back to the castle to be used for the witch's evil purposes. LDL receptors work in much the same way. When the cell sends out the call for cholesterol, forces

FIGURE 13.1

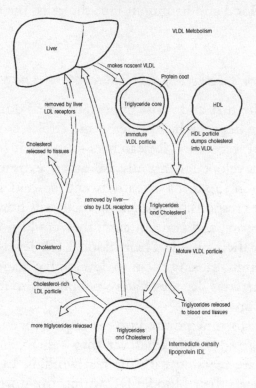

within the cell manufacture these receptors and send them to the surface of the cell, where they lie in wait for the next LDL particle circulating through the blood, which they grab and pull into the interior of the cell. Once inside the cell, the LDL receptor releases the LDL particle and heads back toward the surface to grab another one. The enzymatic machinery within the cell then removes the lipoprotein envelope from the LDL particle and harvests the cholesterol core for synthesis of cellular products. Clearly the more LDL receptors we have scavenging cholesterol from the blood and hauling it into the cells, the better off we are.

Please Don't Take My LDL Receptors Away

Some of the first and most important work done on the relationship between heart disease and cholesterol focused on the LDL receptors. Researchers found that some people who developed heart disease at an extremely early age—often in the teens or early twenties—had a disorder in the genes responsible for telling their cells how to make LDL receptors, and consequently they could not remove LDL from their blood. Their blood LDL levels rose exceedingly high, causing them to develop blockages in their coronary arteries decades before people without this rare genetic disorder.

Their misfortune pointed up the importance for people not so afflicted to do whatever they can to ensure that their cells are teeming with the hardworking LDL receptors that keep their blood LDL within the normal range and reduce their risk of heart disease.

Of Mice and Men

In fact, it seems reasonable to suppose that if we could somehow rev up the production of our LDL receptors our cells could clear the cholesterol from our blood even in the face of a diet high in saturated fat and cholesterol. Recently a team of scientists including Drs. Michael Brown and Joseph Goldstein—recipients of the Nobel Prize for their discovery of the LDL receptor—working at the University of Texas Southwestern Medical Center at Dallas tested this idea in the laboratory.[1]

These researchers developed a strain of mice that produced *human* LDL receptors in their livers at a rate about five times that of the mouse LDL receptors in the livers of the normal mice used as experimental controls. On the normal laboratory diet the mice with the increased number of LDL receptors—the experimental strain of mice—maintained blood cholesterol levels that were 50 percent less than those in the normal controls, a finding that would be expected considering the increased number of LDL receptors. The surprise came when the scientists fed both groups of animals a diet high in saturated fat and cholesterol. As anticipated, the levels of LDL in the blood of the normal mice zoomed upward, while there was *no increase* in the level of LDL in the blood of the experimental mice. In the words of the authors of the study, ". . . increasing LDL receptor expression above its normal level in the mouse *can prevent hypercholesterolemia* [elevated blood cholesterol] *even in the face of a diet that contains large amounts of cholesterol, saturated fats, and bile acids.*" (Emphasis added.)

That's easy, you say, in mice, but can *we* increase the production of LDL receptors in *our* cells? Yes, we can. To understand how, we need to look at the other half of the within-the-cell cholesterol regulation equation. Remember, the cell obtains cholesterol from two sources: it either makes it, or it sends the LDL receptor to fetch it from the

---

[1] Yokode, M., et al., "Diet-Induced Hypercholesterolemia in Mice: Prevention by Overexpression of LDL Receptors," *Science* 250 (November 30, 1990): 1273–75.

blood. We've seen how the LDL receptor works; now let's consider how the cell makes cholesterol.

The Cholesterol Factory

When the signal goes out that the cholesterol level inside the cell is getting low, the cell, along with making more LDL receptors, starts to crank up the production machinery within itself to make more cholesterol. This assembly-line process chugs along, churning out cholesterol and adding it to that brought in by the LDL receptors, until the cell has a sufficient quantity to perform its tasks, then the process slows until the cell runs low again and calls for more. Since the cell's cholesterol comes from these two sources, which are both regulated by the cell, it makes sense that if, for whatever reason, one of the two processes slows down, the other will pick up the slack. This is precisely what does happen. Following this line of reasoning, if we could somehow slow down the rate at which our cells make cholesterol internally, they would have to increase the number of LDL receptors they send to the surface to pull more LDL from the blood. Again, this is exactly what happens; in fact the most potent cholesterol-lowering drug available today—lovastatin (Mevacor)—works on this principle.

The cholesterol synthesis pathway inside the cells is like a production line in a factory. The raw materials are brought in and in a series of steps shaped and fashioned into the final product. There is one step in the line—called the *rate-limiting step*—that determines how fast the production runs and controls how much gets produced. It is at this crucial step—an enzyme with the unwieldy name *3-hydroxy-3-methylglutaryl-coenzyme A (HMG-CoA) reductase*—that the cholesterol drug lovastatin intervenes. It slows down this step and decreases the amount of cholesterol produced. Less cholesterol within the cell indirectly increases the production of LDL receptors that rush to the surface to pluck the LDL cholesterol out of the bloodstream, bringing about a swift and significant lowering of LDL cholesterol in the blood. Unfortunately, it doesn't work its magic without side effects or without expense. Lovastatin has caused liver problems, muscular disorders, gallbladder disorders, rashes, and psychiatric disturbances—to name a few—and at the maximal recommended dose costs in the neighborhood of $200 per month for life. Despite this formidable list of side effects, because it works so quickly and dramatically, it keeps the cash registers ching-ching-chinging in pharmacies all across the country. Wouldn't it be great if there were a way to get the same cholesterol-lowering results without having to resort to drug therapy? There is.

Controlling Cholesterol with Insulin and Glucagon

If you pick up any medical biochemistry textbook and turn to the section on cholesterol synthesis, you will learn that a couple of hormones affect the activity of the rate-limiting enzyme HMG-CoA reductase. What hormones? Our old friends insulin and glucagon. Insulin stimulates HMG-CoA reductase, while glucagon inhibits it. Knowing this, it starts to make sense that people with insulin resistance and elevated insulin often also have elevated cholesterol levels. The high levels of insulin continuously stimulate production of cholesterol, leading to an abundance within the cells. With plenty in the cells, there's no reason to send LDL receptors to the surface to get more, so the amount of LDL in the blood rises and remains elevated.

Glucagon, as is its custom, does exactly the opposite. It inhibits the activity of HMG-CoA in much the same way that lovastatin does and brings about similar results. As glucagon slows down the production of cholesterol within the cell and the supply inside begins to run low, the cell sends its trusty LDL receptors to the surface to harvest LDL cholesterol from the bloodstream, resulting in less LDL cholesterol in the blood. Once again we see how by regulating insulin and glucagon levels we can correct or improve problems that are seemingly unrelated to insulin and blood sugar—in this case blood cholesterol. Our nutritional plan relies on food to balance insulin and glucagon and reduces blood cholesterol levels in exactly the same way that lovastatin does, but without the unpleasant side effects and hefty expense. And that's not the end of the story. This regimen acts in a number of other ways to improve the blood lipid picture, which we'll examine shortly. Before we do, you need to become familiar with one more actor in the cholesterol drama—HDL.

Heroic HDL

If LDL is the villain in the cholesterol drama, then high-density lipoprotein (HDL) is surely the hero. HDL scavenges cholesterol from the tissues, including the linings of the coronary arteries, carries it through the blood, and hands it off to the VLDL particles circulating in the bloodstream, ultimately converting it to LDL. So the transportation of cholesterol is not along a one-way street: LDL carries it toward the tissues for deposition, while HDL gathers it from these tissues and carts it back the other way to the cells of the liver, where it is disposed of. Since both processes occur simultaneously, the amount of cholesterol in the tissues depends on the relative amounts of LDL and HDL in the blood. It's like a freeway leading to and from a major city. At 7:30 A.M. on Monday morning the half heading into town will be congested, but there will still be some traffic on the side heading away from the city. The increased population of the city during the workday, which changes moment by moment, is the sum of the people entering the city minus the ones leaving. If you have a lot of LDL and not much HDL, then the preponderance of the cholesterol traffic is going to be toward the tissues; if, on the other hand, you have a greater amount of HDL, the flow goes in the opposite direction. With these facts, medical researchers have been able to quantify risk for heart disease based on the ratios of these lipoproteins.

My "Bad" Looks Good, but My "Good" Looks Bad

If you have your cholesterol checked in your doctor's office or, more likely in these days of cholesterol madness, at a shopping mall, you will find your results listed under the heading "Total Cholesterol." The number you see there is the sum of all the different lipoprotein envelopes that are carrying the cholesterol—the measurement of all the cholesterol carried in the blood as LDL, VLDL, and HDL.[2] Just as a screening test, total cholesterol isn't too inaccurate because the lion's share (about 70 percent) of it is carried by LDL. If the total cholesterol reading is high, then the odds are that the LDL is high also; conversely, if the total figure is low, the LDL is too. But, there can be exceptions, and that's why most physicians use the fractionated HDL and LDL figures to diagnose and treat our patients.

Medical researchers have investigated and compared the rates of heart disease development to the levels of the individual lipoproteins. You shouldn't be surprised to learn that the higher the level of LDL, the greater the risk of heart disease, and the higher the HDL, the lower the risk. What if both are high or both low? Just such situations do occur, so we prefer to look more at the ratio of the two rather than at either one individually. Two benchmark standards have been established:

1. Total cholesterol divided by HDL should be below 4.
2. LDL divided by HDL should be below 3.

Let's look at a couple of examples to see how this works.

If your total cholesterol is 240 mg/dl (a figure that would have been in the low normal range just a few years ago but today makes people think they can almost feel their coronary arteries clogging with cholesterol) and your HDL is 60 mg/dl, your ratio is 240/60, or 4, which

---

[2] Actually it is a combination of five lipoproteins, but we will concern ourselves only with VLDL, HDL, and LDL.

is okay. If you can raise your HDL to 70 mg/dl even though your total cholesterol stays the same, you are in good shape with a ratio less than 4. Conversely, if you find yourself with a total cholesterol of 180 mg/dl, before you start patting yourself on the back, check your HDL. If it's 30 mg/dl, your ratio of 6 is too high; you need to raise your HDL. Looking at the other ratio, if your LDL is only 120 mg/dl (the upper limit of normal is considered to be 129 mg/dl) but again your HDL is only 30 mg/dl, your ratio is 4, above the benchmark of 3 for LDL/HDL. This is a case where the "bad" (LDL) looks good, but the "good" (HDL) looks bad.

DIET AND CHOLESTEROL QUIZ

Let's consider a scenario involving cholesterol and diet. Using your knowledge of the ratios we've been calculating, decide what you would do. You go to your doctor's office for a physical exam, and he finds that your total cholesterol is 240 mg/dl. He tells you that he has a diet guaranteed to reduce your cholesterol to 200 mg/dl if you will follow it. You do follow the diet and come back to see him in two months. Your total cholesterol is now 200 mg/dl. Are you happy? What if your HDL was 60 mg/dl on your first visit? That makes your total cholesterol–to–HDL ratio 4 (240/60), a good number. What if when you come back in two months your HDL has fallen to 45? Now your ratio is 4.4 (200/45). Your ratio has worsened even though your total cholesterol figure has fallen, because your HDL fell at a greater rate. Your risk for heart disease—the reason you went on the diet in the first place—has now *increased* because your ratio has worsened. Would you be pleased with your new diet?

An interesting hypothetical case, you might say, but what doctor would actually start a patient on a diet that would cause such changes, a diet that would lower HDL more than it would total cholesterol? Well, tens of thousands of doctors put hundreds of thousands of patients on just such a diet each and every day. The diet in the example is the standard high-carbohydrate, low-fat diet that doctors everywhere prescribe for their patients with elevated cholesterol.

The "Controversial" High-Complex-Carbohydrate Diet

As the data on diet and cholesterol continue to accumulate, the evidence indicates that the high-complex-carbohydrate, low-fat diet doesn't live up to its billing as a cholesterol solution. Most studies show that although these diets lower total and LDL cholesterol somewhat, they lower HDL cholesterol by a greater percentage, leading to a worsening of the ratios that are more important than the individual measurements by themselves. A study published in the February 1991 issue of the *Journal of Clinical Endocrinology & Metabolism* illustrates this concept nicely.

The research group led by Dr. Mark Borkman of Sydney, Australia, studied young (average age thirty-seven), normal-weight, nondiabetic subjects of both sexes to determine the effects of diet on various blood parameters. The subjects followed one of two diets—either a high-carbohydrate diet or a high-fat diet—for a three-week period, then followed the other diet for the next three-week period. After each dietary period the researchers examined the subjects and analyzed their blood.

The high-carbohydrate diet was designed to follow the current standard nutritional recommendations and was over 50 percent carbohydrate and under 30 percent fat. It was "based on foods rich in starch and indigestible carbohydrate (whole-meal bread, pasta, rice, and potatoes), fruit and vegetables, nonfat dairy products, and lean meat." (Sound familiar?) The high-fat diet was mainly "full cream dairy products, eggs, butter, and fatty meats, with restriction of starch foods, vegetables, and fruit." Despite this "restriction," the subjects on the high-fat diet managed to consume 31 percent of their calories as carbohydrate, or roughly 175 grams of carbohydrate per day, so this hardly qualifies as a rigorous carbohydrate-restricted diet—an important point because had the carbohydrate been a little more restricted, the results would have been even more impressive.

When the researchers tabulated the results of the study, they found that the total cholesterol dropped from an average of 191 mg/dl on the high-fat diet to about 159 mg/dl on the high-carbohydrate, low-fat diet, a 17 percent decrease; the LDL cholesterol dropped from 139 mg/dl to 111 mg/dl, a 20 percent decrease; and the HDL cholesterol from 42 mg/dl to 32 mg/dl, a 24 percent decrease. The ratios are shown in the following chart.

CHOLESTEROL COMPARISONS STUDY

	HIGH-CARBOHYDRATE DIET	HIGH-FAT DIET
Total cholesterol	159 mg/dl	191 mg/dl
LDL cholesterol	111 mg/dl	139 mg/dl
HDL cholesterol	32 mg/dl	42 mg/dl
Total cholesterol/HDL	4.97	4.55
LDL/HDL	3.47	3.31

If you consider the results of this study and others like it solely from the perspective of what the high-carbohydrate, low-fat diet does to the total and LDL cholesterol, you will conclude that the high-carbohydrate diet lowers cholesterol significantly. But when you throw in the HDL figures, the picture changes considerably. The total cholesterol/HDL and LDL/HDL ratios can be thought of as rough indicators of the flow of cholesterol into and out of the tissues: the higher the number, the greater the flux of cholesterol *into* the tissues—the situation we want to avoid if we are concerned about heart disease. You can see from this table that although the total and LDL cholesterol are lower in the blood of the subjects on the high-carbohydrate diet, the actual flow of cholesterol into their tissues is higher. The authors address this issue in their summary: "These results suggest that practically achievable high carbohydrate diets . . . have net effects on lipoprotein metabolism that may be unfavorable."

These results and others like them have gotten the attention of the medical research community; now the high-carbohydrate, low-fat diet is beginning to be referred to as the *controversial* high-carbohydrate, low-fat diet. Unfortunately most medical researchers have marinated for so long in their antifat, procarbohydrate bias that they can't change their perspective. At meetings and in their writings they continue to promote the standard fare while admitting that it's controversial, but it's the best we have right now. But *is* it the best we have right now? Is there anything better? Absolutely, but before we turn our attention to the way this better diet controls cholesterol, let's fill in one last piece of the cholesterol puzzle.

Most people assume that the lower they can keep their cholesterol, the better; they much prefer a cholesterol of

100 mg/dl to one of 220 mg/dl. As you probably realize, they would be in error. There is an ideal cholesterol range that you should shoot for, one that is as dangerous to go below as to go above, but many health-conscious people continue on in pursuit of ever-lower levels in the misguided notion that they are extending their life spans by conquering cholesterol. These people are making a serious error because they have seen only half of the data.

The Other Half of the Cholesterol Story

The higher your cholesterol, the more likely you are to die with heart disease or stroke. That's the gist of information promulgated by medical research and the cholesterol-lowering drug manufacturers. They demonstrate their data with graphs like those in Figure 13.2.

In truth, mortality from heart disease probably does increase as cholesterol increases and decrease as the level of cholesterol continues to fall—to a point. But this graph is only half the story. Heart disease is not the only cause of death in this country—people do die from other causes. What the multihundreds of millions of dollars in research studies designed to demonstrate a reduction in deaths from heart disease as cholesterol levels decrease *fail to prove* is that reduction of cholesterol to very low levels leads to a decreased rate of death overall. The actual complete graph showing death from all causes (not just heart disease or stroke) as related to blood cholesterol levels looks more like Figure 13.3.

As your cholesterol level falls below a certain point, you jump out of the frying pan of heart disease risk and into the fire of death by all sorts of other diseases. What kind of diseases? Cerebral hemorrhage, gallbladder disease, and many types of cancer, for which falling cholesterol is a marker.

As you can see, the ideal cholesterol level is in the area where the U-shaped curve bottoms out, in the 180 mg/dl–to–200 mg/dl range. Avoid trying to get it lower; don't trade one serious health problem for another.

Putting It All Together

Given what you now know about the various lipoprotein groups, it's clear that you ought to follow a diet that keeps your LDL cholesterol low while keeping your HDL cholesterol high. You should shoot for an LDL/HDL cholesterol ratio of 3 or less, endeavoring to keep your total cholesterol in the optimal range instead of blindly tearing down the path toward ever-lower levels. This is all fine, and other than the last sentence we would find no argument with any of this from even the most vociferous members of the high-complex-carbohydrate, low-fat camp. But how do you do it? How can you corral your cholesterol into its optimum range and keep it there while still eating foods that you enjoy?

Our insulin-controlling diet gives you the means. It lowers LDL and raises or maintains HDL, usually keeping the total cholesterol in the ideal 180-to-200 mg/dl range. By keeping insulin levels low and glucagon levels high, our plan keeps the LDL receptors busy retrieving LDL from the blood and pulling it into the interior of the cells, reducing blood LDL cholesterol levels.

FIGURE 13.2
HEART DISEASE DEATHS VS. BLOOD CHOLESTEROL LEVELS

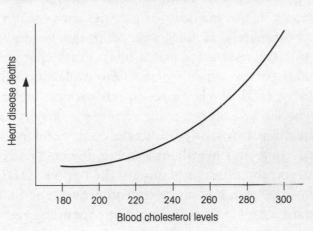

FIGURE 13.3
DEATHS FROM ALL CAUSES VS. CHOLESTEROL LEVELS

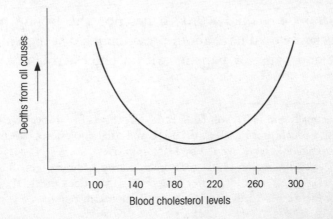

Recall that when Dr. Reaven of Stanford published his findings on insulin resistance and hyperinsulinemia (Syndrome X) one of the features he described was a low HDL. Medical science has yet to provide us with the underlying biochemical reason for this lowered HDL, but it's present in the majority of patients with insulin resistance. Fortunately, as the levels of insulin go down, the levels of HDL rise: we've noted this positive change in patient after patient on our plan.[3] One explanation for the increase of HDL levels we see in our patients is the additional fat allowed on our plan: *dietary fat increases HDL.*[4] Our nutritional structure brings the cholesterol level to its optimal range and maintains it there, lowers "bad" LDL cholesterol, and raises or maintains the "good" HDL cholesterol—the result is an overall improvement in blood lipid status. And it does it on a diet containing red meat, eggs, and cheese—all forbidden on any other kind of cholesterol-lowering diet.

Seeing Is Believing

Reluctant is a mild word to describe the feeling most physicians would have about prescribing a diet high in red meat and eggs for patients with a cholesterol problem.

---

[3] Occasionally the HDL will fall a little, but this fall is always accompanied by a much greater fall in the LDL and total cholesterol, so the ratio of total cholesterol divided by HDL improves.

[4] This is also the reason HDL goes down during a low-fat diet. But because HDL decreases in greater proportion than does the LDL, such low-fat diets can actually worsen those all-important ratios.

We'll admit that it caused us some worry the first time we did it, even though we knew from the research that it *should* work. But the proof of any nutritional regimen's worth is in the laboratory results down the line. And the biochemically correct nutritional plan we developed for our patients with elevated cholesterol succeeded beyond our expectations. We've described this insulin-controlling plan to other physicians who tried a few patients on it very reluctantly at first. As their experiences mirrored ours, and their patients' blood cholesterol levels plummeted just as ours had, these physicians became enthusiastic supporters of the program. Along with the experiences of these colleagues, we often read in medical journals of other physicians who stumble onto a diet that controls insulin and its consequences without really understanding what's happening. They are so amazed at the cholesterol-controlling abilities in the face of what seems to be a diet that would increase cholesterol that they publish their findings.

Much was made of an article that appeared in the March 28, 1991, issue of the *New England Journal of Medicine,* about an elderly gentleman who ate twenty-five eggs per day yet had a normal blood cholesterol level. You may have read this story in your newspaper, because all the wire services picked it up, and several nutrition writers offered their views on the freakishness of it. The consensus seemed to be that this was a special case, like the relative everyone seems to have who smoked four packs a day and lived to be ninety-five. Here are the details:

An eighty-eight-year-old man living in a nursing home ate twenty-five or so eggs per day and had done so for the past thirty years of his life. His physician had documented this fact and reported that despite his eating habits the gentleman's cholesterol had always been in the normal range. The apparent inconsistency of this situation—as far as most physicians are concerned this would be akin to smoking a carton of cigarettes per day for thirty years and having a normal chest X-ray—attracted the attention of a medical researcher at the University of Colorado medical school, who examined this patient and reported his findings. Upon questioning, this slender (6'2", 185-pound) elderly man stated that he followed a standard diet with a wide variety of foods, which he supplemented (for reasons unknown to himself) with a couple of dozen eggs per day. His blood levels of cholesterol were: total cholesterol, 200 mg/dl; LDL, 142 mg/dl, and HDL, 45 mg/dl; his LDL/HDL ratio was 3.16. The body of the article went on to discuss the reasons this man's cholesterol levels were normal despite his intake of 5,000 mg of cholesterol per day (about seventeen times the normally recommended amount). The author concluded that the patient made less cholesterol, absorbed less cholesterol, and got rid of more cholesterol biochemically than the average person, and was thus spared the consequences of his two-dozen-eggs-per-day habit.

We were troubled by this article when we first read it because we couldn't reconcile his normal cholesterol with the diet this gentleman ate. If he were consuming a "normal" diet as the article reported (particularly nursing-home fare), then he was no doubt getting plenty of carbohydrates. His insulin should have been up and consequently his cholesterol as well. After pondering this for a while, it occurred to us that if this man were eating twenty-five eggs a day he couldn't possibly be eating much else. After all, twenty-five eggs represents about 2,000 calories per day, a more-than-adequate amount for a sedentary man of eighty-eight. We corresponded with the author of the article, and indeed, the nursing home confirmed our prediction that "the quantity of these [other] foods is limited."[5] Since the eggs contain no carbohydrate whatsoever and the other foods are limited, it's our guess that this gentleman consumed about 50 or 60 grams of carbohydrate per day along with his eggs, an amount that correlates precisely with Phase II of our plan. Knowing this along with all the mechanisms we have discussed, it's no surprise that this patient's cholesterol stayed within the normal range—he simply went on his own bizarre version of an insulin-controlling diet.

We found another such serendipitous consumption of a diet similar to our plan, this time by multiple patients, reported in the *Southern Medical Journal* in January 1988. In this case a New York physician, H. L. Newbold, M.D., treated a group of patients who had food allergies by placing them on a specific diet to eliminate certain foods thought to cause their allergic problems. In Dr. Newbold's words:

> At the time of the initial visit, each patient was eating an ordinary, varied American diet. All patients had an elevated serum cholesterol. [The average total cholesterol of the study group was 263 mg/dl, with a range of 224–327 mg/dl. The average HDL was 57.1 mg/dl.]
>
> I discovered that each patient could best tolerate beef rib steaks. For varying periods, these patients ate mostly unaged beef rib steaks. Some patients could occasionally tolerate lamb, pork, or chicken in place of the rib steak, but they ate them no more often than once every three or four days. Rarely, they ate cuts of beef other than rib steaks.

---

[5] Personal correspondence with Fred Kern, M.D., the author of the article.

Patients were instructed to have their butchers leave a percentage of fat on the steaks. They were told to eat as much of the fat as they could comfortably tolerate.

These patients were told to supplement their basically meat diet with a small amount of raw fresh vegetables and raw fruits—a restricted version of our program. Before you read this chapter, what would you think of a diet like this one? You would guess it would send the cholesterol levels of these poor patients screaming upward. Almost anyone in today's low-fat world would think that. What happened? Dr. Newbold explains: "After eating a diet high in beef fat for three to eighteen months, the average serum cholesterol fell to 189 mg/dl." The cholesterol levels of these patients declined from 263 to 189 mg/dl while the HDL levels increased from 57.1 to 62.7 mg/dl. Once again we see people going on the "wrong" diet and lowering their cholesterol levels by 28 percent while increasing their HDLs by almost 10 percent—a drop in total cholesterol–to–HDL ratios from 4.6 to 3. Not too bad!

Clearly, as these studies show, you can reduce and control your cholesterol levels without having to resort to the old hidebound, low-fat, low-cholesterol diet. You can partake of a wide variety of fruits and vegetables on our program while at the same time eating the red meat, eggs, and cheese that you may have been avoiding in an effort to lower your cholesterol. Don't be misled by the misguided efforts of your friends and relatives who don't understand the workings of cholesterol metabolism as you do. Continue with your plan and let your lab results speak for themselves.

The Truth About Fiber

Fiber has been touted as a means of reducing weight and the risk of developing colon disorders and cancer, as a remedy for constipation, as a preventer of hemorrhoids, and, thanks to *The 8-Week Cholesterol Cure,* as part of a cure for elevated cholesterol and heart disease risk. After an extensive survey of current medical research literature on the role of fiber in human health, we came to one certainty: no one really knows exactly what fiber is, what it really does, or how it works. But there is consensus on the notion that fiber does improve bowel function by adding bulk to the stool and speeding it more quickly along. These properties prevent or lessen constipation and discourage the formation of hemorrhoids.

The story on cholesterol reduction is less clear, with some studies showing a reduction from fiber intake while others do not. There probably is some benefit here in that fiber may bind with cholesterol in the intestine and prevent its reabsorption.

Fiber does help to stabilize blood sugar by slowing down the absorption of dietary carbohydrates. Slower absorption may blunt the blood sugar rise and the insulin response to it, resulting in a lower, more constant blood sugar level.

Although great hoopla surrounded the news that fiber exerts some protective effect in preventing colon cancer, based on the huge Harvard Nurses Study, in truth, the difference in colon cancer between those women who ate the most fiber and those who ate the least was three cases, an insignificant number.

Our nutritional regimen gives you a wide variety of choices of fruits and vegetables that will provide you with far more fiber—without the metabolically active carbohydrate—than all the bran muffins you could eat. For instance, a bowl of raspberries contains more fiber than ten of the basic-recipe bran muffins described in *The 8-Week Cholesterol Cure* and almost no usable carbohydrate.

Because the fiber content of foods is not metabolically active, you can subtract the grams of dietary fiber from the total carbohydrate content of foods you eat. We call what's left, the Effective Carbohydrate Content of Food (ECC). We've compiled charts of effective carbohydrate grams for a wide range of foods (see Chapter 5).

Peruse those charts and notice that the vegetables giving the best carbohydrate value are the green leafy ones and the cruciferous ones (because they're rich in fiber). The worst are potatoes, corn, and dried beans. Among the fruits, berries of almost all kinds are the best carbohydrate/fiber bargain; bananas and raisins are among the worst.

In fact, using our ECC chart, we find that you could have 1 cup broccoli, 1 cup cabbage, 3 celery ribs, 1 cup green beans, 1 cup lettuce, $1/2$ cup mushrooms, 1 cup zucchini, 1 cup spinach, and 1 cup raspberries spread throughout the day, giving you only 27 grams of metabolically active carbohydrate and 16.3 grams of fiber, most of it of the soluble variety. You could add a couple of slices of light bread and still have eaten only 40 grams of usable carbohydrate and a total of 21.3 grams of fiber—almost 100 percent more than the average American diet. This is hardly stringent in terms of amount of food, vitamin content, mineral content, volume, fiber, or any other parameter.

The ECC charts in Chapter 5 will guide you naturally toward foods that contain more fiber and less starch, because that's where you'll get the most food for the lowest carbohydrate intake. And if you simply can't or won't eat any of the high-fiber fruits and vegetables, and you become constipated, you can always add fiber by using the commercial vegetable fiber powders, such as Konsyl or Nutriflax.

How much fiber do you need? For good health people usually need *at least* 25 grams a day. In the past, restricted-carbohydrate diets have been criticized for not providing enough fiber. Is this a valid concern? Yes, but not with our plan, which provides ample fiber.

The Bottom Line

In America people have become accustomed to thinking of cholesterol as an evil destroyer of health. The average American is not even sure what cholesterol is exactly; only that it's "fat in your blood" and "it's dangerous." In fact, nothing could be further from the truth: cholesterol is absolutely essential for life, and falling levels of cholesterol are a grave sign, often a marker for cancer.

Cholesterol isn't even really a fat; it's a pearly white waxy alcohol with a soapy feel. Every cell in your body requires cholesterol to maintain the structural integrity of its cell membrane, to control the flow of water and nutrients into the cell and waste products out. Your nerves and your brain require cholesterol for normal electrical signal transmission.

Your body uses the cholesterol molecule as a building block for many important hormones: the sex hormones (estrogen and testosterone) and your body's natural steroid, hydrocortisol.

Cholesterol in the bile your liver makes aids in the digestion of fatty foods and helps you absorb fat-soluble vitamins A, D, E, and K from food. Cholesterol gives your skin the ability to shed water.

Every cell in your body can make it. In fact, only about 20 percent of the cholesterol in your blood comes from your diet. Your body (primarily your liver) makes the vast majority (80 percent). To ensure your cells always have plenty, if there's not enough coming in, the cells pick up the slack and make more.

That's why simply cutting back on dietary cholesterol often doesn't cause much of an improvement in blood cholesterol levels.

The standard low-fat-diet approach to treating cholesterol actually causes the cells of your body to have to make *more* cholesterol for vital functions. Control over how much the cells make lies *within the cells* themselves. When the supply in the cell runs low, the cell can either make more cholesterol or send messengers to the surface of the cell to collect some from the bloodstream.

Insulin plays a key role here: it revs up the cells' cholesterol-manufacturing machinery, building up a surplus within the cell, making it unnecessary for the cell to retrieve any from the bloodstream, and thereby allowing excess cholesterol to build up in the blood.

By eating a diet that reduces insulin levels, as our program does, you reduce the signal telling the cells to make cholesterol; they *must* harvest it from the blood to have enough, and your blood cholesterol levels—especially the "bad" LDL—fall rapidly. Even while eating a diet that contains red meat, egg yolk, cheese, butter, and cream, as long as you control your insulin output, your cholesterol will remain in the healthy 180-to-200 mg/dl range with the LDL/HDL ratio under 3. And the extra dietary fat will actually raise the HDL—"good" cholesterol—level in your blood.

Overcoming the Curse of the Mummies

Historical pathology gives descriptions of diseases in all ages that can be exactly applied to diseases of today. . . .

C. G. CUMSTON, medical historian

From time immemorial the fertile valley along the Nile River has produced an abundance of plant life. The river itself teemed with fish in ancient times and provided food and cover for birds, while the lush floodplain provided rich grazing for every sort of wild animal. Out of this flourishing, verdant landscape the early inhabitants, the ancient Egyptians, carved the beginnings of one of the greatest civilizations of all time—pharaonic Egypt.

During the almost 3,000 years from 2500 B.C. to A.D. 395, the Egyptians refined the art of mummification and extended its practice through all social strata. The number of mummies from that period has been estimated by some experts to equal the population of Egypt today. Medical scientists have analyzed many of these mummified remains in such detail that they have been able to determine not only blood type and body size and shape but the presence of specific bacterial or parasitic infections and other diseases and the cause of death. In effect this legion of mummies provides us with a thirty-century-long study of health and disease.

In addition, we have the written history the Egyptians left us. Archaeologists have unearthed tens of thousands of papyrus fragments describing all aspects of life along the Nile in dynastic times. From translations of their meticulous and voluminous records we know how they lived and in what kinds of houses, where and how they worked, how much they were paid, and, most important for our purposes, what they ate.

What the Mummies Ate

The diet of the average Egyptian consisted primarily of carbohydrates. Their staple crops, wheat and barley, supplied a coarse stone-ground whole-wheat flour, which they baked into a flat bread and consumed in great quantity. In fact, during the later periods, the Egyptian army rationed each of its soldiers about five pounds of bread per day, a quantity so impressive that the Greeks of the time called these soldiers *artophagoi*, "the bread eaters."

Egyptian farmers cultivated a wide variety of fruits, such as grapes, dates, jujube, melons, peaches, olives, pears, pomegranates, carob, apples, and nuts, and several varieties of vegetables—mainly garlic, onions, lettuce, cucumbers, peas, lentils, and papyrus. They sweetened their food with honey (since sugar didn't arrive on the scene until about A.D. 1000) and used olive, safflower, linseed, and sesame oils for cooking and medicinal purposes.

The papyrus records tell us that the early Egyptians sat down to dine on a diet consisting primarily of bread, cereals, fresh fruit and vegetables, some fish and poultry, almost no red meat, olive oil instead of lard, and goat's milk for drinking and to make into cheese—a veritable nutritionist's nirvana. Except for papyrus, the Egyptians could have obtained their entire diet from the shelves of any health food store in America.

With such a bounty available, rich in all the foods believed to promote health and almost devoid of saturated fat and cholesterol, it would seem that the ancient Egyptians should have lived forever or at least should have lived long, healthy lives and died of old age in their beds. But did they? Let's look at the archaeological evidence.

What Ailed the Egyptians

We have two ways of estimating the health of these ancient people: searching the surviving papyrus writings of the time for any mention of diseases and examining the actual mummified remains of the ancient Egyptians. Through the science of paleopathology—the application of modern techniques of pathology and other scientific disciplines to the remains of early man, from bone fragments to entire preserved bodies—scientists can determine not only the state of health at the time of death but also the almost indiscernible responses of the flesh to the rigors of primitive life. Obviously the more complete the specimen, the more reliable the analysis. And when scientists can study many fairly intact remains, such as the enormous number of Egyptian mummies available, all from a particular time and place, they can spot disease trends and can speculate with a good deal of certainty about the health status of the population.

Certainly we would expect to find evidence of bacterial and parasitic infections, because at that time there were no antibiotic or antiparasitic medications—those were not developed until the twentieth century. And indeed we do find evidence of widespread infections and infestations. The ancient Egyptians suffered pneumonia, tuberculosis, probably leprosy, and many other less exotic bacterial infections, along with parasites that occur from drinking and bathing in contaminated water.

With no refined sugar in the diet, we would expect that the ancient Egyptians would have perfect teeth, right? Absolutely wrong. Mummies from all socioeconomic strata suffered terrible dental problems. Their teeth were worn down to such an extensive degree that both enamel and dentin were gone, exposing the soft pulp. Without this protective outer surface, the living tissue within the tooth dies, and the empty canal (the area dentists fill when they do a root canal) becomes a source of chronic infection, often leading to abscess formation. The incidence of actual tooth *decay* was not particularly high because the teeth were worn down to the nub before decay could set in.

The Egyptians also had severe gum disease, which most experts believe was caused by two factors—diet and poor dental hygiene. We know little of the oral hygiene habits of the ancient Egyptians, but we can suppose that they wouldn't be any worse than their primitive hunting-gathering ancestors, who weren't particularly afflicted with gum disease, which scientists always find with increasing frequency in societies ascending the ladder of civilization. It stands to reason that the "civilized" diet plays some role in its promotion.

Subsisting as they did on a diet of fresh fruits and vegetables and coarse whole-grain bread, at least we would not expect to find fat Egyptians. After all, the basic Egyptian diet is the very one most experts prescribe for weight loss today. But here is yet another health problem that doesn't correlate with our "healthy diet" paradigm: obesity. Many ancient Egyptians, based on examination of their mummified remains, weren't just a little overweight, but were actually fat. Paleopathologists have described huge folds of excess skin of a type and distribution that indicate the presence of severe obesity. People in that early age probably viewed excess fat much as we do today—not as a thing of beauty. But just as we find the pages of our magazines covered with pictures of slender models, so the ancient Egyptians painted and carved idealized pictures showing their citizens as slender, svelte in their form-fitting pleated linen garments. In view of this discrepancy between the actual and the idealized, it seems unlikely that the Egyptians actively worked to *become* obese—instead, as it does today, it probably just happened to them.

Finally, in view of the low-fat content of the diet, we would anticipate very little, if any, evidence of heart disease, but again, the low-fat, high-complex-carbohydrate paradigm fails the test. The evidence of heart and vascular disease found in the mummy and papyrus chronicles proves that cardiovascular disease occurred extensively throughout ancient Egypt.

When paleopathologists dissected the arteries of the Egyptian mummies, they did not find smooth, supple arterial walls but rather arteries choked with greasy, cholesterol-laden deposits that were often calcified, exhibiting an advanced stage of atherosclerotic disease. Many subjects had arteries that were scarred and thickened, indicating the presence of high blood pressure. Pathologists today find the same diseased changes when examining tissue from a victim of a heart attack, stroke, diabetes, or other disease found in conjunction with late-stage heart disease. In fact it appears that cardiovascular disease was as prevalent in ancient Egypt as it is in America today.

We have further proof that the ancient Egyptians suffered from heart disease. Among the enormous number of papyrus documents that have been discovered are several that were apparently medical textbooks of the time. One in particular, the papyrus *Ebers*, written in about 1500 B.C., describes the pain from heart disease:

> If thou examinest a man for illness in his cardia, and he has pains in his arms, in his breasts, and in one side of his cardia . . . it is death threatening him.

This account perfectly describes the ominous signs of an impending heart attack: pain in the left side of the chest radiating down the arms. Keep in mind that the average Egyptian enjoyed a much shorter life span than we do, and therefore the vast amount of arterial disease found in the mummified remains gives us a fair indication that "illnesses in their cardia" must have threatened death at a relatively early age.

So a picture begins to emerge of an Egyptian populace rife with disabling dental problems, fat bellies, and crippling heart disease. From the evidence, we know atherosclerotic cholesterol plaque and the effects of high blood pressure narrowed their arteries at a young age. Sounds a lot like the afflictions of millions of people in America today, doesn't it? The Egyptians didn't eat much fat, had no refined carbohydrates as we know them today, and ate almost nothing but whole grains, fresh fruits and vegetables, and fish and fowl, yet were beset with all the same diseases that afflict modern man. Modern man, who is exhorted to eat loads of whole grains, fresh fruits, and vegetables to prevent or reverse these diseases.

In the words of Aidan Cockburn (in *Mummies, Disease and Ancient Cultures*), founder of the Paleopathology Association and the first to bring together an interdisciplinary team of scientists to examine mummies with all the sophisticated equipment available today:

> Atheromatous disease of the arteries is . . . a common finding in mummies. Nowadays, a great deal of emphasis is placed on the stress of modern life or on modern diet as factors in the high incidence of this disorder in our present-day industrialized civilization, but the etiological influences were certainly there in the ancient world, and this fact should be taken into account in any theorizing regarding causation.[1]

What does all this mean in the great scheme of things? We think it means that there are some real problems with the low-fat, high-carbohydrate diet. Perhaps, you might argue, it simply indicates that the ancient Egyptians, maybe for genetic reasons, had difficulty dealing with a

[1] Interestingly, cancer was virtually nonexistent in ancient populations of both hunter-gatherers and agriculturalists, so diet may not be a major factor in cancer development. But remember that both protein and fat are crucial for a strong immune system—your first defense against cancer. There's a stronger case for heavy metal toxins as a cancer cause; the tissues of modern man have 10 times more lead than is found in ancient tissues, for instance.

high-carbohydrate diet physiologically and the same disorders wouldn't occur in other groups of ancient people on a similar diet. In fact, they do. Throughout history, when man has turned away from the traditional "prehistoric" diet that evolution designed him to eat to an agrarian (grain-based) one, this decline in health has recurred. We think you will find the following data comparing these two kinds of diets startling as well as fascinating.

The Diet We Were Meant to Eat

Most experts agree that game-hunting was the primary means of sustenance for our ancestors 700,000 years ago. From that time until the beginnings of agriculture (about 8,000 to 10,000 years ago), man lived on a diet composed predominantly of meat of one sort or another. In fact scientists estimate that from 60 to 90 percent of the calories these early people consumed were in the form of large and small game animals, birds, eggs, reptiles, and insects. The forces of natural selection acting over some 7,000 centuries shaped and molded our physiology to function optimally on a diet consisting predominantly of meat supplemented with roots, shoots, berries, seeds, and nuts. Only within the last 100 centuries have we reversed the order to become mainly carbohydrate eaters with meat as the supplement. This dietary reversal—from a diet providing, on average, about 75 percent of its calories from some sort of meat with the remainder coming from plants to one in which only 25 percent of calories come from meat, the rest from other sources—has taken place in approximately 400 to 500 generations, far short of the 1,000 to

10,000 generations deemed necessary by geneticists to allow any substantial genetic changes to take place. We may yet adapt to the high-carbohydrate agricultural diet, but history tells us it will probably take another 10,000 years.

Farming Away Fitness

The change to the agricultural diet created many health problems for early man. The fossil remains tell us that in preagricultural times human health was excellent. People were tall, lean, had well-developed, strong, dense bones, sound teeth with minimal, if any, decay, and little evidence of severe disease. After the advent of agriculture and a change in diet this picture of robust health began to deteriorate. Postagricultural man was shorter, had more brittle bones, extensive tooth decay, and a high incidence of malnutrition and chronic disease—a health picture similar to that of the Egyptians.

The remarkable thing about this generalized decline in health is that it occurred throughout the world. From the eastern Mediterranean to Peru, whenever people changed from a high-protein to a high-carbohydrate diet they became less healthy. In fact archaeologists consider this health disparity so predictable that when they unearth the skeletal remains of a prehistoric society they classify the people as hunters or farmers by the state of their bones and teeth. If the teeth are excellent and nondecayed and the bones strong, dense, and long, the people were hunter-gatherers; if the teeth are decayed and the bones frail and deformed, scientists know the remains are those of agriculturists.

THE DECLINE OF THE HARDIN VILLAGERS

A study by Claire M. Cassidy, Ph.D., an anthropologist with the University of Maryland and the Smithsonian Institution, compares two groups of people arising from the same genetic pool, living in the same area and in roughly the same-size community—two similar groups of people separated only by time and diet. Her paper, published in 1980, documents the health differences between hunter-gatherers and agriculturists (or farmers) as a function of diet. Dr. Cassidy's subjects were the skeletal remains of a group of farmers who inhabited an area identified as Hardin Village, in what is now Kentucky, from approximately 1500 to 1675 and a comparison group of hunter-gatherers who occupied a location called Indian Knoll centuries earlier, around 3000 B.C.

These two groups of people were similar in virtually all respects except diet: they lived in the same part of the country, had the same climate to deal with, and had the same types of wild plants and animals available. Both lived in about the same-size population group and were sedentary or semisedentary, removing the variable of degree of exercise. The farmers ate primarily "corn, beans, and squash. Wild plants and animals (especially deer, elk, small mammals, wild turkey, box turtle) provided supplements to a largely agricultural diet." The hunters, on the other hand, consumed "very large quantities of river mussels and snails. . . . Other meat was provided by deer, small mammals, wild turkey, box turtle, and fish; dog was sometimes eaten ceremonially." Dr. Cassidy sums up the differences: "The Hardin Village [farmers'] diet was high in carbohydrates, while that at Indian Knoll [hunters'] was high in protein."

She evaluated the skeletal remains of these two groups for bone and tooth changes indicative of iron-deficiency anemia, growth arrest from disease or malnutrition, and decay, and was able to determine the effects of the different diets on these otherwise similar peoples. She found the life expectancies for all ages lower and infant mortality higher among the farmers. Iron-deficiency anemia was nonexistent among the hunters but identified in 8.2 percent of the farmers. Growth arrests among the hunters were periodic and of short duration, possibly due to regularly occurring food shortages at certain times of the year, while growth arrests among the farmers were random and of much longer duration, indicating chronic malnutrition. More children suffered infection in the farmer population, with evidence of infection in the long bones thirteen times more common in farmers than hunters. Tooth decay, widespread among the farmers, rarely occurred among the hunters.[2] In Dr. Cassidy's words, "the agricultural Hardin Villagers were clearly less healthy than the Indian Knollers, who lived by hunting and gathering." She attributes this disparity in health to the difference in diet: "The health data provide convincing evidence that the diet of the agriculturists was the inferior of the two. The archaeological dietary data support this conclusion."

Dr. Cassidy is not alone in reporting this phenomenon. Many scientific papers have been written on this subject, and they present even the most passionate believer in the

---

[2] The farmers had an average of 6.74 decayed teeth, while the hunters had only 0.73. Interestingly, no hunter children had tooth decay, whereas some farmer children had developed cavities by the second year of life.

superiority of the high-carbohydrate diet with some food for thought. As Dr. Kathleen Gordon, like Dr. Cassidy an anthropologist at the Smithsonian Institution, writes in one such paper: "Not only was the agricultural 'revolution' not really so revolutionary at its inception, it has also come to represent something of a nutritional 'devolution' for much of mankind."

The Thrifty Gene: Store That Fat!

The anthropological record provides plenty of evidence that the change to a high-carbohydrate diet caused a general decline in health of people designed to eat a high-protein, carbohydrate-restricted diet. Why? What is there about a high-carbohydrate diet that causes the trouble?

There has been discussion in the scientific community for years about the so-called "thrifty gene." First used with reference to diabetes, this phrase has come to mean the genetic material that has been passed along to us by our prehistoric ancestors that allows us to better survive hunger and privation. Since periodic famines, brought on by game scarcity, heavy winters, droughts, or other natural disasters, were a part of prehistoric life, it makes sense that the people best suited to survive these deprivations would live to reproduce. Obviously this happened. Natural selection culled the weak and left a population that had the biochemistry and physiology necessary to squeeze every possible calorie from the food at hand and store it efficiently. This energy efficiency or biological thriftiness was precisely what we needed to survive in prehistoric times—but what about now?

When we eat a meal, we know that we are going to eat again in a few hours, but our enzymes and hormones don't. When the food comes in and is broken down into its components by our prehistoric digestive enzymes, it is absorbed into the blood and attacked by our primordial digestive hormones. Each calorie is put to work to meet the body's immediate demands with the remainder being stored as fat to be called on as needed. When the next meal comes along in four hours instead of four days, this whole process repeats. Since we eat meals regularly, we end up storing too much fat, which creates a new set of problems probably never experienced by prehistoric man.

The primary hormone involved in this entire process is insulin. Insulin is our main anabolic, or bodybuilding, hormone and is called into action each time we eat—especially if we eat or drink a food containing carbohydrates. Insulin increases the storage of fat, drives the sugar from the blood into the cells, and in general performs all the energy-conserving functions that allowed our ancestors to survive. Unfortunately, in our plentiful time of high-carbohydrate intake insulin works to our detriment. When levels of insulin become too high, as they do on our modern diet, this hormone causes us to retain sodium (and with it excess fluid), leading to high blood pressure; it causes our bodies to increase the production of cholesterol; it causes some damage to the arteries; it makes us store fat in a particularly unhealthy way; and it even can start the entire process leading to atherosclerosis and heart disease. All this treachery from a hormone that allowed us to survive prehistoric times.

The Bottom Line

Modern nutritional wisdom would predict that the diet of the ancient Egyptians—high in complex carbohydrates, low in fat, no refined sugar, almost no red meat—should have brought health, fitness, and longevity to the Egyptians of old. But it didn't.

Translations of the ancient Egyptian papyrus writings and modern examination of their mummified remains by pathologists tell us quite a different tale. The evidence speaks of a people afflicted with rotten teeth and severe atherosclerosis, suffering from elevated blood pressure and dying in their thirties with heart attacks. And contrary to the paintings of the willowy svelte figures in pleated linen that adorned their tomb walls, the large skin folds of the mummies tell us that their ancient low-fat, high-carbohydrate diet left them obese as well.

The Egyptians are not the only ancient people whose health suffered because of a diet consisting mainly of complex carbohydrates. An anthropologist examining skeletal remains of early man can tell immediately whether the bones and teeth belonged to a hunter-gatherer (mainly protein eater) or a farmer (mainly carbohydrate eater) simply by their condition. The hunters grew tall, with strong, well-formed bones and sound teeth, and the remains of the farmers usually show skeletal signs of malnutrition, stunted growth, and tooth decay.

For 700,000 years humans ate a diet of mainly meat, fat, nuts, and berries. Eight thousand years ago we learned to farm, and as our consumption of grains increased, our health declined. Genetic evolutionary changes take a minimum of 1,000 generations—or another 8,000 to 10,000 years to adapt.

Our metabolic machinery was designed to cope with an unpredictable food supply. We had to store food away for the lean times ahead. The hormone insulin did this for us. Unfortunately, a diet heavy in carbohydrate also sends our insulin levels soaring, and our body interprets this as a need to store calories, to make cholesterol, and to conserve water—all important to our survival way back then. Some of us inherit this conservation ability—a *thrifty gene*—in great measure. People who have this trait gain weight easily and have a more difficult time losing their excess, and the current nutritional low-fat, high-carbohydrate prescription leads to overweight and weight-related health problems even more quickly among them.

Appendix

Sources and Resources

Purveyors of Wild Game

Denver Buffalo Company
1120 Lincoln Street
Denver, CO 80203-9790
Phone: (800) BUY-BUFF; (800) 289-2833
Fax: (303) 831-1292
catalog available

Game Exchange/Polarica
105 Quint Street
San Francisco, CA 94124
Phone: (800) 426-3872
catalog available
    or
73 Hudson Street
New York, NY 10013
Phone: (800) 426-3487
catalog available

Game Sales International
2456 E. 13th Street
P.O. Box 7719
Loveland, CO 80537
Phone: (800) 729-2090

Cates Family Farm
5992 CTH T
Spring Green, WI 53588
Phone: (608) 588-2836

Coleman Natural Product
5140 Race Court Unit 4
Denver, CO 80216
Phone: (800) 442-8666

Prepackaged Nutritional Meal Replacement Products

If you would like more information about some of the high-quality-protein meal replacement products we use in our practice and how to incorporate them into your new nutritional strategy, call (800) 925-1373 or check our website at **www.eatprotein.com**.

Other Food Sources

The Soys Bluebook
P.O. Box 84
Bar Harbor, ME 04609
Resource guide to manufacturers and distributors of soy products worldwide.

Newsletter

We are in the process of preparing a newsletter for our patients. For subscription information, send your name and address to:
Newsletter
Colorado Center for Metabolic Medicine
7490 Clubhouse Road, Suite 103
Boulder, CO 80301
or check our website: **www.eatprotein.com**

Pertinent Worthwhile Reading

Neanderthin: A Cave Man's Guide to Nutrition
Ray Audette, Ph.D., Paleolithic Press
This interesting and well-written book adopts a true caveman and almost mystical approach to nutrition: if a caveman could hunt it or gather it to eat it, so can you. An approach more restrictive than we think necessary, but an interesting perspective from a bright and creative writer. Available for $12.00 plus $3.00 shipping and handling from:
Paleolithic Press
6009 Laurel Oaks
Dallas, TX 75248

Dr. Bernstein's Diabetes Solution
Richard K. Bernstein, M.D.
Little, Brown and Company Inc.
Dr. Bernstein, a long-suffering type I diabetic, has a fascinating history. He developed his methods of treatment

by experimenting on himself during his predoctor days,. when he was an engineer. He realized the benefits of the carbohydrate-restricted diet and tight control of blood sugars but was unable to penetrate the medical establishment despite his astounding success because his methods were not consistent with accepted medical wisdom. Rather than tilt at windmills, the 45-year-old Mr. Bernstein enrolled in medical school to give himself credibility. He wrote his first book while in medical school and since obtaining his M.D. degree he continues to write and has a private practice specializing in the treatment of diabetes. If you or someone you care about has either type of diabetes, get Dr. Bernstein's book. It contains a wealth of information on all aspects of diabetes care and is written by someone who truly knows his subject. We can't recommend this book highly enough.

The Zone
Barry Sears, Ph.D.
HarperCollins, 1995
Currently available in bookstores and written by a close friend of ours, this book looks at nutrition from an eicosanoid-modulating perspective. Although Dr. Sears takes a somewhat different approach from ours, the underlying science is fundamentally the same, and his book has great chapters on nutrition and chronic fatigue syndrome, cancer, heart disease and other chronic illnesses, and sports performance.

Motivational Tool

For $59.95 (plus $2.50 shipping), you can have an anatomically correct photograph of yourself at your ideal weight. If you have trouble imagining yourself thin, this photo on your refrigerator may be a powerful totem. Send a front-on whole-body shot plus a check to Sound Feelings, 7616 Lindley Avenue, Reseda, CA 91335. Call (818) 757-0600 for an order form. For more information, e-mail Sound Feelings: **info@soundfeelings.com.**

Bibliography

To access our complete research bibliography and learn more about the wealth of medical literature upon which we based our program, please check our website: **www.eatprotein.com.**

Becoming a Patient

For more information about becoming a patient at our clinic, check our website: **www.eatprotein.com.**

INDEX

and selenium, 182
sensitivity, 105–6, 122
serum test, 53–54
and vitamins, 175
working overtime, 34–37
See also Hyperinsulinemia
Iodine, 179
Ion channel, 179
Iron, 59, 177–78, 179, 198
Italian restaurant, 129

Japanese sushi/Teriyaki
restaurant, 130
Jenkins, Dr. David, 142
Jensen, Arthur R., 306
*Journal of the American
Medical Association*, 172
*Journal of Clinical
Endocrinology &
Metabolism, The*, 378
Junk food, 40–42, 125, 212

Kaplan, Dr. Norman, 298–99,
300
Kern, Dr. Fred, 387n
Ketoacidosis, 313
Ketones, 148–150, 309–10
Ketosis, 148, 149–50
Kidney function tests, 55
Kidneys, 36, 49, 59, 101,
138, 145–46, 182,
316–17, 318, 329
Kuter, Stan, 200, 201, 202–3,
206

LA, 345
Laboratory tests, 53–63
complete blood count, 59
hemoglobin A_1c, 57–58
lipid profile, 56
serum insulin, 53–54

SMA–24 or chemistry
profile, 54–56
thyroid panel, 59–63
12-lead electrocardiogram,
58
urinalysis, 59
Lean body mass (LBM),
92–93
in Phase I Worksheet, 117
in Phase II Worksheet, 119
Leprosy, 397
Letter on Corpulence
(Banting), 16
Light-headedness, 138
Linoleic acid, 10, 336–42,
345, 357
Lipid Levels, 61
Lipid profile, 56
Lipoprotein lipase, 304, 305
Lipoproteins, 366–73,
374–80
Liver, 35, 49, 97, 102, 309,
329, 364–68, 371, 375,
392
function tests, 55
Lovastatin (Mevacor),
372–73
Low-calorie, high-
carbohydrate, low-fat diet,
92–93
Low-fat, low-cholesterol diet,
44–45, 388
Lunch, 109, 153
in Daily Meal Outline, 126
menus, 217–23
in Phase I Intervention,
116
in Phase II Intervention,
118
See also meals (light and
speedy)

Macadamia oil, 101
Macronutrients, 7–8, 10
Macrophages, 322
Magnesium, 181, 185
Mahdah (Asian sage), 16
Main dishes, recipes for, 254–87
Males *See* Men
Malnutrition, 404, 407
Manganese, 185
Margarine, 341–43, 353, 358
Maximum Achievement (Tracy), 211
Meals (light and speedy), recipes for, 233–42
Meat, 172, 176, 350–51, 387–88, 401–3
in Phase I Worksheet, 117
in Phase II Worksheet, 119
in protein equivalency charts, 154–57
See also Muscle meats; Organ meats; Red meat
Men, 68
body fat for, 64, 72–75, 121
body weight, ideal, for, 83
body weight, lean, for, 75
hip and leg pattern for, 68
Menstrual cramps, 334
Menus, 216–23
Merrill, A. Roger, 188
Metabolic system, 45
correcting disturbances of, 103
and food plan, 103, 134–37
healing of, 50
and insulin, 24, 28, 32–37, 180
Mevacor. *See* Lovastatin

Mexican restaurant, 130
Micronutrients, 7, 100, 169, 171, 184
Milk, 176, 363
Minerals, 100, 177–84
chelates, 178–79, 185, 186
RDA for, 170
supplements, 179, 181, 184–86
See also Iron
Mitochondria, 303–4
Molybdenum, 179, 185
Monounsaturated fat, 101, 343, 352
Monounsaturated fatty acids, 345
Montaigne, Michel de, 360
Mot, Linda (pseud.), 325–26
Mummies, Disease and Ancient Cultures (Cockburn), 400
Muscle growth, through exercise, 188, 195–99, 205
Muscle meats, 176, 182
Myocardial ischemia, 321

National Center for Health Statistics, 38
National Cholesterol Awareness Program Step Two Diet, 21
National Health and Nutrition Examination Survey, second (NHANES II), 38
National Research Council's Committee on Diet and Health, 39–40
Nervous system, 363
Netzer, Corinne T., 95

Roasts, 352
Rudman, Dr. Daniel, 190
Running, 200, 202

Safflower oil, 345
Salads, 91
  recipes for, 249–54
Salt, 28, 49, 138
  mineral, 178
  potassium, 145
Saturated fat, 101, 341, 345, 350–53, 371
Scavenger cells. *See* Macrophages
Schwarzenegger, Arnold, 187, 302
Scurvy, 172
Seafood, 176, 181
  See also Fish
Sears, Dr. Barry, 331
Seeds, 175, 182
Selenium, 182, 185
Serum insulin test, 53–54
Sesame oil, 101, 343, 345
Sex hormones, 362, 392
Sinoatrial node, 320
Skin rashes, 97
Sleep, 204, 350
  stage III, 192
  stage IV, 191–92
Sleep apnea, 124
Sleeplessness, 150
SMA-24 or chemistry profile, 54–55
Smooth muscle cells, 317, 322
  arterial, 35, 36
Snacks, 91, 99, 109, 112–15, 116, 118, 126, 153, 197, 209, 217–23
  recipes for, 240–41, 253

Sodium, 58, 138, 178n, 182, 316, 406
Soft cheese, in protein equivalency charts, 154–57
Soft drinks, 152
Soups, recipes for, 242–49
Southern Medical Journal, 387
Soybean oil, 344
Starches, 52, 91, 176, 180, 390–91
  controlling, 107–11
Steaks, 97, 351
  See also Rib steaks
Stefansson, Vilhjalmur, 9n, 17, 148, 172
Stillman, Dr. Irwin, 17
Strength, muscular, 197–98
Stress, 332, 340–41, 358
Stroke, 25, 174, 381, 399
Stryer, Dr. Lubert, 149
Sugar, 10, 41–42, 49, 52, 91, 143, 151–52, 180, 289, 328–29, 397
  controlling, 107–11
Sunflower oil, 345
Sweets, 152–53, 289
Syndrome X, 300, 384

Tarnower, Dr. Herman, 17
Testosterone (hormone), 362, 392
Thiamine, 169, 176
  See also Vitamin B$_1$
Thin So Fast (Eades), 14n, 202, 314
This Slimming Business (Yudkin), 17
Thompson, Vance, 16

ABOUT THE AUTHORS

MICHAEL R. EADES, M.D., author of *Thin So Fast,* and MARY DAN EADES, M.D., author of *The Doctor's Complete Guide to Vitamins and Minerals*, live in Little Rock, Arkansas, where they practice bariatric (weight loss) and general family medicine. They are the founders of Medi-Stat Medical Clinics.

REFRAMING
THE PATH TO
SCHOOL LEADERSHIP

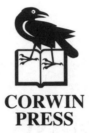

**CORWIN
PRESS**

The Corwin Press logo—a raven striding across an open book—
represents the happy union of courage and learning. We are a
professional-level publisher of books and journals for K-12
educators, and we are committed to creating and providing
resources that embody these qualities. Corwin's motto is "Success
for All Learners."

REFRAMING THE PATH TO SCHOOL LEADERSHIP

A GUIDE FOR TEACHERS AND PRINCIPALS

LEE G. BOLMAN
TERRENCE E. DEAL

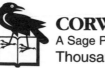

CORWIN PRESS, INC.
A Sage Publications Company
Thousand Oaks, California

For information:

Corwin Press, Inc.
A Sage Publications Company
2455 Teller Road
Thousand Oaks, California 91320
E-mail: order@corwinpress.com

Sage Publications Ltd.
6 Bonhill Street
London EC2A 4PU
United Kingdom

Sage Publications India Pvt. Ltd.
M-32 Market
Greater Kailash I
New Delhi 110 048 India

Printed in the United States of America

Library of Congress Cataloging-in-Publication Data

Bolman, Lee G.
  Reframing the path to school leadership: A guide for teachers and principals /
Lee G. Bolman, Terrence E. Deal.
      p. cm.
Includes bibliographical references (p.   ).
  ISBN 0-7619-4606-3 (c)
  ISBN 0-7619-4607-1 (p)
  1. School management and organization. 2. Educational leadership.
I. Deal, Terrence E. II. Title.
  LB2805 .B58 2002
  371.2--dc21
                                                2002000165

This book is printed on acid-free paper.

06 07 08 09 10 9 8 7 6 5

Acquisitions Editor:	Robb Clouse
Associate Editor:	Kylee Liegl
Editorial Assistant:	Erin Buchanan
Copy Editor:	Karen Slaught
Production Editor:	Denise Santoyo
Typesetter:	Siva Math Setters, Chennai, India
Cover Designer:	Michael Dubowe

Contents

Acknowledgments

Many of the ideas in this book were stimulated by our research on school leadership under the auspices of the National Center for Educational Leadership, funded under grants from the U.S. Department of Education. Our friends in Washington, David Stevenson and Ron Anson, were steady sources of both support and constructive criticism, and we are very grateful to both. We also owe much to our colleagues in NCEL for their ideas and encouragement. Ideas from Susan Johnson's work on the school as a workplace and from Carol Weiss's work on decision making are echoed in this book. Reva Chatman's doctoral thesis, "Fresh Roses," a novel about beginning teachers, and Tracy Kidder's wonderful chronicle of teacher Chris Zajac in *Among Schoolchildren* gave us both inspiration and a deeper understanding of classroom life. William Greenfield, Thomas P. Johnson, Ann Lieberman, Gayle Moller, Emmanuel L. Paparella, and Carrie Sedinger all provided very helpful comments and suggestions on earlier versions of the manuscript. Homa Aminmadani and Linda Corey provided terrific administrative support.

Our spouses, Sandy Deal and Joan Gallos, provided more than the usual support and love—without which writing would be dreary, if not impossible. Each also brought her own special expertise. Sandy Deal's extensive experience as a clinical psychologist greatly strengthened the teacher–student interactions in the book. Joan Gallos used her work on gender issues in the classroom and in adult life to provide many helpful insights; Joan's feel for good storytelling also strengthened this work in many ways. Many educators in the United States and abroad have been *our* mentors and guides, and we have learned more from them than we can ever say.

About the Authors

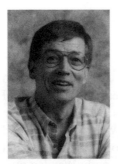

Lee G. Bolman is the Marion Bloch/Missouri Chair in Leadership at the University of Missouri-Kansas City. An author, teacher, consultant, and speaker, he has written numerous books on leadership and organizations with coauthor Terry Deal, including best-sellers *Leading With Soul: An Uncommon Journey of Spirit (1995, 2001)* and *Reframing Organizations: Artistry, Choice, and Leadership (1991, 1997),* as well as *The Path to School Leadership (1993)* and *Becoming a Teacher Leader (1994).*

Bolman holds a BA in History and a PhD in Organizational Behavior from Yale University. He lives in Kansas City, Missouri, with his wife, Joan Gallos, and the two youngest of his children, Christopher and Bradley.

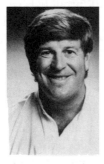

Terrence E. Deal is the Irving R. Melbo Professor at University of Southern California's Rossier School. He is an internationally famous lecturer and author who resides in San Louis Obispo, California, with his wife, Sandy. He has written numerous books on leadership and organizations. In addition to those written with Lee Bolman, he is the coauthor of *Corporate Cultures* (with Alan Kennedy, 1982) and *Shaping School Culture* (with Kurt Peterson, 1999).

Bolman and Deal's books have been translated into more than ten languages.

Introduction

I f you're a teacher or principal who wants to become a better
leader, we wrote this book for you. It's intended as a portable
companion, a mentor that is available anytime you need advice or
counsel. You can take it with you, look it over after hours, consult it
when trouble arises, and use it to stimulate a reflective dialogue—on
your own or with colleagues. The book is filled with the words and
wisdom of two seasoned veterans: Margaret Juhl, a master teacher,
and Brenda Connors, a wise and warm veteran principal. Though
they are fictional characters, they are deeply rooted in the real-world
life of contemporary schools. They've been there, and they know
what they're talking about because of wisdom gleaned from experience. They are exemplars for the countless teachers and principals
who are blessed with unusual leadership skills and savvy.

A unique feature of this book is its focus on the intersection
between life as a new teacher and the challenges faced by a novice
principal. Though teachers and principals work in the same build-
ings, they often occupy very different worlds. Absence of mutual
understanding and appreciation only exacerbates the inevitable tensions any working relationship will produce. The better each party
understands the other's reality, the easier it will be for them to find
mutually acceptable ways to fulfill the interests of both the school
and its students.

Novice teachers and principals often bounce from one unpleasant surprise to another. Yet the unending stream of challenges and
pitfalls are normal and highly predictable—if you know what to look
for. The purpose of this book is to help you decipher what is really
going on in schools to avoid the sinking feeling of being caught off
guard. The key to becoming a highly effective teacher or principal is

1

to develop powerful habits of mind—profoundly practical ways of thinking about schools and classrooms. Most professionals painfully learn these lessons in the school of hard knocks—through trial and error. This book offers a quicker, less painful route to achieving the same goal.

Your first challenge as a new professional is to get the lay of the land. You need a way to make sense out of a confusing and messy terrain so that you can master what's going on and figure out your options. In diagnosing any situation, you will draw on past experience and learning. These have given you mental lenses that you rely on to define and frame reality. Even when your lenses are off target, you're stuck with them, because they're all you've got. Without them, your world would be a senseless blur. For a concrete example, study the following image.

好

Unless you read Chinese characters, the image makes no sense. If you saw it somewhere, perhaps on a menu in a Chinese restaurant, you would probably overlook it. But that's only because you can't decode it. If you could read Chinese, you would recognize it immediately as a very common word. Take another look, and you'll notice that it is composed of two separate characters. Each of these can be a word by itself, and each is a simplified picture of a type of person. Look at the character on the left. What kind of person could it represent? How about the character on the right?

The character on the left is a woman. You can see legs, a body, and a neck. The one on the right is a child. You can see it holding its arms out as if to hug the woman. You might imagine that woman-child together would mean *girl* or *daughter.* But the logic of Chinese script isn't often literal. Together, the two characters form the word *hao,* which means good. To the ancient Chinese, and maybe to you as well, portraying a woman and a child together seems like a pretty good thing.

The key point is, if you don't have good mental tools for decoding everyday life in schools, a lot of things might as well be written in Chinese. They won't make sense, and you probably won't pay them much attention. The trouble is, you'll be ignoring the vital clues you need to understand what's going on and what you need to do.

Your prior training has provided concepts to help you understand many day-to-day specifics—individual students, teaching methods, curriculum, budgets, maybe even school law. But you probably have received less help in understanding leadership or in viewing schools as complex systems. University education typically gives short shrift to broadening your vision, sorting out social dynamics in your classroom or school, or working with others. The solution of how to transform schools from the isolating and under-rewarding environments they so often become therefore looms as an overwhelming mystery.

The two of us spend much of our time working with people in so-called "leadership positions"—administrative and managerial roles existing in every organization around the world—armies, businesses, hospitals, or governments. The sad truth is that would-be leaders fail more often than they succeed. Because almost no one sets out to flunk the test, we have to ask why so many do. We have repeatedly found that administrators and executives are more successful when they can look at things from more than one angle. The best leaders use multiple frames or lenses, each offering a different perspective on common challenges. The ability to use multiple frames has three advantages: (1) each can be coherent, focused, and powerful; (2) the collection can be more comprehensive than any single one; and (3) only when you have multiple frames can you *reframe.* Reframing is a conscious effort to size up a situation from multiple perspectives and then find a new way to handle it. In times of crisis and overload, you will inevitably feel confused and overwhelmed if you are stuck with only one option.

Think about how to deal with a particularly difficult student or parent. Sometimes, when trapped in an inappropriate approach, you become immobilized, and the student or parent controls the situation. Other times, you may plunge mindlessly forward into reckless and misguided action. You fly off the handle and make things worse. When we don't know what to do, we do more of what we know—we're only digging ourselves into a deeper hole.

We have identified four frames that are commonly used by teachers as well as administrators (Bolman & Deal, 1997):

1. The *political frame* points out the limits of authority and the inevitability that resources are almost always too scarce to fulfill all demands. Schools and classrooms are arenas where individuals and groups jockey for power. Everyone is caught up in this swirling

political vortex. Goals emerge from bargaining and compromise among competing interests rather than from rational analysis. Conflict becomes an inescapable by-product of everyday life. If handled properly, it can be a source of constant energy and renewal.

2. The *human resource* frame is a favorite among teachers and principals. It highlights the importance of individual needs and motives. It assumes that schools and classrooms, as other social systems, work best when needs are satisfied in a caring, trusting work environment. Showing concern for others and providing ample opportunities for participation and shared decision making are among the ways to enlist people's commitment and involvement. Many teachers and principals have found that involving others in shaping decisions gives them a sense of ownership in what happens each day.

3. The *structural frame* emphasizes productivity and posits that classrooms and schools work best when goals and roles are clear and when efforts of individuals and groups are highly coordinated through authority, policies, and rules as well as through more-informal strategies. Holding people accountable for their responsibilities and setting measurable standards are an important part of this rational approach.

4. The *symbolic frame* centers attention on culture, meaning, belief, and faith. Every school or classroom, as does every human group, creates symbols to cultivate commitment, hope, and loyalty. Symbols govern behavior through shared values, informal agreements, and implicit understandings. Stories, metaphors, heroes and heroines, rituals, ceremonies, and play add zest and existential buoyancy to an enterprise. The school becomes a joyful way of life rather than a sterile or toxic place of work.

In dealing with leadership challenges, most educators rely primarily on the human resource or structural lenses. Yet, many of the situations you face are highly charged politically and emotionally packed symbolically. Even young and inexperienced educators have to use power to get things done and create symbols to anchor meaning and hope. A school or classroom is a jungle and a cathedral as much as it is a family or a production system. If you sometimes feel that each day spawns an endless series of ambushes and pitfalls, reframing can help.

In our teaching and consulting, we have presented these ideas to thousands of professionals worldwide. As they learn and apply the frames, they regularly notice three things:

1. The frames are powerful, memorable tools.

2. The frames help people see things they once overlooked and come to grips with what is really going on.

3. When individuals reframe, they see new possibilities and become more versatile and effective in their responses.

This book offers the same lessons to principals and teachers. In a series of intimate and intense dialogues between a newcomer and a seasoned veteran, the novice comes to see troublesome situations more clearly, to anticipate trouble before it arises, and to develop more comprehensive and powerful leadership strategies. Join us for a bumpy, exhilarating ride through a year at Pico School. Meet Joan Hilliard, a new teacher who struggles with the same challenges every new teacher confronts. Also get to know her boss, Jaime Rodriguez, a new principal who barely squeaks through his first year. We deliberately made both characters highly committed and talented young professionals who persist in the face of obstacles and learn from their mistakes. Both are blessed with very helpful colleagues (as well as a few daunting opponents). We have all seen plenty of pessimistic accounts of what's wrong with schools. We wanted to provide a more optimistic view—a hopeful image of the possibilities for classroom and school leadership.

OUTLINE OF THE BOOK

Chapter 1, "A New Teacher's First Day," takes Joan Hilliard through her first exciting but troubling day at work. In Chapter 2, "Getting Started on the Right Foot," Hilliard reflects on her interactions with veteran teacher Margaret Juhl regarding the disastrous opening faculty meeting with new principal Jaime Rodriguez. As players get to know each other, they need to go beyond personalities to see new possibilities for building more effective relationships.

Chapter 3, "A New Principal Finds a Wise Friend," brings the rookie principal and a wise veteran, Brenda Connors, together. Connors helps Rodriguez sort through the confusion of his new job to get a better understanding of what is happening and what he can do about it.

In Chapter 4, "The Old Guard and the New Principal," Rodriguez is dismayed to find that his efforts to take charge and set directions are generating far more conflict and opposition than support or appreciation. In Chapter 5, "The Tracking Wars: School Politics at Work," Hilliard and a group of her colleagues become enthusiastic about building the school's commitment to the district's new inclusion policy. They are disappointed by resistance from other teachers. Margaret talks to Joan about political dynamics in schools and explains how to map them to be more effective. In Chapter 6, "Sagging Morale," the appearance of a vicious, anonymous newsletter alerts Rodriguez to significant morale problems among the teachers. Brenda Connors guides him through basic human resource frame issues: individual needs, morale, participation, and empowerment. Chapter 7, "Student Discipline: Who's Really in Charge?" explores often-neglected issues of school structure. When an effort to revise the discipline policy gets hopelessly bogged down, Connors helps Rodriguez see that the process was unintentionally designed for failure. After clarifying goals, roles, and accountability, the school finally develops a policy that works. Chapter 8, "Standards," looks at the standards movement and its impact in the real world of schools and classrooms.

In Chapter 9, "The End of the Year: Symbols and Culture in Schools," Rodriguez wonders why he is still haunted by his predecessor's ghost. Connors helps him understand the symbolic issues of meaning, faith, and culture. Key members of the school's informal network develop a powerful and moving ceremony of celebration and transition, freeing the school to move forward. In Chapter 10, "'I'm Just a Great Teacher!'" Joan wonders why many of her veteran colleagues have lost the spark and spirit that first brought them to teaching. They lament years of low pay, lack of respect, and bureaucratic frustrations. They come to realize that, at a deeper level, they face a crisis of meaning and faith. In developing a celebration of teaching to open the fall term, they reenergize themselves and create a transforming experience for Pico's teaching staff. In Chapter 11, "Teaching and Leading: Finding a Balance," the collapse of Joan's relationship with her longtime boyfriend, Larry, becomes the catalyst for a schoolwide discussion about how educators can balance commitments to career, family, and private life.

Chapter 12, "A Talk About Values," relates the four frames to ethics and moral leadership. Rodriguez and Connors explore values embedded in each of the frames and discuss the challenges of dealing with the dilemmas that arise from ethical conflicts. Chapter 13, "The Essence of Teaching: Leaving a Legacy," begins when Margaret Juhl is stricken with breast cancer. The entire Pico community rallies. Her bout with mortality leads to a dialogue between Margaret and Joan about the purposes and values underlying teaching as a profession. In Chapter 14, "Passing the Torch," Joan Hilliard confronts tragedy and loss, looks deep within herself, and finds the inner strength to rededicate herself to her calling. The story comes full circle as Hilliard and Rodriguez become mentors for another generation of school leaders.

The dialogues between Hilliard and Juhl and Rodriguez and Connors are much like those we have had many times over the years with fellow educators. Our role is typically to listen and pose questions rather than to provide answers. Good questions help people to see things in new ways and recognize promising leadership opportunities that are there all along. When school leaders can reframe situations, they become more confident and certain. They feel less anxious and overwhelmed. Most important, they are more effective and get things done.

We hope you will find the conversations both lively and informative. We grounded the book in the real world of schools and in the experiences of practicing teachers and administrators. The book offers a return to an old-fashioned approach to learning a craft. The educators in these pages, even the savvy veterans, are far from having all the answers to the mysteries of school leadership. But they are grappling with many of the same questions and issues important to you. Hopefully, you will find yourself identifying and relating their experiences to yours. Even better, you'll be able to think about what you can learn from both their triumphs and their stumbles. In the process, you will probably find new ideas and insights to help with the challenges you face. We hope that the dialogues will stimulate you to think more deeply about yourself and your leadership. Teachers and principals are among America's most important leaders. Ask a random sample of adults to name the most important leader they have ever known. Many will light up as they remember a caring and gifted teacher or principal who inspired them. Above all, we hope that the book will help you to find new paths to confidence and success, as well as to deepen your contribution to students and others who count on you for guidance and inspiration.

PART I

A Pair of Rookies

CHAPTER ONE

A New Teacher's First Day

J oan Hilliard could feel the smile on her face as she stepped from
her car. They weren't the best wheels in the country, but they
were hers, a token of four years spent working in a brokerage firm.
Joan had always wanted to be a teacher, but she had finished college
at the wrong time. To her great disappointment, she couldn't land a
teaching position. She had still wanted her own classroom but
decided that any job was better than nothing. The brokerage firm had
paid well, and she felt better for the experience. She had learned
about herself, how to work with other adults, and what life at work
was all about. Above all, she felt more confident. She had learned to
cope in a demanding and stressful environment. That experience had
to help in a classroom full of kids.

She was delighted to get a teaching assignment at Pico School.
It looked like a friendly place from the outside. The surrounding
neighborhood had declined from its earlier glory, but the school had
green lawns, well-trimmed shrubbery, and lots of large, lattice-paned
windows. Built in the 1940s, the school had much of the architec-
tural charm that Joan remembered from the schools of her childhood. As she walked through the arched entryway, she noticed the
vaguely familiar smells of new wax and summer mustiness. As she
turned down the corridor leading to the principal's office, she
noticed a tall, broad-shouldered man with hands on hips, scrutiniz-
ing the sheen on the floor. She guessed correctly that this was the
custodian, admiring his work before hundreds of student feet turned
it into a mosaic of scuff marks.

As she moved closer, the man looked up and smiled as if he had
expected her. "You must be Joan Hilliard. Welcome to Pico. I'm Bill

Hill, the chief custodian. Let me know if I can help you get settled. I'll stop by occasionally to see how you're doing and let you know what's going on."

"Is this the way to the principal's office?" asked Joan, slightly puzzled about what the custodian might have to offer that would be of interest to her.

"Straight ahead, second door on the left," Hill replied. "You were a stockbroker, huh? Not as fancy here. You'll have to buy most of your own supplies. Of course, our kids are a lot different from the adults that you've been working with. They need a lot of discipline, and a lot of caring, too. My own philosophy is that . . ."

"Thank you very much, Mr. Hill. I'm sorry I can't chat longer, but I don't want to be late for my meeting with Mr. Rodriguez."

"Oh, don't worry, he's new, too. I just hope he's as good as our old principal, Mr. Bailey. We worked together for years. Wonderful man. Anyway, you run along. We'll have plenty of time to talk later. It's good to have a new player on our team."

Joan continued down the hall, all the while trying to make sense out of her encounter with Bill Hill. "You'd think he ran the place. He'll probably read what I put on the board before he erases it. At my old job, the custodians never gave advice on how the market was doing."

As she opened the glass door labeled "Principal's Office," Joan's reverie was interrupted by a cheerful voice. "Yoo-hoo, Ms. Hilliard, welcome to Pico!" The voice belonged to a smiling, gray-haired woman wearing a "Pico Pride" T-shirt over a pair of faded blue jeans. "I'm Phyllis Gleason, the school secretary. Mr. Rodriguez got called to the superintendent's office unexpectedly. He'll fill you in on the school and your assignment when he gets back. In the mean-time, he asked me to show you around. Would you like a cup of coffee before we start?"

"Sure, why not?"

As Phyllis went off in search of coffee, the door to an office marked "Assistant Principal" opened, and a short, square-shoul-dered, graying man walked out. He looked at Joan, frowned, and asked, "Who are you?"

Both his tone and crew cut reminded Joan of a Marine drill sergeant. She was surprised at how nervous she felt. "Oh, uh, I'm sorry. I'm Joan Hilliard, and I . . ."

"Oh, yeah!" the man interrupted, with the commanding tone of someone who expected to be listened to. "I heard about you. No teaching experience. Just what we need. You sure as hell didn't learn anything about classroom control from a bunch of stockbrokers. Most of them don't even know anything about the market, much less about handling kids." With that, he marched forcefully out of the office just as Phyllis returned with the coffee.

Joan must have looked as crestfallen as she felt, because Phyllis seemed to understand immediately what had happened. "Oh, you met Mr. Shepherd."

"I didn't exactly meet him," Joan replied. "He didn't bother to tell me who he is. Is he always so, um . . .?" Joan paused, looking for a discreet way to phrase her question.

"Gruff? Oh, don't take it personally. His bark is worse than his bite. He's the same with everyone."

"He's the assistant principal?"

"Yes, been here 10 years. Some people thought he might be the next principal. But the superintendent felt that Mr. Shepherd should do what he does best. He's *awfully* strong on discipline."

Did Phyllis intend praise or veiled criticism of the assistant principal? Joan wasn't sure. She decided not to press the issue. She wondered if the principal would be as abrupt as Sam Shepherd. She was disappointed to find that the secretary was taking charge of her orientation. As Phyllis started to lead her around the building, Joan wondered if the tour would simply be a time filler. But her doubts gradually turned to awe and admiration. Phyllis seemed to know everything and shared it all in loving detail, as if she had witnessed everything firsthand. With unflagging enthusiasm, Gleason introduced Joan to everyone they encountered, and Joan was impressed with the warmth of the responses. Joan was even more amazed by Gleason's ability to field questions on just about everything—schedules, materials, children, parents—you name it.

"They treat her like the school oracle—knows all, tells all, whatever she says is the way it is," thought Joan to herself. "Maybe Phyllis is really in charge around here." It was only as they neared the end of the tour that Joan realized how much of her own background and ideas about teaching she had shared with Phyllis. "She seems as interested in my thoughts about teaching as Bill Hill did," mused Joan.

Phyllis stopped in front of a door with an opaque window marked 208. She took Joan inside a spacious classroom and said, "This is your room this year. What do you think? Maybe it's a little plain compared to what you're used to. But within these four walls, you're the boss."

"It's great! Lots of windows and plenty of wall space and bookshelves. The walls are a little bare, but we'll take care of that in no time." Joan's mind was flooded with a thousand thoughts. She had waited a long time for this moment. She tried to imagine the empty desks filled with students. Her students. Her classroom.

Phyllis waited for a few moments while Joan took it all in. "I'll leave you alone for a while to think about what else you'll need. Whatever it is, I'll try to get it for you."

"Thanks, Phyllis," said Joan. Then a question occurred to her. "Who had this room before me?"

"Oh, well, him," Phyllis replied. "He didn't stay long. Nice young man. Smart, too. But he had a little trouble with discipline. The noise and the fights were the biggest problem. It *was* entertaining to walk by his classroom. Never a dull moment. But don't let that worry you. I'm sure you'll be different. Just remember not to smile before December. And anything you need to know, come to me." Phyllis smiled once again and started back to the principal's office, turning her head only to acknowledge Joan's "Thank you."

After her rescheduled meeting with Jaime Rodriguez, Joan mulled over her morning's encounters. Nothing was quite what she had expected. Why did the secretary and the custodian loom so large in the affairs of the school? How many people would be looking over her shoulder and giving her advice on how to teach? She thought about raising her concerns with Jaime Rodriguez but thought better of it. He seemed friendly and genuinely pleased that she was joining the Pico faculty, but she didn't want to sound like an idiot. Still, the two had formed an almost instant bond as they realized what they shared—both were new and nervous. Joan could hardly believe her luck in finding a principal who seemed so supportive and easy to work with.

The day's thoughts were still spinning in Joan's mind as she walked to her car for the drive home. Just as she was opening the front door of her car, she heard someone calling her name. She turned her head and saw a group of teachers chatting in the parking lot. One of them, a male who fit Joan's stereotype of a veteran football coach, came over. "Joan Hilliard?" he said as he walked over and offered his hand. "I'm Phil Leckney. My classroom is just down the hall from yours. Welcome to Pico. Some of us are headed over to Andy's Café. Would you like to join us?"

Joan felt torn. She had promised to meet her boyfriend, Larry, in half an hour. After hesitating, she replied, "Well, I can stay for only a little while, but I'd love to."

The conversation at Andy's reinforced Joan's feeling that she had come to the right school. Her new colleagues laughed heartily when she told of her encounters with Bill Hill and Phyllis Gleason.

"To understand Bill," Margaret Juhl responded, "come in some morning at 7:30 and go to the cafeteria. You'll see the free breakfast kids. And you'll see that Bill is a big brother for just about everyone in the room. He knows all the students and a lot of the parents, too. Bill grew up a few blocks from here. He probably knows more people in the neighborhood than anyone else at Pico."

"Well, it might be a draw between him and Phyllis," Phil Leckney chimed in.

"True," said Margaret. "She's sort of a combination of Dear Abby, Diane Sawyer, and General Patton. The key thing to remember is the line from the old song, 'You can get anything you want, at Phyllis's restaurant.' "

Joan joined everyone else's laughter. As the group quieted down, Joan was caught off guard by a question from Vivian Chu. Chu, another veteran, had not said much until she turned to Joan to ask, "You met with Mr. Rodriguez today, didn't you? How did it go?" Joan felt every eye at the table turn to her. It dawned on her that her colleagues were as curious as she was about Pico's new principal.

As Phil Leckney put it, "He's an unknown. Phil Bailey was a great guy. Not Mr. Superprincipal, maybe, but he was pretty supportive, and he let us teach. New principals are all alike. They want to save the world and change everything. They don't understand the idea that if it ain't broke, don't fix it. How hard will it be to break this guy in?"

No one seemed to know the answer. The consensus was that they would learn a lot more the next day at the opening faculty meeting of the new school year. Then the conversation shifted to Joan's experience in the business world. Her colleagues peppered her with questions about what she did, what it was like, and, to her embarrassment, how much money she made. It almost felt as if they wished they had tasted another career themselves to find out if the grass was greener somewhere else. The conversation at Andy's was so engrossing that Joan was startled to look at her watch and notice that she was a half hour late to meet Larry. Bidding her colleagues a hasty farewell, she rushed off. On balance, she felt, it had been a great day. She just hoped that Larry was not too miffed that she was late.

CHAPTER TWO

Getting Started on the Right Foot

S o, when are you going to be through today?"
The edge in Larry's voice was jarring. He was still in bed, and Joan was just putting the final touches on her teaching costume.

"I'm not sure, Larry," she said carefully. "Margaret and I are meeting with the principal to talk about his opening sermon. You remember, I told you about it."

"Oh, yeah. Rodriguez did his vision thing, and Margaret cut him off at the knees."

"Well, not quite," said Joan, as she thought back a few days to the first faculty meeting of the new school year. She remembered it vividly. She knew that Rodriguez had wanted to get off on the right foot as much as she did. She had entered the first faculty meeting with optimism and excitement. After a few preliminaries, Rodriguez began to speak about his vision for the school. Joan had initially felt excited about his image of a child-centered school in which all students were expected to succeed and to achieve at their full potential. In her previous job, there had never seemed to be any real sense of mission beyond making money.

Rodriguez had seemed tense, but he delivered his message with conviction, even fervor. Joan soon realized, however, that many of her colleagues didn't share her excitement. Some looked bored; others appeared openly resistant. A few rows behind her, she could hear Phil Leckney making snide comments to those nearby.

When Rodriguez finished, he asked for questions. At first, none came. The silence was oppressive. Joan could not remember when she had felt more tension in a room. The stony silence broke only when Margaret Juhl asked, "Shouldn't you get to know this school and how we do things before you preach about how we should teach?"

Joan was startled by Margaret's bluntness and felt pained when she glanced at Jaime Rodriguez. He looked stunned, almost frozen in place. Joan wished she had the courage to go over and give him a hug. "He looks like he needs help," she thought to herself in the seconds before another young teacher, Carlos Cortez, leapt to his feet and spoke with obvious anger in his voice.

"The man just got here and you people don't want to give him a chance. Mr. Rodriguez is saying things someone has needed to say for a long time. I'm getting pretty tired of people who think this school is so perfect that we can't improve." Cortez's outburst triggered a series of sharply worded exchanges between older and younger teachers. Joan began to wonder what she had got herself into. She had never seen anything like this in her old firm. The climate there had been competitive, even cutthroat, but people never went for the jugular. She was relieved when Rodriguez quickly moved to adjourn the meeting.

After the meeting, Joan asked Margaret Juhl to explain what had happened.

"Well," said Juhl, "I'm still sorting it out myself. Jaime is probably feeling a little shell-shocked, wondering what hit him. And he may be pretty angry at me."

"Aren't you worried about that?" Joan asked.

"Only if he stays angry. He could make life difficult for me if he wanted to," Margaret replied.

"Do you think maybe you should apologize, or something?" Joan asked.

"Of course not. He may not know it yet," said Margaret with a smile, "but I was doing him a favor."

"That was a favor?" Joan asked incredulously.

"You were there. You saw all those stony faces. He meant well, but his speech flopped. He didn't have a clue about what was going wrong. It may take a little while, but I hope he'll realize that I was telling him what he needed to hear—why the teachers didn't like his opening salvo."

"But, what if he doesn't listen?" asked Joan.

"We'll know soon," answered Margaret. "He called me and asked for a meeting."

"And what about Carlos?" Joan looked worried.

"I'll talk to Carlos. He may think I'm leading a charge to undermine the district's first Hispanic principal. The truth is, I want Jaime to succeed as much as Carlos does. If you really want to torpedo an administrator, you don't do it with a frontal assault. It's safer and more effective to kill them softly behind the scenes. Silent resistance and passive aggression are deadly. You may have seen it happen in your last job. Rodriguez was digging himself into a hole. Someone had to tell him. And remind him about the first law of holes."

"What's the first law of holes?"

"When you're in one, stop digging!" said Margaret with a laugh. "Anyway, if I talk to Carlos one-on-one about how we can help the new principal succeed, I think we can have a meeting of the minds."

"I don't know," said Joan skeptically. "He seemed pretty upset."

"Joan, when I was younger, I used to pussyfoot around disagreement and conflict. I was afraid of getting people angry or upset. But I slowly realized I was just sweeping things under the rug until the lumps got so big we tripped over them. Teaching is not an exact science. We're not always going to agree with one another. And if we're at loggerheads about things we care about, how in the world can we talk about our disagreements without having anyone feel anything?"

"Maybe that's why everyone's trying to ignore the tensions between the Latino and Anglo teachers?" asked Joan.

"Exactly. People are hoping that if we ignore it, it will go away. But we know it won't. In the meantime, we hurt the kids as much as we hurt each other. The same thing happens with all the other conflicts we try to brush aside. They pile up and then blow up. That's not my idea of a healthy school. How can you deal with anything if you can't talk about it? In the long run, it's more productive to get things out in the open."

"Just the same, you really left Jaime hanging," said Joan. "He looked crushed after you went after him."

"I know—it was painful for both of us. But the one thing worse than hearing something straight is getting no feedback at all. If you looked around the room, you saw crossed arms and people rolling their eyes. It wasn't even subtle. There were a lot of unhappy folks in that audience. If that stays hidden, teachers think their new principal is a jerk, but he doesn't know it. Down the road, he notices that the teachers are resisting everything he's doing. So he blames us, and we blame him. We think he's a tyrant, and he thinks we're dinosaurs."

"So everyone blames someone else, and the school gets stuck. But why did you convene a meeting at Andy's Café without Jaime? Weren't you being less than open yourself?" asked Joan.

"I knew teachers needed to talk about what happened. When I spoke up, I was speaking for a lot of other people. You remember the conversation at Andy's?"

"Hard to forget. Venting, criticism, anger. But after a while the tone started to shift. You could see some teachers almost starting to feel sympathy for Jaime."

"Exactly," said Margaret.

"Were you nudging the conversation in that direction?"

Margaret smiled broadly. "Sure I was. I could do that because people trust me. They saw me stand up to Jaime, and I've stood up for teachers before. By the end of the evening, people were a little more willing to give him another chance. That's what I hoped for."

"But I still feel bad for him," said Joan. "He's new like me. I don't know if I could handle being picked apart like that in public. It's bad enough that my boyfriend criticizes everything I cook. The first few days with my class, I've done more things wrong than right. If someone aired my dirty laundry in public, I'm not sure I could take it."

Margaret's face softened. Her voice was warm and gentle. "I know. Jaime may feel the same way. I remember how much support I needed as a new teacher. But I also needed someone to level with me when I was screwing up. Do you want to keep feeding Larry stuff he hates? If I have suggestions for your teaching, do you want to hear them?"

"If you can help me teach better, maybe I could even tolerate public humiliation. But I'd still feel lousy. I'll bet Jaime is pretty upset."

"Sure, he is. Building an open relationship takes more than firing a beginning salvo. You have to follow up. That's what I'm planning next."

As Joan took her last sip of coffee, Larry interrupted her long reverie. "Earth to Joan! Earth to Joan! You've been staring at the coffee pot for the last five minutes. I thought you were bringing me a cup."

"I'm sorry, honey. I guess I was still thinking about the school. Anyway, I'm sure the meeting today can't last beyond 5 o'clock. How about pizza? My treat?"

"Sounds great, only if the pizza isn't topped with pepperoni *and* Pico."

"I promise," said Joan laughing. There were still moments when Larry was as delightful as she remembered him in graduate school. But he had seemed more supportive of her career when they were both in the same business. Now that she was teaching, he seemed to expect that *her* workday should last from the time *he* left in the morning until *he* got home at night. Joan couldn't help wondering if they would ever make it over the long haul.

CHAPTER THREE

A New Principal Finds a Wise Friend

As Jaime Rodriguez looked from his office into the empty school yard, he mulled over his first days as principal of Pico. It had been much rockier than he'd expected. He'd hoped to impress his faculty with his dedication and vision, but he was all too aware that he had missed the mark. He was grateful for one thing. He'd found a coach just when he was going under for the third time. He had run into Brenda Connors as the two of them were leaving a meeting at the district office. Connors asked him how it was going. Rodriguez hesitated, trying to figure out whether she really wanted to know. But he'd been impressed with her during the meeting. She seemed to be the kind of principal he hoped to become: caring, confident, professional, wise, and sensitive.

Avoiding the temptation to give a pat answer, he asked, "Do you want the truth?"

"Nothing but."

Jaime hesitated, but finally decided to plunge in. "To tell you the truth, if I didn't have a new house and a big mortgage, I might pack it in."

Connors's response was warm and direct. "That's about how I felt. Almost 20 years ago, but still seems like yesterday. How about a cup of coffee?"

"How about something a little stronger?"

"I think I know just the place," Connors said with a knowing smile.

Once they found a comfortable table and ordered drinks, Connors opened the conversation. "I asked how things were going because I still remember my first week on the job. I thought no one could be so scared and confused and still survive. Everything was blowing up in my face. Angry teachers. School in chaos. I felt pretty hopeless as a leader. But then I got a gift. The assistant superintendent then was a grizzled old character named Harold Sawyer. Everyone called him "Buzz." He was a couple of years from retirement. He scared me at first. He seemed so demanding and impatient. I was afraid he was dumbfounded that a principalship could go to someone with so little talent.

"At the end of the first week, he dropped by my office. I froze. I was afraid he'd come to tell me to pack up my desk and get out before I did any more damage. I was petrified. But I'll never forget his words. 'You know,' he said, 'This used to be my office. I was principal here for 12 years. The first couple, I didn't have a clue what in hell I was doing. If the staff hadn't carried me along, the parents would have ridden me out of town on a rail. You'll probably learn quicker than I did. But being a new principal is a lot like flying in a fog with no radar. If you're interested, I could give you a few tips.'"

"I'd have hugged that man if I weren't so afraid of him. It turned out he really meant it. He was the life preserver that got me through the first year. He became one of my best friends. Even after he retired, we kept in touch . . ." She paused and lowered her head. ". . . until he died a couple of years ago."

Rodriguez thought he saw a trace of tears in her eyes.

"I miss him. Anyway, Jaime, if you'd like someone to talk to, I'm volunteering."

"If you're offering a life preserver, I need it. But it's hard to believe your first year was that rough."

Connors smiled. "In a few years, I'll bet a young principal tells you the same thing."

Rodriguez mulled over that first conversation with a smile. Connors's warmth and insights had been of much more value than the drink. She encouraged him as he tried to explain why his first days had been so unsettling. What surprised him most was that she could make sense out of things that he couldn't figure out.

When he had entered the Pico principalship, Rodriguez wanted to take charge and set high standards for both staff and students. He was counting on his interpersonal skills to win people over. He'd always been good at building relationships, even with those who saw things differently. He felt he could do the job at least as well as other principals he had known. Above all, he felt excited about the contribution he hoped to make. Schools were under fire, and Rodriguez wanted Pico to set an example of what was possible.

But that was before his first faculty meeting. When he entered the meeting room minutes before the official starting time, he was disappointed to find no one there. His discouragement grew as teachers slowly drifted in. He was particularly offended by some who registered hopes that the meeting wouldn't last very long.

Rodriguez opened the meeting by talking about his vision. He'd done his homework—hours of it. He shared his dreams of a child-centered school that set high standards for all students. But he was discouraged to notice many teachers frowning or crossing their arms. Some were staring out the window or at papers in front of them. After he finished, he asked for questions. A long silence ensued. Then Margaret Juhl hit him with her question. Rodriguez was stunned. He'd been expecting praise and enthusiasm, not a frontal attack. It had never occurred to him to have a Plan B. He was caught flat-footed and helpless. Before he regained his balance, a small war broke out between his critics and defenders. Fearing things were getting out of hand, he'd moved quickly to adjourn the meeting. He left feeling like a failure.

The next day, he got another surprise when the superintendent called him promptly at 8 A.M. "Jaime," he said, "You've got good ideas—raising standards, a child-centered school. I'm 100% behind you. But you have to be careful not to move so fast that you get the faculty upset."

"Welcome to the big leagues," he thought to himself. "How did word get to the superintendent that fast? What's going on here?" Only later did he learn about the informal gathering at Andy's following the faculty meeting. It was clear he had not been on the guest list. Presiding at that meeting was Margaret Juhl. Jaime knew she was a 22-year veteran of the Pico faculty. He'd heard that most of the senior teachers respected her, and many parents revered her. She had also served for a number of years as the representative of the teachers' union.

He knew he'd got off on the wrong foot. But how? Where had he gone wrong? His discomfort increased over the next several days with a steady stream of reminders from teachers about his predecessor, Phil Bailey. He got tired of hearing, "That's not how Mr. Bailey would have done it." He began to wonder who was running the school—him or Phil Bailey's ghost.

As he poured all this out in the first conversation with Brenda, she listened attentively, occasionally offering a comment or question. The more they talked, the better Rodriguez felt. Things started to make more sense. She could see things in ways that he couldn't. She helped him see the difference between power and authority. She explained that new leaders always undergo some form of initiation ritual or "hazing." She reminded him that people need time to adapt to change and reassured him that comparisons to Phil Bailey were a normal part of transition, not a sign that Jaime would never be accepted.

Rodriguez remembered asking Brenda at the end of their conversation if they could meet again. "I got a lot of help when I was a new principal," she had replied. "I owe it to Buzz to return the favor."

That night, Rodriguez slept better than he had in weeks.

Leadership Lessons

Seeing and Solving Barriers to Entry

Like other new educators, Joan Hilliard and Jaime Rodriguez arrived at Pico School brimming with hope and enthusiasm. Starting a new job or a new career is one of life's great moments. The road ahead promises adventure, opportunity, and independence. Long-delayed dreams can finally be realized. Everything seems possible. Bumps? Obstacles? Who wants to think about problems when the world is brimming with possibilities? Yet there are always land mines lurking just below the surface. Too often, we discover them only when they blow up in our face. Enthusiasm and optimism can quickly erode into a mire of disappointment and disillusion.

Newcomers will always encounter bumps on the road. Joan's and Jaime's experiences offer guidelines for spotting and dealing with pitfalls with the least amount of wear and tear.

Expect to be tested. When you enter someplace new, you're busy trying to find your way, whereas the natives are actively trying to figure you out. They want to know what you are bringing to the school. Will you fit in? Might you be a troublemaker? A threat? Joan Hilliard was tested multiple times in her first few hours at Pico. The custodian, Bill Hill, tested her flexibility and receptivity when he told her he'd be stopping by to see how she was doing. Sam Shepherd, the assistant principal, tested her resilience and self-confidence with his challenging and chilly greetings. Joan could easily have responded in ways that caused her new colleagues to see her as difficult and rigid or, conversely, as weak and easy to manipulate. Pay attention to these tests. They're important clues about people's expectations and about yardsticks they use to evaluate one another.

Study cultural clues. As soon as Joan walked into Pico School, she began to notice clues about how the school worked. Many of them were surprises. Joan wisely paid attention to what she was finding— and tried not to take too much for granted.

When you walk through the front door of any school, it will speak if you watch and listen. What do you notice when you enter the building? How does the place look? How does it smell? Joan noticed the clean floors, the smell of fresh wax, and the custodian appraising his work. What sounds, if any, strike you? Walk around to get the lay of the landscape. Notice artifacts—banners, photos, trophy cases. Is there a sign that says, "Welcome"? Or merely one that says, "All visitors must report immediately to the principal's office"? What's on the walls? Photos of students? Random graffiti? Notice what people wear. Is the principal in a dark suit? Or an aloha shirt? Pay particular attention to how people greet you. Joan's frosty encounter with the assistant principal was offset by warm welcomes from Bill Hill and Phyllis Gleason.

If you pay attention, your observations will yield thousands of clues to penetrate fog-shrouded cultural practices. But there's more you can do. When you're new, finding your way around will be a lot easier if you get some help from local guides.

Find guides: mentors, priests, and storytellers. There's a cast of characters in every workplace who can be recruited as mentors and guides. Locate informal priests or priestesses. You won't always find them in a big corner office. They may be typing away in a small cubicle, like Phyllis Gleason, or polishing floors, like Bill Hill. They're often old-timers who came in with the furniture. They can tell you how things came to be and instruct you in cultural mores and norms. Be reverent, pay attention, and you'll find a storehouse of knowledge and wisdom. You can also make friends whose counsel and support could be a big help somewhere down the line.

Look, too, for storytellers—individuals like Phyllis who dramatize everyday exploits and perpetuate school lore. Listen to their tales and read between the lines. Phyllis Gleason's casual comment about Joan's predecessor, who couldn't control his class, was a gentle warning about possible trouble ahead. You'll get important lessons on how to get ahead and what to avoid. You'll hear things you'd almost never find in policy manuals. Stories make lessons real and memorable. Even though unofficial, the lessons are often right on. They will often tell you about heroes and heroines—the living logos who exemplify what the organization stands for. At Pico, Phil Bailey, the former principal, and Margaret Juhl, the veteran teacher, both exemplify this role.

On the other hand, you might find that the heroes in your school are folks who toe the line and kiss up. If that's what gets rewarded, but it's not your style, you've learned an important lesson. Maybe you're in the wrong place.

Connect with grapevine gossips. Gossips are always privy to the latest scoop—even things that are supposed to be confidential or hush-hush. Hear them out, and you'll often get the best briefing going. Their accuracy isn't perfect, but they're reliable informants about current issues, concerns, hopes, and fears. If you hear a story about how the principal was upbraided by the superintendent in a hallway conversation, the details may be distorted, but you can be pretty sure something interesting is afoot. Rumors of impending layoffs may be exaggerated, but you'd be wise to prepare for rough seas. However, gossip is a two-way street. You have to give in order to receive. Don't be too cautious about divulging a few things yourself. Chances are the truth will be less harmful than what the gossips make up on their own. A few minutes over coffee with your local gossip is often worth more than a multitude of meetings and memos. Information is power. Being up to date and in the loop gives you a real advantage over people who rely solely on the official channels to keep on top of things. And if there are things you'd like people to be talking about, there's no better place than the grapevine to get the word out.

PART II

The Political Frame

CHAPTER FOUR

The Old Guard and the New Principal

T he morning after his meeting with Brenda Connors, Rodriguez found himself still mulling over their conversation. He particularly remembered Connors's advice about school politics. At first, he had protested, "I don't want politics in my school. A principal shouldn't have to be a politician."

Connors had not challenged him directly. She simply asked, "What do you make of the superintendent's phone call?"

"It's a puzzle. I've got some clues but I don't know how to put them together."

"Who might have a pipeline to the superintendent?" she asked.

"I wish I knew."

"Well, let's try to scope Pico's political terrain. Who are the influential people who might not be on your side?"

Rodriguez was embarrassed to realize that he had not thought much about potential opposition. He paused before responding. "Well, there's Sam Shepherd, the assistant principal. He was passed over for my position. He still thinks he's the right man for the job. He knows how to crack the whip, but he's more like a warden than a school leader. Most of the black and Latino parents feel he doesn't respect them or their kids."

"Who else?" Brenda asked.

"There's Margaret Juhl. She's a veteran. Teachers and parents respect her. She nailed me at the first faculty meeting. After I talked about my vision for the school, she pretty much told me I had no right to tell teachers how to teach. It felt like a slap in the face. The room got very tense."

Brenda nodded understandingly. "I know Margaret. She definitely has a mind of her own, and she's not shy about telling you what's on it. But she's a pro. Spend some time with her. She could be an asset and an ally."

Jaime groaned. "Do you think I'm a glutton for pain?"

Brenda smiled. "No. But Margaret's a very important player. Do you know what Lyndon Johnson said about people like that?"

"No, what?"

"It's a lot better to have them inside the tent peeing out, than outside the tent peeing in."

They both laughed.

"O.K. I've got your point. I'll talk to Margaret."

Then she asked, "So far, you've focused only on the professional staff. Are there other influential players?"

Rodriguez thought for a minute. "There's Bill Hill, the custodian. People say he's the eyes and ears of the school. Seems to know just about everything that goes on. He's not bashful about sharing it. Then there's the secretary, Phyllis Gleason. I think she came in with the furniture. She probably knows more than I'll ever know about the school. I really need her. But I don't get the feeling she's delighted having me as her new boss."

He stopped, and frowned. "The more I think about it, the worse it seems. I'm new. I got off on the wrong foot. And I have a lot of opposition."

"Who are your allies?"

Rodriguez hesitated for a moment. "Beats me."

"What about your younger staff?"

"Well, some of them are pretty frustrated. They think the school's too conservative, that it doesn't really respond to kids. There are three Latino teachers in the school, and I know they were glad to see me get the job. One of them, Carlos Cortez, came to my defense after Margaret Juhl jumped me. He tells me that the Latino teachers resented Phil Bailey for never doing anything to celebrate Cinco de Mayo."

"What's your relationship like so far with Phyllis?" Connors inquired.

"I think she's still comparing me to Phil," Rodriguez responded, "but the assistant superintendent says that she loves the school and is absolutely loyal."

"Talk to Phyllis and Bill. When you've got a mystery, you need some clues. They might be able to help you get a better picture of what's going on. And what you might need to do next."

"What do you mean?"

"One of the things they never teach in graduate school is how to map the political terrain. My first year as a principal, we had *big* budget cuts. Talk about a jungle! When there's a drought and the water hole starts to dry up, the animals get desperate. I realized that I had to figure out who the key players were. I had to know what they wanted and how much power they had. So I went around and talked to some people and asked questions. Then, I actually drew a map on a piece of paper. On the right side, I put the real conservatives, the people who were probably going to resist almost any change I came up with. On the left, I put the people who I was pretty sure I could count on. Then, in the middle, I put the folks who were neutral and might go either way. There were a lot of fence-sitters, and that told me something right away."

"They were the swing voters?" Jaime asked.

"Exactly. As I put folks on the map, I put them higher or lower, depending on how much power I thought they had. Then I thought about how we could negotiate, instead of going to war. When a new principal comes in, all the unresolved issues get opened up. The different interest groups are all jockeying to hold on to what they have and see if they can get more."

Rodriguez felt uncomfortable with all the talk of power and politics. He liked to think that he was an educator, not a politician. But Connors made sense. "So, you're saying I need to figure out who's with me and who's against me. I need to draw my own map. I'll talk to Phyllis and Bill tomorrow."

While shaving the next morning, Rodriguez began to rethink his situation. Before arriving at Pico, he had images of leading a motivated and harmonious faculty. Seeking help from the secretary and the custodian had not been in his official game plan. But it was beginning to look as if he needed them more than vice versa. They might be able to point out barriers and gateways on Pico's political road map. He felt both excited and apprehensive about his new course.

His apprehension dissipated quickly in the first few minutes of his meeting with Phyllis Gleason. She agreed to meet as soon as he asked, though with little apparent enthusiasm. Rodriguez felt awkward at the beginning, but after a few pleasantries he got right to the point. "Phyllis, how long have you been at Pico?"

She responded instantly. "It'll be 26 years next March."

"So you've had plenty of opportunities to learn how things work here."

"Yes, I have."

"Could you teach me?"

Gleason smiled broadly. "I'm glad you asked. You know, Phil Bailey asked me the same question when he was new. The first thing to understand is that, except for some young teachers, this place has been pretty stable. Most of the old-timers have been together for years. They're friends. They stick together, particularly when threatened by an outsider."

"Like me?" asked Jaime.

"Like you. You jumped into a sermon about high standards and children as if the old-timers had never thought about those things. In their minds, that's exactly what they've been doing for years."

Jaime squirmed as he realized the errors of his opening speech. He listened carefully as Phyllis Gleason shared her years of experience. Things started to fall into place. Gleason helped by pointing out that Rodriguez had things in common with some teachers. He and Margaret Juhl had graduated from the same teachers' college, albeit at different times. Sam Shepherd and Rodriguez were both Rotarians. Many of the black and Hispanic teachers had been waiting for a long time for someone to champion concerns about better instruction for students of color.

Later that morning, in the maintenance office, Bill Hill confirmed much of what Gleason had told him. He added more. Hill had grown up in the local community. He knew most parents and community leaders. His friends were on the school board. He knew most students by name. He was in the cafeteria every morning. He befriended "free breakfast" students and served as a big brother for many of them. Rodriguez could see Hill's love for the school went well beyond his official duties as custodian. At the meeting's end, Hill gave Rodriguez the names of two parents who, he said, would be more than willing to host an informal coffee hour to help Rodriguez get better acquainted.

As Rodriguez mulled over the morning, he was surprised at how productive it had been. He had not anticipated how important Gleason and Hill were or how much they would appreciate being recognized and valued. Both were delighted to feel they had something to teach their new principal. Rodriguez felt a little less overwhelmed. He felt he had made two allies. He even looked forward to reaching out to others who might not be so receptive. He focused on Margaret Juhl. She could be a big help as an ally or an endless pain as an enemy. He knew he had to reach out.

At their breakfast meeting a few days later, Rodriguez arrived feeling tense. Juhl's abrupt opening did not help.

"So, what's on your mind?" she asked. Her tone seemed brusque.

"Well . . . ," he said, grasping for the right words. "You've been at Pico a long time and are highly respected. I thought you might be able to give me some lessons—teach me a few things."

"Look, I'm close to retirement, breaking in a rookie principal is a lot of work. But I'll give you one clue. Phil Bailey had confidence in his staff. He let us teach. He did not blunder in with sermons insulting our professionalism."

Rodriguez's first impulse was to snap back or to look for a way to speed up her retirement. But he recalled his counsel from Brenda Connors. "Very few school leaders know how important it is to learn how to facilitate your opposition. Otherwise, your opponents agree to your face then stab you when your back is turned." Rodriguez figured this might be a good time to take her advice to heart.

"Insulting teachers is the last thing I intended," he said, speaking slowly. "I know how important all of you are. I want us to work together to improve things."

"Why not get to know what we're already doing before telling us how to do it better? Did you think they dropped you into a disaster area waiting for a messiah to ride in and fix things?"

Rodriguez winced. He tried again. "Of course not. Pico is a great school. I'm lucky to be here. I hear you—people felt I was talking down to them. I don't have all the answers. That's why I wanted to meet with you. I need your help. Not just for my sake, but for the sake of our school and kids. Everyone tells me how much you care. If we agree on that, I know we can work together."

Margaret looked at him for a long time. She finally responded. "You're right, I do care about this school. The question for me is whether your deeds are going to match your words. If they do, I'm willing to give you a chance."

As the discussion continued, the climate was still strained. But Rodriguez continued to listen and probe Margaret's views of where the school had been and where it needed to go. Eventually, they revisited Jaime's speech at the opening faculty meeting.

"I guess I was so eager, I jumped the gun," Jaime said. "I hadn't thought enough about how others might feel. Pico has a lot of experienced teachers. I'm sure they believe they're doing a good job. I'm the new kid on the block. They have a lot to teach me. I should have said that. I'll admit, your question floored me. But maybe you were just giving me a dose of my own medicine."

"I wasn't trying to make you look bad," said Margaret. "I was trying to warn that you were in danger of driving off a cliff!"

"That's clearer to me now. It's also becoming obvious that I'm better off with people who tell me the truth. It would be worse to have people talk behind my back or stick it to me when I'm not looking. Thanks, Margaret. To be honest, I didn't expect this kind of conversation with the teachers' union rep."

"Well, I'm not wearing that hat right now. I want a cooperative relationship wherever it's possible. I *will* fight as hard as necessary to represent the teachers when I'm wearing my union rep hat. In either case, I'll be straight with you."

Juhl confirmed her promise a few days later when she called to give Rodriguez a gentle warning about Sam Shepherd. She even offered hints for how Rodriguez might approach his assistant principal. Though she never said it explicitly, Rodriguez sensed that she saw Shepherd as a negative force. "Are you aware," she asked casually, "that he's only two years from retirement?"

A meeting with Sam Shepherd a day later ended when Shepherd walked out of the meeting. Shepherd had not said much, until Rodriguez asked for his support. Then he snarled that he wanted no part of turning a well-run school over to the inmates.

As the door slammed, Rodriguez realized he had to act. Everyone would be better off if Shepherd moved on. Before his next meeting, Rodriguez did his homework. He touched base with Phyllis Gleason and Bill Hill to learn as much as he could about Shepherd. At an informal meeting, he listened to parents' complaints about Shepherd's rigid and authoritarian treatment of students. Even more important, he had another long talk with Margaret Juhl about Shepherd's personal agenda. A week later, when he walked into their second meeting, Rodriguez got right to the point. "I know you don't like me very much."

"You said it, I didn't," Shepherd muttered.

"I also understand that you don't think the school is big enough for both of us," Rodriguez continued. "I agree, and so does the superintendent. We want to offer you some options. I have a memo for you that lays out two of them. Option one is that you move to Hillview as assistant principal. It's your neighborhood, and you might find the principal and kids there more to your liking. You might like the other option even more. The district is willing to offer an early retirement package. I hear you've wanted to run a hunting camp for a long time. This might provide the down payment."

Shepherd looked stunned. He mumbled, "I've got to think about it," and walked out, this time without slamming the door. The next day, his letter of resignation was on Rodriguez's desk.

Connors had been right, Rodriguez thought to himself. You need to map the political terrain before making your moves. A person's position on the organizational chart may not tell how much they know or how much influence they wield. He thought back to something he'd read in graduate school about sources of power, and it suddenly made sense. Some people at Pico, like Phyllis Gleason, had power because of their information and know-how. Others, like Bill Hill, were influential because of their friends and allies. Sam Shepherd was powerful because of his control of rewards and his ability to coerce. Phil Bailey still had lingering personal power based on memories of his genial warmth. Rodriguez himself had the authority built into the principal's role, but that wasn't really enough to do the job. His know-how as a principal was unproven, and he was just beginning to build his own alliances. He had the potential for substantial power as a result of his influence over agendas and symbols. But his first effort to put them into action in his vision speech had flopped. He now had a much clearer sense of what had happened and what he needed to do next.

By going out and talking to people, asking questions, and listening, he was able to discover areas of shared interest that made it much easier to work with most of the people in the school. Building coalitions had turned out not to be as hard as it seemed at first. But sometimes, as with Shepherd, it was necessary to take decisive steps. The key was to do it in a way that did not create a martyr or a victim around whom others would rally.

Rodriguez looked forward to his next weekly visit with Brenda Connors. For a change, he had a triumph to report. Her congratulations felt much better than the condolences she had given him in their previous consultation. His exhilaration was tempered, though, when Connors told him to remember that winning a battle was not the same as winning the war. He felt she was probably right but wondered what she meant. When he asked her, she smiled and said, "Let's wait and see how things go from here. But remember, a school and a kindergarten classroom have a lot in common. Like an ocean, you never turn your back on them."

CHAPTER FIVE

The Tracking Wars

School Politics at Work

Joan was almost at the end of her rope. There could not have been a worse day for Roscoe, a teacher's worst nightmare, to act out. As usual, he had managed to draw his sidekick, Armando, into his latest mischief. The pair were artists at ruining a teacher's afternoon. Joan had tried just about everything short of wringing both of their necks, with little success. Nothing she had learned in college or business had prepared her for this. Her classroom was reasonably orderly most of the time. Right now it was careening straight toward chaos.

Joan wondered if she would have enough energy to finish planning tomorrow's lessons and meet Larry for dinner later that evening. She was only two weeks into the term, and school was already spilling over too much into their relationship. Evenings were becoming another vexing challenge instead of a warm and welcome escape. At her last job, the workday started early but always ended in time for dinner, and she rarely took work home. Just as she was asking herself whether a long run or an after-school glass of wine would be more therapeutic, she was heartened when Margaret Juhl walked into her classroom. It was Joan's first adult hello of the day.

"Rough day?" asked Margaret.

"Worse than that," replied Joan. "I've been through one of Roscoe's romps—with accompaniment from Armando. They literally destroyed this afternoon. I always believed in inclusion until Roscoe came along. He's a rocket without a guidance system. When he loses it, he's simply uncontrollable. It's been hell! I figured kids couldn't be that much tougher than some of the adults I worked with. But an angry client is a lot easier than this."

Margaret smiled. "I get at least one child like that every year. Deep down, you love them, but they can drive you nuts. When you get through to them, you feel wonderful. But when you can't, it breaks your heart. In the meantime, you've got to keep ahead of it. If you get behind, you have a year of misery ahead of you."

"Too late. I'm afraid I'm already behind," responded Joan with a dejected look. "What makes it even harder is that Roscoe is a natural leader. When he goes off the deep end, the other lemmings are right behind. And Armando thinks that he's Sancho Panza, following his master to the end."

"I don't know how many times I've seen a pair like that. Experience helps you put things in perspective, but each year brings a new set of Roscoes. Your training never really prepares you for it."

"Well, it helps just knowing I'm not alone," said Joan with a smile. "Everything has been feeling so overwhelming and stressful. I'm beginning to wonder if I'll ever make it through the year."

"The headaches never go away completely. The heartaches don't either. But that's part of what teaching is all about. Good teachers learn to put them in perspective. Just between us chickens, some people never do. They either get out or burn out. You remind me a little bit of me. My first year teaching, I got lucky. An amazing lady came into my life. She knew more about teaching than I ever hope to know. She taught me a lot, and I've learned a few things since. Some of it might even help with Roscoe."

"I can't believe it," sighed Joan. "They say your first year is like being tossed into a swimming pool. You sink or swim on your own. I could sure use some help. Maybe I shouldn't even ask this, but do you also give advice on love lives?"

Joan hesitated until she saw Margaret smile warmly. Then she continued. "I've been going with a guy named Larry ever since I was in college. Things were going fine until I started teaching. He can't seem to understand why I don't have as much time for him anymore. I'm afraid he's about ready to tell me that either Pico goes or he does. How do I convince him that things will get better? Right now, I'm supposed to meet him for dinner in an hour, and I've got a million things left to do."

Margaret laughed gently. "Well, I'm not much of an expert on how to deal with Larry, because I'm still single. But let me meet this Larry sometime. Right now, though, let's talk about Roscoe."

A week later, Joan was out sick for a day. That was bad enough, but there was worse to come. Jaime Rodriguez found her on the way to her classroom the next morning. His news was bad. Roscoe and Armando had been so unruly that the substitute teacher had left muttering that she would never take that class again. Joan could not help feeling miffed by Jaime's suggestion that she attend an in-service seminar on strategies for dealing with exceptional youngsters. Was Rodriguez blaming her? Did he think she had somehow failed? Joan decided it was time to develop her own homegrown strategy.

Following Margaret's advice, Joan began by trying to learn more about Roscoe from someone who knew him well. Joan knew just the person to ask. Heidi Hernandez was one of the brightest and most cooperative students in her class. Heidi was wise beyond her years, though she tended to perform below the incredible potential that Joan saw in her. Heidi often stayed after school to talk to Joan about her own dream of going to college and becoming a teacher—even though no one else in her family had graduated from high school. Joan knew that Heidi and Roscoe lived in the same neighborhood. Equally important, she felt she could trust Heidi.

As class was ending on a sunny Thursday afternoon, Joan struck up a conversation. "You know Roscoe pretty well, don't you, Heidi?" she asked.

"Sure," said Heidi. "He lives right down the street from me. Sometimes we walk to school together. Sometimes, he's real nice. Other times, he's just plain mean."

"Why do you think that is?" asked Joan.

Heidi hesitated for a moment. "This won't get Roscoe in trouble, will it?"

"No, it won't," Joan replied. "I'm Roscoe's teacher as much as I am yours. Maybe you know something that would help me be a better teacher for him."

Heidi screwed up her face and thought for a moment about what Miss Hilliard had said. Then she appeared to relax and started to talk freely. "I think about him a lot, Miss Hilliard. His mom doesn't fix dinner for him the way my mom does. His father gets mad a lot, and he's always yelling. You may not know this, Miss Hilliard, but Roscoe really likes being at school. He thinks you're the best. I think he really wants you to like him, but he doesn't think he's smart enough. When he acts weird in class, at least he knows you'll pay attention to him."

As she thanked Heidi, Joan tried hard not to show the emotion she was feeling. She knew what she wanted to do next. The next day, she worried all day about how her meeting with Roscoe would turn out. As luck would have it, Roscoe was on reasonably good behavior. He seemed surprised when Joan asked him to stay for a while after the final bell had sounded.

"Come on, Miss Hilliard, what'd I do? Armando was causing all the trouble. Make him stay after school."

"You didn't do anything wrong," Joan assured him. "I just want to talk to you."

"About what?" asked Roscoe suspiciously.

"About you," said Joan.

Roscoe reluctantly agreed to stay. At first, he just stared at his feet, shifting his weight from leg to leg, with a sullen scowl on his face. He seemed afraid that Joan wanted to punish him for something. But as Joan began to ask how Roscoe felt about things, he sat down and looked up at her. He seemed to be looking for clues in Joan's expression. Then he started to talk in a low whisper, and Joan was surprised at what came out. He confirmed many of the things that Heidi had said a day earlier. He did not come right out and say it directly, but he hinted that Joan might be one of the reasons that he enjoyed coming to school. "You're pretty nice," he said. "My last teacher sent me to the office all the time. She said I was a pain. You don't do that, even when I'm bad."

"You know, I like you, Roscoe," Joan replied. "You have a lot of spirit. But let me ask you a question. Do you think you're doing as well as you could in school?"

Roscoe blushed and looked down at his scuffed shoes again. "I don't know," he said. "Maybe not."

"Would you like to do better?" asked Joan.

He looked up, shrugged his shoulders, and said timidly, "I don't know if I can."

"I'm sure you can, and you just said so yourself. Maybe we could make a deal. I help you, and you help me. If we work together, you might be surprised at how well you do."

Roscoe smiled for the first time during their conversation. "You think so? O.K., Miss Hilliard, it's a deal." Then his expression changed to a look somewhere between earnest and impish. "But talk to Armando, too. He's always getting me in trouble."

Over the next few weeks, the results were mixed. Roscoe was not always true to his word, but he did try—and he did improve. At times, it seemed that he simply could not control himself. At other times, Joan could see him doing his best to resist the temptation to do something disruptive. But even when Roscoe was doing his best, Joan realized that he needed more help if he was going to keep his promise for very long. At lunch one afternoon, she told Margaret what had happened with Roscoe over the last few weeks. "It's an improvement, but I still feel I need to do something more."

"Didn't Jaime offer to send you to that conference on classroom management? I went a few years ago. Even for someone who's been teaching a long time, it's pretty useful. It gave me some neat ideas that really help with all students, especially those with special needs. You might get some good ideas on ways to structure your classroom."

Margaret's endorsement convinced Joan to tell Rodriguez that she would take his suggestion to attend the conference. She had anticipated that the biggest hurdle would be persuading Larry that it was worth her being away on a Saturday. She dreaded one more harangue about being married to her work. The fates were kind for once, though—Larry had to be away on business that weekend.

Joan almost flew to school the Monday morning after the conference. The program had been even better than she had expected. She had learned that she was not alone in her struggle to manage students like Roscoe, and she came away with at least a dozen new ideas. She also came away convinced that many of the issues went beyond her classroom and needed changes in schoolwide policies. She was bubbling with enthusiasm when she turned in her expense report to Phyllis Gleason. Phyllis accepted the report with her usual cheerful efficiency but added an unexpected bit of cautionary advice.

"Joan," she said, "you look just as eager as some of the other teachers who've returned from conferences with a bag of new tricks. Just don't be disappointed if everyone isn't as excited about your new ideas as you are."

Carlos Cortez shared none of Phyllis's caution when Joan talked to him later that morning. Joan had expected Carlos to be supportive. She was thrilled that he was as excited about revising Pico's tracking system as she was. In fact, he quickly arranged for an informal afternoon meeting at Andy's Café with several other young teachers. Everyone there agreed that something needed to be done.

"We're labeling too many kids and shunting them off into special classes or classes for slower kids. That just about guarantees that they'll fall farther and farther behind. And it's particularly the minority kids who get labeled," said Carlos. "The district's new inclusion policy is a step in the right direction. It's way overdue, really. But there's too much foot-dragging."

"What bothers me is that they're trying to be inclusive without giving teachers the support they need," Joan replied. "Here I am in my first year. I've got some very challenging kids, and I really need some help. I've been wondering, 'Why me?' Am I wrong, or do some of the older teachers figure out ways to get those students assigned to someone with less seniority?"

"I've seen the same thing," replied Carlos. "If you believe in inclusion, you wind up with all the students that other teachers don't want. We really need everyone to get behind the policy and make it a schoolwide commitment. Otherwise, we're just creating a new form of tracking."

Everyone at the table agreed with Joan and Carlos. When they left Andy's later, they had all made a commitment to make the district's policy a part of Pico's philosophy and practice. Carlos and Joan went to work with enthusiasm to develop a presentation to Pico's faculty.

Their optimism grew when they talked to the principal. He applauded their initiative and encouraged them to move forward. When they made their presentation to the faculty, they had expected some questions and criticism, but they were stunned by the outpouring of anger and resistance that swept quickly over the meeting.

Phil Leckney led off by questioning whether younger teachers understood what they were getting into. "Look, guys," he said, "I've been to a lot of conferences too. The eggheads in the universities always have some great new idea to save the world, but I've had a lot of years in the trenches. Those professors aren't talking reality. A lot of them have never taught in a public school classroom."

Vivian Chu, always known as a staunch advocate of high academic standards, jumped in to support Leckney. "When we say that all children should learn, we sometimes wind up focusing all our attention on the children who aren't and forget those who are. The district has already cut funds for gifted and talented. Who's standing up for them? We have to provide a challenging education for our brightest kids. If we don't, their parents will pull them out, and we'll lose kids who provide a model for everyone else. Then, there's all those kids in the middle. Sometimes they're the forgotten majority."

Leckney's and Chu's views received immediate support from a number of veteran teachers. Even Margaret Juhl and Jaime

Rodriguez seemed powerless to turn back the tidal wave of staunch resistance. The meeting ended in a stalemate, and a visibly shaken Joan grabbed Margaret on the way out of the room to ask in a trembling whisper if they could talk later. Margaret asked Joan to give her a call in the evening.

On the telephone that night, Joan got right to the point. "Could you believe that today? We're trying to help students who aren't being served. A lot of those teachers are locked in concrete. They put their own convenience ahead of the needs of the kids."

Joan was surprised by Margaret's candid response. "I wish that you had talked to me before the meeting. I could have predicted the response that you'd get."

Joan was as surprised as she was disappointed. "Are you saying we should have just kept quiet? Whose side are you on, anyway?"

"I'm on your side, because I think you're right," said Margaret, "but I understand where the others are coming from. This issue is not just about students. It has a lot to do with the same thing you're concerned about—managing differences. You remember how the battle lines were drawn between you and Roscoe. The standoff began to change when you took time to understand his side of things. You've got a similar situation here. But instead of a difference between two individuals, we now have a potential war between two groups. People are starting to rally the troops to make sure their interests triumph. You have a political problem. You need a political strategy."

"This isn't about politics, it's about students. Why should I need a political strategy?" Joan asked skeptically.

"It may sound cynical, but it's also realistic. We have two groups with different beliefs, and both are struggling for what they think is right. But we'll all lose if the school turns into a battleground."

"So, are we supposed to just back down?" asked Joan with more than a hint of annoyance in her voice.

"One of the things they never teach you in graduate school is how to understand political tugs and pulls. But you must have run into this kind of thing in your old job."

"Sure, but the office politics was one of the reasons I wanted to get out of there and into a classroom. In a brokerage, people are always looking for an edge, always trying to outproduce everyone else. I figured schools would be different."

"Not as different as you thought," Margaret replied. "When I was in my second year of teaching, the teachers' union went out on strike. First time in the history of the district. I went out with most of the teachers, but some of the veterans reported for work. I couldn't believe the hatred on the picket lines—the yelling and the name-calling. I'll never forget talking to one teacher a couple of days before the strike. She told me that no matter what happened, she was coming to work. She said that the students were more important than a few more dollars in her paycheck. After it was over, a lot of her old friends wouldn't even talk to her—they avoided her in the halls. It took a *long* time for the school to recover. I knew I had to learn more about conflict and why it was so hard for people to deal with."

"So what did you do?" asked Joan with curiosity.

"I asked around, and somebody finally told me about a book that had a couple of chapters on organizational politics. I was skeptical until I read them because I figured, 'Hey, I'm a teacher. This sounds like the stuff principals read when they want to know how to manipulate us.' But I devoured that whole book because suddenly a big lightbulb came on. As teachers, we all work in organizations, and half the time we can't figure out what's going on, because no one ever teaches us anything about how they work. We get a lot of stuff about psychology, teaching methods, curriculum—the stuff that's important in the *classroom*. But they don't teach us about *schools*."

"But why is that important if what you care about is what you do in the classroom?" asked Joan.

"Two reasons," said Margaret confidently. "The first is that the classroom is sort of a miniature organization in its own right. I was surprised when I started to think about it that way. Some things fell into place that never made sense before, and I started to see a lot of new possibilities for teaching and classroom management. Think about the struggle between you and Roscoe. People had tried plenty of coercion and punishment before, and he just kept getting more resistant. You started to get somewhere when you negotiated with him. The second reason is that how the school and the district work as an organization makes a big difference in your classroom. The debate over the inclusion policy is just one example."

"I'm still not with you," replied Joan with a puzzled look. "What's the connection between organizations and the inclusion policy?"

"Look at it this way. From a political perspective, a school is a collection of coalitions—a bunch of different groups, like teachers, administrators, students, and parents. Each group has its own beliefs, its own values, and its own interests. Every group wants certain things, but there's almost never enough to go around. For instance, a lot of parents would like the school to revolve around the needs of their own child. As a teacher, you want to do everything you can for their child, but you also have to respond to all the other children in your class."

"But that means parents aren't really a coalition. They're a bunch of individuals," protested Joan.

"Sometimes and sometimes not," said Margaret. "Coalitions come and go, depending on the issue at hand. On some issues, the Pico teaching staff is really united, but right now, the inclusion policy is not one of them. Instead, you've got a couple of coalitions forming within the teaching staff, each based on different beliefs, different backgrounds, and different experiences."

"Maybe, but so far I don't see that you're telling me anything I didn't already know."

If Margaret detected the impatience in Joan's voice, it seemed not to bother her. She continued cheerfully, "O.K., but here's where I think it really starts to get interesting. If you want to understand what's really going on around something like the inclusion debate, you need a political map."

"A political map?"

"You want Pico to make a full commitment to the district's inclusion policy. Some people agree, others don't. To make a map, you start by asking who the key players are: Who are the people who are likely to make a difference in how the issue gets resolved?"

"O.K., there's the teachers. Some are with us, some are against us, and some haven't made up their minds."

"Right, and that last group could turn out to be very important," said Margaret. "Who else?"

"Jaime Rodriguez, and he's with us. We know that Dr. Hofsteder, the superintendent, is on our side. Then there are parents, but a lot of them probably haven't thought very much about the issue. Once they hear about it, they'll probably break into different camps, depending on how they think it affects their own children."

"Now we're making progress," said Margaret. "As you're talking about the players, you're also talking about their interests and what stake they have in the issue. If you go around and talk to a few people and ask some questions, you'll probably have an even better understanding. Then, you're ready to create your map."

"I'm beginning to see the map of the inclusion debate. The good news is we have some powerful allies, like the principal and the superintendent. But the opposition is pretty strong, too. So, we can probably win, but the war could be pretty gruesome."

"Once you understand that, you can start to think about other options besides armed combat."

"Like what?"

"Negotiation, for one."

Deep down, Joan felt very uncomfortable with all the talk of power and combat. She really wanted to believe that a teacher could remain above the sordid world of politics. Yet Margaret made sense. "I don't know. Negotiation sounds like what you do when you're buying a used car, not when you're trying to help kids."

Later that night, Joan wrestled with Margaret's closing suggestion—befriend your enemies. "You could start by meeting with Phil Leckney," Margaret had suggested. Joan wondered if she and Leckney could even have a civil conversation. Yet Margaret was right. It wouldn't help to tear the school apart. Joan also wondered why Margaret had suggested talking with Phyllis Gleason before the meeting with Phil. But the most persuasive thing that Margaret said was, "If you're going to be consistent with your philosophy for dealing with differences among kids, don't you want to practice what you preach in dealing with your colleagues?"

To Joan's surprise, her meeting with Phyllis was a lot like her earlier meeting with Heidi Hernandez. From Phyllis, Joan learned a lot about Phil Leckney and the other teachers who were on his side. Joan got a clearer sense of how much they could do to block the ideas that were so important to her and her allies. Phyllis also helped Joan get a better understanding of what "the opposition" was really concerned about. For example, Leckney was not so much against the new proposal as he was against anything that would make it difficult to stay on top of an already challenging group of students.

Margaret's offer to facilitate the meeting between Joan and Phil Leckney had turned out to be a good idea. It was clear that Margaret had been in similar situations before. She opened the meeting by focusing on the issue rather than on personalities or the feelings people had about one another. She also set some ground rules for the conversation. Both groups, she said, were committed to a quality education for Pico's students, but they had different views on how to do it. She suggested that they start by having both Joan and Phil each talk about their own views, insisting only that they focus on what they wanted for students, instead of what they didn't like about the other's stance.

As they talked, Joan was surprised to find more areas of agreement than she had expected. As the conversation deepened, Leckney acknowledged some of the challenges that he and others were grappling with. "It's changed an awful lot since I started," said Phil at one point. "When I was young, I felt like I came to teach and the students came to learn. That's not how it is anymore. The neighborhood's more run down. We've got a lot more poverty, a lot more single-parent families, more and more kids who barely speak English. We never used to have to worry about weapons or drugs in the school. Maybe I should have been trained as a social worker or something. It's tough enough managing the students I've got."

As Joan acknowledged her own struggles with classroom management, she and Phil felt a bond for the first time. She learned from Phil that part of the opposition to her proposal came because it seemed to require that every teacher add to their burdens when they were already feeling overwhelmed. Many of the teachers were genuinely doubtful that the new approach would be an improvement. They all remembered other "improvements" that had flopped and made things even worse. They feared, in fact, that the proposal might overwhelm teachers and lead to an overall reduction in the quality of instruction at Pico.

Margaret then raised the possibility of a pilot project as a way to learn more about how the new approaches might work. That would give the teachers who believed in the proposal a chance to experiment with it and let others have a chance to wait to see whether their fears and concerns turned out to be justified.

The meeting ended on a high note. Joan and Phil agreed that they both believed in the importance of student achievement and classroom management. Even though they disagreed on the impact of the district's inclusion policy, Phil agreed to support the idea of the experiment. Joan, Carlos, and a small group that called itself the "True Believers" formed to develop plans for the experiment. On learning of the group's name, some of the veterans playfully chose to label themselves the "Wise People." When one of them teasingly suggested that "True Beginners" would have been a better name for the other group, Carlos retorted immediately, "Does your group spell *wise* w-h-i-t-e?" The zingers hit home, but there was laughter on both sides. Joking and teasing became a playful way to acknowledge the tensions and build linkages between the two different groups.

With enthusiastic backing from Jaime Rodriguez and no serious opposition from their colleagues, the "True Believers" plunged into the effort with great enthusiasm. Unknown to everyone at the time, the inclusion issue was only the tip of the iceberg in a larger problem of student discipline at Pico. While the pilot project moved ahead, new clouds formed on the horizon.

Leadership Lessons

Map the Terrain, Hone Your Skills

Educators often view politics with a mixture of distaste and dread. They hope that their school will somehow climb beyond the petty world of conflict and self-interest to the sunlit path of reason and collaboration. Like it or not, though, politics won't go away. The question is not whether schools will have politics but what kind of politics they will have. Those who ignore and avoid politics simply leave the field wide open for the less squeamish. It makes much more sense to understand the political landscape and to develop the skills that enable you to be a productive and effective participant.

Schools are political because of two essential features. The first is they are inevitably coalitions of different individuals and groups with enduring differences in background, beliefs, and agendas. People differ by role (for example, parents, teachers, administrators, students), by discipline or grade level (counselors, special education teachers, resource teachers), by race and ethnicity, by social class, and by ideology (for example, beliefs about how best to teach reading or mathematics). The second essential feature is scarce resources. There is never enough money, time, or human energy to do everything or to give everyone all they want. Choices have to be made. Money spent on athletics can't be used to buy textbooks, and vice versa. Someone has to teach in the grade levels where high-stakes tests are mandated, even if no one really wants to. A principal can't review a budget, calm an angry parent, discipline a wayward student, and lobby the superintendent all at the same time.

The interplay of different interests and scarce resources inevitably leads to conflict between individuals and groups. Sometimes competing differences can be fairly easily resolved through reason and data.

More often, they are rooted in deeply held preferences, values, or beliefs. It's like asking Catholics and Baptists to agree about papal authority: There's little that the two groups have in common. In such cases, power and political sophistication become critical.

In coaching the new professionals, Connors and Juhl posed three central questions:

1. *Who are the key players?* Who are the people, or groups, who care about the issue at hand? Will they care enough to support or oppose you? Who will, or might, make a difference in how things turn out? Whose help is necessary? Whose opposition is too important to ignore?

2. *What is the interest of each of the key players or groups?* That is, what stake does each player have in this issue? What does each player want, and what can you do to help them get at least part of what they care about?

3. *How much power does each player have?* Who is likely to have the greatest influence over how this issue plays out? What are the sources of power for each key player? Who could become a valuable ally if their power was mobilized? Are there any "sleeping dogs" better left undisturbed?

The answers to those questions make it possible to draw a map—a two-dimensional figure in which the vertical axis represents power and the horizontal axis represents position, or interest.

Once you have a map, you're in a position to make much more informed choices about what to do. In developing an approach, you can consider the strategies that are typically employed by effective and constructive politicians:

1. *Clarify your agenda.* You are clear on your agenda when you have both a vision of where you want to go and a strategy for getting there.

2. *Build relationships and alliances.* Work on building relationships with the key players. Spend time with them, and find out how they think, what's important for them, and what they would like from you. The better your relationships, the more likely you are to build support and defuse opposition.

3. *Soothe and learn from the opposition.* Talk to potential opponents. Listen to them, ask questions, and listen some more. Make sure that you understand how they think and what they care about. Acknowledge the importance of their perspectives. Encourage them to engage in a dialogue with the people with whom they disagree.

4. *Deal openly with differences.* It is tempting but dangerous to ignore conflict or to sweep it under the rug in hopes that it will go away. Usually it just festers and gets worse. People need a chance to voice their concerns and to hear other people's as well. Otherwise, differences too easily descend into personal animosity, backstabbing, and street fights.

5. *Negotiate.* When you know what you and other key players want, you're ready to talk about options and possibilities for "win–win" solutions. Optimism and persistence can work wonders when guided by the question, What can we do that works for as many people as possible?

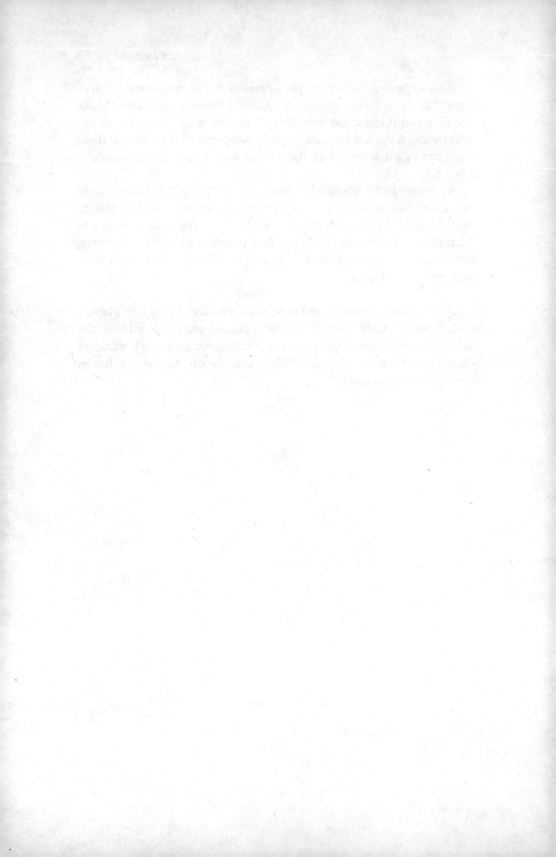

PART III

The Human Resource Frame

CHAPTER SIX

Sagging Morale

The controversy over the inclusion policy gradually subsided. Life at Pico flowed smoothly over the next few months. Even so, Connors warned Jaime to expect more turbulence. As the holiday break approached, he wondered if she had been too pessimistic. Suddenly, he was blindsided by a new and powerful storm that seemed to come from nowhere. Rodriguez always prided himself on his people skills. He found it hard to believe that teacher morale could drop so precipitously. The signs were unmistakable: teachers coming late to faculty meetings, not showing up for parents' night, or resisting playground and cafeteria duty. Rodriguez was particularly stunned by an anonymous newsletter that viciously attacked him, complete with not-so-subtle ethnic slurs. At the end of January, he knew it was time for another long talk with Brenda Connors. Swallowing his pride at having to admit that he should have paid more heed to her warnings, he called and scheduled a dinner later that week.

He and Brenda met at a popular restaurant not far from Connors's school. Over the appetizer, Rodriguez briefed her on the latest crisis. She did not seem very surprised, but made no mention of her earlier warning. Connors noted that sags in teacher morale following the holidays are not unexpected. But then she asked a more pointed question: "How's *your* morale?"

Rodriguez thought carefully before replying, "Pretty bad. Maybe it's just a slump after the holidays, but that newsletter really got to me. It's hard to believe anyone would do something like that. It had to be someone on the staff. I'd really like to think that my staff members are mature professionals, but referring to me as the 'Tortilla Kid' is a pretty low blow."

"Why might someone do something like that, Jaime?" asked Brenda.

"Racism, what else?"

"I was the first black principal in three different schools, so I know something about racism. Sure, there's racism everywhere. But I've learned that if you stop there, it doesn't help very much. It's a label, not a solution. You have to go deeper to find out what's eating at people. Someone has to be pretty frustrated to go that far. The way I see it, people are a lot like plants. Plants have certain needs, like light, water, nutrition, and warmth. When their needs are met, they grow and develop their potential. If not, they shrivel and get distorted."

"If you're saying a principal has to be a gardener, I agree. That's sort of what I try to do. I spend a lot of my time trying to make sure that my teachers get the things they need," Rodriguez responded.

"How do you do that?"

"One of the most important things I've done is to continue a precedent that Phil Bailey started: I'm out visiting classrooms as often as I can."

"What do you do when you make those visits?"

"I always look for things that can help my teachers do a better job. One thing I learned in school is that my job is to be an instructional leader, not a paper pusher. I always talk with teachers about ways to improve instruction. I want to give them the suggestions and feedback they need to create the kind of school that we all want."

"One way that people are different from plants is that they can often tell you what they need, if you pay attention. Are you sure what you're giving them is what they want from you?"

Jaime realized immediately that he wasn't sure if he knew what they wanted. "I don't know," he answered. "Maybe I need to find out."

"Remember that each individual is unique," Brenda replied. "Some of your teachers may appreciate what you're doing, because they want feedback to help them teach better. But others might be looking for a sign that you care or a pat on the back. They might not welcome what you're offering them. Someone could even be upset enough to write a newsletter in retaliation. They might be trying to get back at you: 'If you make my life miserable, I'll return the favor.'"

"But if someone is that upset, why don't they just tell me? I've said any number of times that I'm always available. I've asked them to come to me first when they're upset about something I've done."

"Having your door open does not always mean having an open door. Someone once told me about what he called the mystery-mastery model. He said that people have a tendency to protect themselves. One way is blame someone else when things go wrong. But they rarely tell the person they're blaming, because that's risky. Maybe it's human nature to protect yourself and other people from the truth sometimes. But I've always liked the adage that if life gives you a lemon, try to make lemonade."

"I've got the lemon. What do I do with it?"

"Maybe you can turn this newsletter into an opportunity. It could be a chance to open up the conversation between you and the teachers. Right now, you're not getting what you need, and some of them aren't either."

"You're probably right, but where do I start?"

"When I've run into this kind of situation, I've had good luck with bringing in a neutral third party to help get the conversation going, but that might not work here."

"Why not?"

"Because of where the school is right now. You're still new, and the faculty is pretty suspicious. They might not trust an outsider, particularly someone you bring in. It might be better if you and your teachers take this on together. You'll need to make sure that the faculty supports and feels involved in the process."

"So how would you begin?"

"Suppose you start by talking to some of the people you trust. Ask them what they think is going on and how it should be approached. When you think about a school as a family, it's important to remember that you don't always have to come up with the solution by yourself. Families often work better when everyone shares the responsibility for solving important problems."

"I know what you're saying is right. That's what I try to do at home. But as a new principal, I feel I have to take charge and show people I'm the leader."

"Jaime, in my first year as a principal, I worried about losing my authority and teachers' respect. So, I tried to prove how strong I was. It backfired. People could tell that I was insecure. I learned from Buzz Sawyer that sometimes the best thing you can do is to let other people know how you're feeling. If your school is a garden, you don't have to be the only gardener. Your needs are as important as anyone else's."

"Maybe I've been trying too hard to be superhuman?"

"Exactly. One other point. Sometimes, people want feedback. Other times, they just want support and love. When your wife asks you how she looks in a new dress, she may not be hoping for a detailed critique. She may just want some reassurance."

The next day, Rodriguez met Margaret Juhl at the mailboxes just as she was leaving school. He asked her if she had a minute and invited her into his office. After asking a few questions about her request for more science supplies, he got to the point. "Margaret, it's no secret that we have some unhappy people here. And you know I'm upset about that newsletter. You've always been honest with me. What do you think is going on?"

"I'm as surprised by that as you are. Things seemed to deteriorate really fast after the holidays. Some of our regular moaners started the ball rolling, but it seems like it became infectious, and now almost everyone is mad about something. The newsletter must be from someone who's pretty mad, but didn't feel they could say it directly. I think it's been building for a while."

"What would you think about setting up some informal meetings with small groups of teachers to try to talk about what's going on?"

"I'm not sure. It's been a long time since we've done anything like that. Some informal meetings might get people talking more openly. But I don't think you should initiate it."

"Who should?"

"It would be a lot better if it came from the faculty," Margaret replied. "Let me see what I can do."

"Thanks, Margaret. Is there anything I can do to help you?"

"If you get invited to a meeting, just show up and stay cool," was Margaret's reply.

Rodriguez was surprised when an invitation came from Phil Leckney. He and Leckney were not close, even though Rodriguez had gone out of his way to help with discipline problems in Leckney's classroom. As Rodriguez arrived at Leckney's home, he was reassured by Leckney's warm greeting and hospitality. He had gone to a lot of trouble to arrange the event. The real surprise for Rodriguez came after dinner. The conversation began awkwardly, as if everyone had something to say but was afraid to say it.

Rodriguez tried to get the ball rolling. By talking about what he was feeling, he hoped to get other people to open up as well. "I really want to thank Phil for setting up this meeting. I think everyone knows I was pretty upset by the newsletter. But I'm not looking for someone to blame. I'm really hoping that we can talk about what's happening and what we can do about it."

After another brief silence, one of the veteran teachers responded, "You want to know what's wrong? I'll tell you. You've been here six months, and all I've gotten from you are kicks in the butt. It's like you come in every day trying to figure out what I'm doing wrong. Did it ever occur to you that I'd like to hear if I'm doing anything right?"

Rodriguez felt every eye in the room turned to him, waiting for his response. Then it came to him that he felt the same way. "I know just what you mean, because that's how I feel. I can understand how you're looking for a pat on the back, because so am I. You're wondering if I see you doing anything right, and I'm wondering if the faculty thinks I'm doing anything right."

"So we feel you're tearing us down," said Margaret, "and you feel that we're tearing you down. It's like the saying that if you feel like a molehill, you try not to let anyone else be a mountain."

The tension broke, and there was an air of relief, even excitement, as people realized they were all feeling starved for support and encouragement. Several teachers shared their own stories around this theme, and the conversation gradually became more open and animated. Rodriguez was still startled when Leckney suddenly interrupted someone else to blurt out, "I've got something I want to get off my chest. I feel even worse than all these other people. You made me look like a wimp in front of my students. That's why I put out that newsletter."

Rodriguez felt a rush of feelings: a mixture of anger, admiration, sorrow, and even a surprising impulse to protect Leckney. After counting slowly to five in his mind, Rodriguez asked Leckney, "But why a broadside like that?"

"Because that's what you've done to me for the past six months," said Leckney. "You seem to save all the warm fuzzies for your Mexican friends."

Carlos Cortez jumped in. "What warm fuzzies?" he asked. "You're crazy if you think he does special favors for his so-called Mexican friends. He does the same thing to us. I'm still looking for my first compliment from the so-called Tortilla Kid." Even Rodriguez started to laugh at that point, though he was not sure why.

The laughter broke some of the tension, but everyone knew the reference to "Mexican friends" had touched a nerve. Rodriguez chose his words carefully. "Phil, I appreciate your honesty. I didn't like the newsletter, and I particularly didn't like the part about the 'Tortilla Kid.' Frankly, I thought the whole thing was a cheap shot. But it took guts for you to tell me now that you did it. And I hear what people are saying—I've been making your lives miserable, and you've found ways to return the favor. We've been working on two different wavelengths. You felt that I was trying to catch you doing something wrong. All I was thinking about is 'How can we make this school better?' "

"I care about that, too," replied Leckney. "But constant criticism doesn't help me teach better."

"I know how that feels. I understand that I haven't been telling you about all the good things you're doing. What I'm learning tonight is that we all want a place where we feel accepted and cared for. We have some work to do to create that. Even though some of us are Latino, some are black, and others are Anglo, we're all professionals, and we all have the same job. If we work together, we can do it."

Joan was quiet during much of the meeting. She felt numbed by all the tension. She was relieved, though, to feel a new spirit of cooperation as she left Leckney's home on her way to a nearby coffee shop to meet with Margaret. As she drove to the restaurant, she found herself thinking more about her seesaw relationship with Larry than about the school. Margaret had finally met Larry the week before. He seemed genuinely captivated by her stories about teaching. He even shared his own stories about teachers who had been important to him. Afterwards, he had given Joan the supreme compliment. "Honey, I may be out to make a fortune. But in your new career, you're destined to make a difference."

It felt like a breakthrough at the time, but Larry was soon back to his unsympathetic self. Joan had been stung by his harsh tone a few nights later as they met at the pizza shop. "First of all, you're late. Second, all you want to talk about is what's going on at that freaking school. I'm getting fed up!"

Joan felt embarrassed, guilty, and angry all at once. But she resisted the temptation to strike back. She tried the same advice that had seemed to help with both Roscoe and Phil Leckney. "Do you feel I'm putting the school ahead of you?" she ventured.

"It's pretty obvious, isn't it?"

Joan tried to reassure him, to convince him how important he was to her. He listened and seemed to calm down a bit. For a while, it appeared as if they were finally making some headway. But then the conversation ran into an invisible roadblock neither knew how to get around. "At least we have an icy truce," Joan thought afterwards. But she doubted that the war was over. Then she pulled into the parking lot of the restaurant and spotted Margaret's car.

As soon as they sat down, Margaret sensed Joan's preoccupation. "What's on your mind?" she asked as casually as she could.

"Larry, more than anything."

"I enjoyed meeting him."

"Oh, he felt the same way. Afterwards, he sounded as if he was really beginning to understand why my work is so important to me," Joan said with a sigh.

"You don't sound that pleased."

"I was, but it didn't last. Now he's back to grumping again."

"What about?"

"I don't have time for him. I can't let go of my work. I'm putting everything else ahead of him." She paused. "Maybe he's right."

"It sounds like you both need things that you're not getting from the other."

"I know that," Joan said with annoyance. "We talked about that. It seemed to help for a while. But I don't think we really resolved anything. It's a little like dealing with Roscoe."

"Teaching and relationships have a lot in common. What's your biggest concern about Larry?"

"That he doesn't understand me. He doesn't listen. He doesn't really care about my needs."

"And how is that different from what concerns him?"

Silence fell over the booth. Joan saw it right away but hated to admit it. She and Larry felt pretty much the same thing about one another.

"Here's what often happens," Margaret continued. "Something goes wrong in a relationship. We get upset, and we start to blame the other person. Then we start trying to fix whatever we think is wrong with them. We pressure them, try to manipulate them, tell them what they're doing wrong."

"That's pretty much what I'm getting from Larry."

"How well is it working?"

"It just makes things worse."

"Could he feel you're doing the same thing to him?"

"Probably," Joan admitted.

"So there you are. We try to get the other person to change. It doesn't work very well, but then we blame the other person for being defensive and not listening."

Joan was squirming. Margaret's words were hitting all too close to home. "So," Joan asked, "what's the alternative?"

"Communication. Listening. Working together. Start with the things you have in common. Such as, you want him to care about you, and he wants you to care about him. If you can say that to each other, then you can start talking about what each of you can do to help the other."

"It seems so obvious," said Joan ruefully. "Instead of being honest about what I want from Larry, I've been criticizing him for not giving it to me. And he's doing the same to me. What's crazy is that we're at war because we both feel the same way."

"It happens all the time," replied Margaret. "It's easy to forget that a relationship is always a two-way street. You need to be open with Larry about what you're feeling, but you also need to make sure you understand where he's coming from. When Larry said he was fed up, you could have told him he wasn't half as fed up as you were. Instead, you asked him if he felt you care more about the school than about him. You had a hunch about what he was feeling, and you checked it out. That's when the conversation shifted, right?"

"Yeah. For a little while, anyway."

"It was a good start," said Margaret. "You have to keep at it. You're not likely to see a miracle cure with Larry, or with Roscoe."

Joan felt herself breathe a sigh of relief. She could feel her shoulders and arms relax. She sipped on hot chocolate and thanked Margaret for listening and caring. Meanwhile, across town, the telephone was ringing in Brenda Connors's home. An exhausted but elated Jaime was on the other end of the line. "Thanks," he said. "You gave me the nudge I needed. I learned how big a gap you can have between what you think you're doing and what your teachers think you're doing."

"I had to learn that the hard way myself," Connors replied. "We all carry around these pictures of ourselves the way we'd like to be. But we don't always live up to our ideas, and a lot of times we don't know when we're not. The people around see what we do, not what we think we're doing. I've had a lot of painful lessons about the gaps between what I'm doing and what I think I'm doing. The only way I've found to get those lessons is to get honest feedback from others."

"That's exactly what happened for me," said Rodriguez. "And you're right about one thing. Feedback can sting."

"Sure. That's why people don't always ask for it. But it's a case of pay now or pay later. Procrastinate, and the price goes up. The truth often hurts in the short run, but it seems to bring dividends over the long haul."

"Well, I've got the pain. I hope I'll see the gain as well."

Leadership Lessons

Build Relationships
and Empower Yourself

Even highly educated professionals bring their needs and their humanity with them when they come to work. They still need to feel safe, to belong, to feel appreciated, and to feel that they make a difference. School administrators sometimes make the mistake of sucking up as much responsibility and power as they can, often with plenty of encouragement from their constituents. Our colleague, Mari Takahashi, compared schools in the United States and in Japan. She found that in the United States, principals tended to feel the weight of just about everything on their shoulders. In Japan, staff and students felt a responsibility to make the principal's job easier. U.S. principals worked much longer days, with much of their time devoted to fighting one fire after another. Japanese principals arrived later and left earlier—they couldn't stay too late in the afternoon, because teachers felt they could only go home after the principal had left.

The following guidelines can help principals and teachers respond to some of the perennial relationship challenges in schools:

Empower yourself and others. When leaders try to do everything themselves, they leave everyone else frustrated and disempowered. The school bogs down because nothing gets done unless the boss does it or approves it. Connors encouraged Rodriguez to open up communication and share the responsibility for making the school a better place. Staff began to feel that their needs were finally being recognized, and feelings of ownership started to spread. Likewise, Juhl demonstrated how to combine caring, honesty, and effective listening to build open, collaborative dialogues.

Open up communications—ask questions and tell the truth. Spend time with people—particularly with the people who seem to disagree with you. When we're at odds with someone else, we often avoid them and stop listening to them. The problem is that when we shut down, they shut down as well. When conflict arose between Rodriguez and the faculty, Connors encouraged him to get closer rather than to withdraw and to work at understanding the sources of the discontent. Loving your enemies is a remarkably durable and practical maxim. Listen to others. Attend to their feelings, concerns, and aspirations. And tell them the truth. It's familiar advice that almost everyone endorses. But it's easier to practice than preach. The primary barrier is fear. We'd say what we think—if we weren't afraid of the consequences. Much of Margaret Juhl's ability to be helpful to both Jaime Rodriguez and Joan Hilliard came from her willingness to risk telling the truth to her boss as well as to her friends—even when she knew they might not like what she had to say.

Ask for feedback. Without feedback, both principals and teachers become blind to how they're seen and out of touch with how well they're doing. But the people around us often withhold their perceptions because they're afraid of how we'll respond. Asking is the easiest way to get honest feedback. This takes persistence and skill in framing the right questions. But keep at it and you'll expand your learning opportunities. If you simply ask a friend or colleague, "What did you think about my lesson/classroom management/speech," the first response you get will often amount to vague reassurance ("Seemed fine to me"). Not much help. Follow up with more specific probes: "What do you think worked best?" "What could I have done to make it better?" "How do you think the students reacted?" Persistence makes your requests clear and credible.

Take initiative to empower yourself and others. Much of Margaret's Juhl's leadership at Pico School comes from a combination of her experience and her willingness to take initiative on issues that she could just as easily avoid. She doesn't sit around waiting for someone else to fix problems she sees. She can't jump on every challenge that comes along. As most teachers do, she's got too much to do and too little time to do it. But she doesn't let that become an excuse for inaction. By taking initiative and looking for allies who share her concerns, she helps to make Pico a better school.

As Juhl does, you can help your school by looking for chances to contribute, learn, and have fun. Schools almost always have more things to be done than people to do them. Look for opportunities, and grab the most promising ones.

PART IV

The Structural Frame

CHAPTER SEVEN

Student Discipline

Who's Really in Charge?

February was turning into Rodriguez's best month yet. The postholiday morale crisis and the anonymous newsletter led to a series of informal meetings with faculty. The process was challenging but, in the end, exhilarating. Morale was up. So was trust. People were talking to one another. Rodriguez was on a high. Until the bubble burst. This time the hot button was student discipline.

In the old days, Sam Shepherd had been tireless in his efforts to bring offenders to justice. He had been police officer, judge, and jury, all rolled into one. When teachers sent offenders to Shepherd, the outcome was never in doubt. He kept the lid tightly clamped on the pressure cooker while he was there. But after he left, the steam began to overflow. Teachers were complaining about not being backed up. There were more fights on the playground and in the lunchroom. Some parents were getting worried about their children's safety.

Rodriguez knew something had to be done. He also knew he could not do it himself. This seemed to be a perfect opportunity to try out the district's new shared decision-making program. The superintendent, Mildred Hofsteder, was a strong advocate for decentralizing responsibility and involving faculty and parents in decision making. Every school had been asked to establish a faculty-parent council to serve as an advisory body to the principal. Because discipline was an issue of great interest to both parents and faculty, it seemed like an ideal task for the newly formed council to work on.

Meanwhile, Joan Hilliard was pleasantly surprised to learn that, as a first-year teacher, she had been elected as the council's first chairperson. Carlos Cortez had persuaded her to become a candidate, and Joan was delighted when Phil Leckney also rose to support her. When she asked Phil about it later, his explanation was simple. "I supported you for two reasons. The first is that your business experience might be useful. The second is that not too many people wanted the job. I might as well tell you that some people may support you because they think you'll be a pushover. But I know you better than that."

At the first meeting of the council, Jaime Rodriguez charged the group with looking into the worsening discipline problem. He offered them two alternatives as a way to focus their discussion. One was to hire an administrator to replace Sam Shepherd. The other was to develop a new schoolwide approach that would involve everyone—the principal, the faculty, and even parents and students—in implementing a shared discipline code. Joan was happy to have the issue on the agenda, but she wondered why Rodriguez hadn't talked to her before presenting the two options. She worried her position as chairperson would be undermined if other council members felt the principal was actually running the show.

In subsequent meetings, her fears were confirmed. The council represented various segments of the Pico community, including teachers, parents, and students. The group was diverse, particularly in ideas about discipline. Despite Joan's best efforts, the council soon bogged down in conflict and trivia. There were debates between liberals and conservatives, teachers and parents, those who wanted a single, schoolwide discipline philosophy, and others who wanted discretion for individual faculty. Rodriguez attended every meeting and often behaved as if he were chairing the council. Joan learned that some individuals were meeting privately with Rodriguez to lobby his support for their private agenda. Joan sensed that she was rapidly losing her ability to be effective as a chair. The question was, What could she do about it? She once again called on Margaret Juhl.

"It's not just you," Margaret said reassuringly, "the same thing is happening in lots of schools. Everyone's talking about empowering teachers and sharing decision making, but people are also telling principals that they're supposed to be strong instructional leaders. So principals often feel in a bind. They don't want to step on teachers' toes, but they feel accountable. As teachers, we often fall into the same trap by waiting for the principal to take the lead. That makes it very confusing. You're supposed to be chairing, but the principal is always there. It's like a dance where no one's sure who's leading, who's following, and what rhythm you're supposed to be listening for. Some people are trying to waltz, and others are doing hip-hop. Shared decision making is a good idea, but it's tough to make it work."

"But why is it so hard?"

"It's basically a structural problem. No one's sure who's in charge. Is it you or the principal? People tend to figure that the principal is the real boss in a school, so they look to him for direction and answers. Jaime feels the pressure, and he does what a lot of administrators do: He shoulders the load. No one's at fault, but it won't fix itself. You'll have to do something to clarify the situation."

"Like what?" asked Joan.

"Well, Jaime's learning fast. I think maybe you just need to get his attention."

"How?"

"Send him a brief note telling him you're quitting."

"You're kidding! I want to be chair. I think I have something to contribute."

"I agree, and so does Jaime. He needs you as the chair at least as much as you need to be in the role. Trust me, as soon as he gets that note, he'll see you."

"Then what?" asked Joan.

"Tell it like it is, and don't pull any punches. Just make sure that Jaime understands you're not blaming him, but you don't want to be part of a two-boss system that confuses everyone."

Joan was doubtful that the gambit would work, but she had enough confidence in Margaret's intuition to give it a try. Besides, she said to herself, I don't have a better idea. Her confidence in Margaret was soon reinforced. Within 24 hours of her sending a note to Jaime, he wrote back asking for a meeting as soon as possible. Joan went to Phyllis Gleason to make an appointment.

"Boy, does he want to see you!" said Phyllis with a knowing smile. "You don't need an appointment. Go right in!"

Jaime literally bounced out of his chair as soon as Joan walked in. He offered her the warmest greeting she could remember in a long time. Then he got right to the point. "Joan, I hope you'll reconsider. If you quit now, I think it will set the council back."

Remembering Margaret's advice, Joan knew she didn't want to give in until she was sure Jaime understood the problem. "Well, let me tell you why I resigned. For me, it's been a no-win situation. I've felt responsible for everything because I'm the elected chairperson, but everyone assumed you were really in charge. Every time I tried to do my job, you did something to remind people that you were really running the show."

Joan had feared Jaime would be surprised or even offended at her candor. Instead, he smiled reassuringly. "I think you're right. After I got your note, I talked to a colleague that I trust, Brenda Connors. She told me the same thing. So we agree," Rodriguez replied. "We need to clarify the council's role as well as that of the chairperson. I've got an idea about how we can do it, but I need your help."

"Well, here we go again. You always have the answers. Aren't you interested in my ideas?" asked Joan.

Rodriguez seemed briefly taken aback, but then he smiled again, and openly acknowledged that she had a point. "Look, Joan, I'm new and you're new. We both have a lot to learn. And right now you might not rate me as one of the most promising students you've seen."

It was Joan's turn to smile. "Now we're getting somewhere. But I'm not going to be the chair unless we clear up the confusion about who's running the show."

"Can I offer a suggestion?"

"Sure, if it's really a suggestion and not a command. You have a lot more experience under your belt than I do, and I want to learn from you. But sometimes your suggestions sound more like marching orders."

"Okay, okay, I get the message. You're the captain on this team. You and the council make the decisions. Actually, my suggestion was based on something that Brenda told me about. You decide whether it's a good idea or not. It's a process called CAIRO. It sounds like the capital of Egypt, but it's really a straightforward way of trying to bring structural issues to the surface."

"How does it work?" asked Joan, willing to hear him out.

"Well, CAIRO is an acronym. Each of the letters stands for a different kind of responsibility that someone can have in a decision. For example, someone, or some group, is ultimately responsible for making it. They get the *R* in Cairo, because they're responsible; the monkey is on their back. A *C* goes to anyone who needs to be consulted. *A* designates someone who has to approve the decision. If someone just has to be informed about the decision, they get an *I*. And they get an *O* if they're out of the decision loop."

"O.K., I know what you're talking about. I ran into something similar in my last job. So, you set up a chart, like a matrix, with the different people along one dimension and the different responsibilities along the other."

"Exactly."

Joan liked the idea, but worried Jaime would try to take too much responsibility for implementing his "suggestion." She stated her concern directly. "If we do it, I need to manage the process."

"That's a deal! Let me know if you want me to help. And tell me the next time you think I'm stepping on your toes."

At the next meeting, Joan led the council through the CAIRO exercise. She explained the CAIRO acronym and distributed a matrix. First, she asked everyone to fill it out individually. Then they shared their individual perceptions. It was an eye-opener for everyone. It turned out that there were at least three different ideas about how the discipline policy was supposed to be developed. Implicitly, Rodriguez believed that it was his decision in the final analysis. Many teachers felt that the responsibility ultimately ought to be theirs, as most of the implementation would fall into their laps. Many parents felt that the council should make the final decision. The group broke into laughter when a parent commented, "This looks a lot like the way my family works."

Afterwards, Hilliard went to Rodriguez and said, "You know, the exercise helped. But I realized something even more basic today. The way the council is set up almost guarantees failure. It's the wrong group to hammer out something as complicated as a new discipline policy. The council is too big, it's too diverse, and it's got too much to do and too little time to do it. The CAIRO exercise showed we have too many people who think they have the *R*. But if you think about it, only some on the council have a big stake in this policy. I think we should make them a group with responsibility for preparing a draft. They could consult with you, with the teachers, with the community, and with students. Then, if I understand how this site-based management is supposed to work, the council should retain final approval rights."

Jaime closed his eyes and clasped his hands to his lips. It was clear that he was thinking hard about what Joan had said. "Maybe you hit the nail on the head. Maybe I set this up wrong to begin with. I was talking to Brenda Connors about this. She told me that a group needs to be clear about four things: what it's supposed to do, what authority it has, who it's accountable to, and what it's accountable for. You're right—a smaller group with a clearer task has a better shot at coming up with a workable policy. The council already has too much on its plate."

"Exactly. So the council can make its job easier by delegating this task. But they have to give the subgroup a clear charge."

"I agree. Is part of the charge to make sure that the major players all feel that they were heard in the process?"

"Sure," said Hilliard. "Let me develop a plan. I'll check it with you and with some of the council members. If enough people buy in, I'll get someone to bring it to the council."

At the council's next meeting, Hilliard arranged for a parent to propose a new design for dealing with the discipline problem. The parent said at the outset that the proposal had emerged from conversations among a number of people concerned about making the council work better. "The idea that we've come up with," she said, "is to create a task force. Their job is to develop a proposal and bring it back to us. They will consult with the entire school community and develop an approach that's fair, consistent, and workable for faculty, parents, and students. Then they'll come back to us. We can either approve the policy, modify it, or send it back for more work. Once we approve, the policy goes to Mr. Rodriguez, who says he expects to support our decision."

Several council members glanced at Jaime, wondering whether they could believe what they had heard. Jaime acknowledged the glances and said simply, "The only thing I want to add is that I fully support this approach."

A teacher responded immediately, "That just makes so much sense. We've been beating our heads on a wall and getting nowhere. I think it's a great idea." After discussion and some modification of the proposal, the council approved it. A task force of three teachers and two parents went to work with enthusiasm. After holding many meetings with different parts of the school community, they came back to the council two months later with a proposal that soon drew broad support. The council approved the new policy unanimously, and everyone was optimistic that the whole effort was a giant step forward for the school.

The council did not stop there. One parent had commented pointedly, "Before we get too smug, remember that we've been through things like this before with the PTA. We make decisions, but nothing gets done. Someone called it the 'Pico pile,' the scrap heap of policies and programs that get approved but never really happen."

"You're raising a really important issue," Rodriguez commented. Who has the *R* for implementing the new policy? Otherwise, it might fall through the cracks or into my lap."

"That makes sense," said Hilliard. "We need to be clear about that so the new policy doesn't wind up in the Pico pile. Is this something the council should do, or should we ask the discipline task force to work on it?"

Rodriguez smiled to himself as the council decided to work through the implementation issues. He felt that he had helped move the process forward without taking over. He planned to tell Brenda that evening.

The success of the discipline task force had many ripple effects. Later that night, Brenda Connors smiled to herself after another telephone conversation with Rodriguez. "He's learning fast," she thought. "He has terrific people skills, but I knew he needed to get a better handle on structure. I used to have the same problem. I figured if I cared about people, structure wasn't that big a deal. In a way, Jaime is catching on faster than I did." She gave herself a pat on the back for helping to speed up his progress.

During a long lunch break on a Saturday shopping excursion, Joan recounted the details of the discipline policy process to Margaret. Margaret seemed very pleased. "I hope you feel as proud as I do about what you've accomplished. Maybe it's your business experience. Even though you're a rookie teacher, you're becoming a model of what it means to be a teacher leader."

Joan beamed with pleasure. "Well, I really owe it all to you."

"Maybe I helped, but you really owe it to yourself. You brought a lot with you, and you learn fast. I think you're in line for rookie of the year. I just hope our colleagues can learn from your example. We're going to run into other issues just as tough as the discipline policy. If shared leadership is going to work at Pico, more teachers have to believe they can take some initiative."

"One reason for them to do it is that it helps in the classroom as well," replied Joan. "In working out the confusion in the council, I realized that I have similar issues in my classroom."

"Which ones?" asked Margaret.

"Well, I was doing to my class what Jaime was doing to the council—taking on all the responsibility. I was training them to be passive learners, always waiting for my next instructions. I did all the work, and all they had to do was sit and watch. It's not easy, but I'm trying to show them the difference between the *R* and the *C* in CAIRO. I'm trying to structure tasks where I have a *C*—they should consult me for ideas and suggestions—but they have the *R*. They're accountable for the decisions they make."

Margaret thought for a moment, and then said, "Of course. Whether we're talking about empowering teachers or empowering students, the basic issues are the same. I've got an idea! You and I should do a schoolwide in-service on CAIRO and how it relates to relationships between students and teachers. We'll try to get parents involved too. What do you think?"

"I'd love to! I learn so much every time we talk, but we haven't had that many opportunities to work together. The rookie and the veteran—we might make a great team."

"We already make a great team. The rookie is turning into a pro."

Joan savored that comment throughout a quiet evening at her apartment. Larry was on another weekend business trip. Sometimes Joan was almost relieved when Larry was away midweek, since she usually had so much work to do anyway. But a Saturday night alone was a different matter. She wanted to call him, but once again he had neglected to mention where he would be staying. There were too many hotels in Atlanta for her to spend the night trying to track him down. "Oh, well," she thought to herself. "Maybe it's just as well. If I tried to explain why I'm feeling so good about my conversation with Margaret, he might just tune me out anyway."

The ringing of the phone interrupted her reverie. "Sorry I couldn't call earlier, honey," said Larry's familiar voice, "but the meeting ran late. Anyway, I wanted to tell you that I love you. What's happening?"

CHAPTER EIGHT

Standards

T he tension in the faculty lounge could be cut with a knife. The superintendent of schools, Mildred Hofsteder, rarely visited Pico. When she did, there was always trouble, at least in the memories of many teachers. Today she was here to attend the afternoon faculty meeting. There was none of the usual banter as teachers filed in. Dr. Hofsteder stood at the front, flanked by Rodriguez and an older man with gray hair, a gray suit, and a generally gray look.

"Bureaucrat. Probably from the State Department of Education," Phil Leckney whispered to Joan.

"We're really in for it," she replied.

Jaime opened the meeting with brief introductions of the guests before yielding to the superintendent.

Hofsteder wasted no time in getting to the agenda. "As you know, the legislature has passed new state standards for reading and math. Naturally, we will be complying with this new mandate. At the end of each year we will be testing students in grades four through eight to assess our progress. As the law requires, scores will be reported for each school and the school-level results will be available to the public. Dr. Samuels from the Department of Education will brief you on the details."

Samuels droned earnestly into his presentation and soon lost much of his audience.

"What's he saying?" Joan asked Phil.

"Dunno. The guy only speaks bureaucratese."

But Samuels seemed to warm to his subject when he shifted to the topic of accountability, and his next words snapped the audience back to attention.

"The State Department wants to be sure that schools understand the seriousness of our new process for promoting educational excellence. There will be no free rides for underperforming schools, principals, or teachers. All children should be learning. If they're not, then we'll move resources to schools that can provide the educational support the students need."

By the time he finished, Samuels had left most of the teachers feeling indicted and threatened. His request for questions brought only silence. Joan looked over to Margaret Juhl, half expecting her to leap to the school's defense, but even Margaret sat tight-lipped. Jaime looked almost ill. He squirmed but finally regained his composure and thanked the guests for coming to Pico. Hofsteder and Samuels exited, leaving a very quiet room behind them. Only when they were out of earshot did the real meeting began.

"Good God!" Leckney gasped. "They want us to create school councils. They've put in tougher evaluations for teachers. They instituted a new drug program. We're supposed to be working more closely with business. Now they're going reduce our teaching to a bunch of items on a multiple-choice test. Maybe I'm getting too old for this sort of thing, but come on! I'm a professional. Treat me like one!"

Rodriguez was surprised at the intensity of his reaction. "That's pretty strong even for you, Phil. What bothers you so much?"

"When you've been teaching as long as I have, you see a lot of things come and go—alternative this, new that, authentic something else. We get fads from the business world. Glorious ideas from the universities. Pet projects from politicians. How do you ever build anything if you keep throwing out what you did last year? How is one more fad going to help?"

"I know that the fad of the year is a big problem in education. You all keep reminding me that we have a Pico pile filled with new programs that fell by the wayside. I know it won't solve all our problems," Jaime responded. "But I think you all know the reality. We have a mandate from the state and the district that we can't just ignore."

"But that doesn't mean we have to like it," Phil responded, to nods of assent from many of his colleagues.

"No, but we're going to be better off if we can figure out the most productive way to deal with it. How about if we kick this one around a little before we just dismiss it as worthless."

"Okay," Phil responded in a more modulated voice. "But you're going to have to do a lot more to convince me that this isn't one more flash in the pan they are trying to stuff down our throats."

Jaime was feeling the heat. He knew Samuels's presentation had been a disaster, leaving most of the faculty feeling angry and insulted. But Samuels had gone, and the new state requirements were still in place, backed by a formidable coalition of the governor, the state legislature, and the school board.

"You're right," he said, "we're all dealing with layers of history. We have a trash heap full of all the stuff that comes in and gets tossed out, but hangs around anyway. When I started here, I thought I had answers to the school's problems. All I did was convince most of you that I was the problem. We're all tired of these solutions that are mandated from above. But we can't just give up."

Vivian Chu jumped in with support. "Jaime's right. We all know that some of our kids are falling through the cracks. And we don't have very good ways of identifying those who do. We also know that behind our classroom doors we do pretty much what we want. Remember what's his name? The one who used to teach in Joan's room? His classroom was like a movie theater. All he did was run the projector and keep the kids entertained. I don't know why he didn't sell popcorn. Maybe we do need a little more accountability."

"It's not a matter of being more accountable or giving up. It's what we have to give up in order to be more accountable." Margaret Juhl rose to her feet and spoke with unusual fervor. "We all know what's at the heart of teaching, and that's never going to be measured on a multiple-choice test. Most of you are like me. You became teachers because you wanted to make a difference. And I believe that I do. You can't always measure it with test scores, but over the years I have gathered a lot of testimony from students and parents. If we move on this standards and testing thing, we need to make sure that we don't gut the soul of what we do. We're not here just to dispense information. We're here to shape young lives. Who we are is as important as what we teach."

Nodding heads and affirmative responses showed that, once more, Margaret had hit the nail on the head.

Jaime responded, "I agree, but we're still going to be held accountable for short-term results. It's not just my butt on the line. Pico's reputation is also at stake. However those test scores come out, they'll be in the newspapers. Right or wrong, a lot of people will be judging us on those numbers. Let me propose that we do two things. Get one group working on the latest research on teaching for results. Vivian, would you be willing to chair that one?"

Vivian nodded assent.

"Margaret," said Jaime, "how about if you chair another effort to work on building evidence around the important intangibles we all value. Joan can bring this matter to the parent council to get their support. What do you think?"

Nodding heads told the story. Even Phil Leckney seemed to be willing to go along. But the banter at the bar later that night painted a less optimistic picture. It wasn't going to be that easy.

As usual, Phil led the initial charge. "Jaime's caught in the middle. He's trying to save his butt by foisting all this off on us. I wish we had a stronger leader, someone who would go to bat for us."

Joan jumped in. "Wait a minute, Phil. You're right, Jaime's getting squeezed like an orange. But we're in the same vise. And speaking of leadership, where were you, Margaret? We all expected you to take the bureaucrat on. Why didn't you speak up while he and the superintendent were here?"

"Over the years, I've learned not to attack when there's nothing to be won. Taking on Samuels might have made us all feel good, but what good would it have done?"

"Shouldn't the bureaucrats hear how teachers really feel?" asked Leckney.

"That wasn't his mission. He was a messenger, sent to read us the riot act. He did his job. If we took him on, we'd get him annoyed, embarrass the superintendent, and make Jaime squirm harder than he already was."

"So now what do we do?" asked Joan.

"Face reality. Pressures for standards and accountability aren't going away anytime soon. So we're in a dilemma. We have to work with the prevailing policies, but we also have to do what's right for our kids. It's a dance. Good teachers have done it for years. They'll still be doing it long after I'm retired."

"Retirement is sounding pretty good to me," Phil volunteered.

"Phil," said Margaret soothingly, "you know your wife says that the day you retire, she's moving out."

"You've got a point, but why should I stay if I'm going to be spending most of my time teaching to the test?"

"Phil, I wouldn't stay either if that were the price," said Margaret. "The tests are one way to keep score. Not the only way. To my mind, not the most important way. I want my kids to learn what they need to learn. If they do, they'll probably do all right on the tests. But the test that matters is whether I help them have productive and happy lives. If they do better on that one than on a bunch of multiple-choice items, I figure I've been a success."

"Dangerous thinking, Margaret," Phil responded.

Margaret smiled. "Old-timers like you and me are dangerous. We're the kamikazes who can keep the pot stirred and help strike a balance between testing and caring. There are a lot of people in this community who've been touched by what we do. If we play this right, we'll get a lot of support from them and from our kids and parents. That's why Jaime's committees make good sense. It lets us buy some time and get our ducks lined up."

"I hope they're not sitting ducks," Phil sighed.

Everyone laughed. And then Joan pitched in, "Only time will tell."

Leadership Lessons

Align the Structure With the Work

In a classroom, a school, or any other group, people like to know where they're headed, who's in charge, what they're supposed to do, and how their efforts relate to others'. Putting eager students or talented teachers into a confusing system wastes their energy and undermines their effectiveness. Structural arrangements demand continual attention just as human needs do. Teachers sometimes figure that the job of social architect is reserved for administrators. Bosses are supposed to develop policies, provide direction, and make sure everyone's on the same page. Sometimes administrators live up to expectations. Often, they don't. If administrators aren't picking up the ball, someone had better, or there will be frustration all around.

Clarify roles. On any team, people need to know how their work relates to others'. Without coordination and teamwork, the best individual efforts produce a poor outcome. Maybe you remember a time you made an inspired effort that flopped because someone got in your way or didn't come through. It's frustrating for everyone. If you're in a situation where people are constantly stepping on others' toes or pointing fingers of blame, try an experiment. Choose an issue or task where there is continual confusion or conflict. Apply the CAIRO concepts. Create a matrix listing responsibilities in the far-left column. In the remaining columns, place individual roles across the top. Now have everyone individually assign a letter to each person for every responsibility. Give *R* to the person who's responsible—the one with the monkey on his or her back. Now assign letters specifying that person's (or group's) relationships to others. Give an *I* to anyone to be kept informed, a *C* to anyone who needs to be consulted, an *A* to anyone who has approval rights, and an *O* to anyone essentially "out of the loop." CAIRO goes beyond an organization chart to pinpoint exactly what people are expected to do and how they relate to others. Any employee can initiate the activity. Administrative blessing isn't essential, though it certainly helps.

The CAIRO exercise done collectively usually produces several important discoveries. It shows that people often have very different views of how things are supposed to work. It reveals who's overloaded or underused, how many levels of approval someone needs before taking action, and who appears to need to be in control. The exercise often clarifies why people are always at each other's throats and why important things rarely get done.

Design groups for success rather than failure. Groups are a basic feature of schools. Every classroom is a group, and teachers often group students for instructional purposes. Teachers and administrators participate in a variety of teams and groups, both large and small. Whether you're the leader or a member, you won't have a very good experience in a group that doesn't know where it's going or what it's supposed to do. Make sure the group is clear about Brenda Connors's four keys to success:

1. What are we supposed to do? (What's our goal? What's the task we're charged to do?)
2. What authority and resources do we have?
3. To whom are we accountable?
4. What are we accountable for? (What are we supposed to produce? A policy? An implementation plan? A written report? An oral presentation?)

Groups need to know what they are supposed to do, how their success will be judged, and who will do the judging. Student groups need to know if they're accountable simply to each other, or to the teacher. When principals appoint a faculty committee or task force, they need to be clear what it's supposed to do and what authority it has. Is it supposed to make a decision, or simply make recommendations? What authority and resources does the group have? Groups with manageable tasks, sufficient authority, and clear accountability have a higher probability of success.

Set or clarify goals. Deep down, we're all goal directed. Teachers or students rally to a cause they know about and care about. No one gets energized by goals they don't know, can't understand, or don't believe in. The trick is to set specific, measurable goals that set up a clear, challenging, reachable target.

Shape a structure that fits. In schools and classrooms, a lot of structure is already in place—curricula, assessment procedures, legal mandates, and much more. Some is helpful. Some gets in the way. How do we decide what arrangement of roles and relationships we need? A workable structure has to fit the task and the people who will do it. Structure is definitely not a matter of one-size-fits-all. A top-down structure with clear rules and specific procedures works for routine, repetitive tasks like ordering supplies, issuing pay-checks, and scheduling classes. But the same system breaks down in handling more complex and open-ended tasks, particularly ones that require skill and discretion. There can be value in standardized cur-ricula and proven teaching techniques if they are offered as tools that teachers can adapt to their specific circumstances. But efforts to improve schools by imposing "teacher-proof" methods have conti-nually run aground in the face of the unpredictable and unique features of individual teachers, students, and classrooms.

Structure can work for or against us, though we're much more likely to notice when it misfires or gets in our way. There are good rules—and bad ones. Brilliant meetings and disasters. Sometimes people in authority know what they are doing; others haven't a clue. More discretion sometimes pays off big. Other times, it produces mammoth screwups. Schools have good and bad goals. The good ones are displayed as virtues. Shadier ambitions are hidden. A work-able balance between public virtues and the "real objectives" pro-vides a reasonable focus that people can honor and accept. Finding the right balance is an ongoing challenge. It doesn't do any good to label all structure as bureaucracy and red tape. We need to make the formal system work for us. That's not the sole province of anyone. It's an ongoing dance. When the dance goes well, it shapes arrange-ments that generally work. Not all the time, or for everyone. But for most people most of the time. It only happens when teachers and administrators stop blaming and learn to dance the same steps.

PART V

The Symbolic Frame

CHAPTER NINE

The End of the Year

Symbols and Culture in Schools

Jaime Rodriguez and Brenda Connors met for dinner at a sidewalk café on a beautiful evening in May. For Jaime, it was a chance to thank Brenda for all her help. For her, it was a chance to congratulate a star pupil on a very successful first year. That done, Rodriguez turned to a lingering issue—the ghost of Phil Bailey. "You know, even though I feel good about what we've been able to do this year, I don't understand why there's still so much talk about Phil. It's like his ghost runs the school. One thing I'd like to do before the end of the year is exorcize his haunting presence."

"Maybe an exorcism might work," said Brenda, "but there's another way to think about it. It's human nature to form attachments. We get attached to things and people that are important to us. We even bond to things we don't like—like devils or scapegoats. We blame them for problems we don't understand. When an attachment is broken—if you lose a job, get divorced, or move to a new city—you feel the loss. Think about your own experience. How do you feel when you lose something you care about?"

"A lot of things," replied Rodriguez. "I feel sad, angry, confused, depressed, ambivalent, you name it. I see it in people around me. I remember what my mother went through after my father's death. It was real tough."

"Sure. A death in the family might be the biggest loss of all. But you can feel loss even with something that doesn't seem important. Remember the caboose at the end of the train? It isn't there anymore.

A little electronic box does the job today more efficiently than the old caboose and its crew," Connors pointed out.

"But," Jaime objected, "I used to love waving at the caboose when I was kid."

"That was a long time ago, but you still miss the caboose. Phil Bailey is Pico's caboose, and you're the electronic box. Most cultures have figured out that ceremonies help people deal with loss. When people die, we have wakes, flowers, funerals, and mourning periods. When people get married, we have an elaborate ceremony and a big party."

"Marriage is a loss?" asked Rodriguez.

"There's something lost and something gained in any major change. People get married for love and companionship, the desire to have children, and lots of other positive things. But marriages get into trouble because people have trouble letting go of old identities and old relationships. That's why there are so many jokes about in-laws. It can take years to make transitions. Phil Bailey was at Pico a long time. It's not surprising that people still miss him. Change is a little like what happens when a trapeze artist has to let go of one bar before grabbing the next. It's scary to let go, but there's more danger in hanging on too long."

"Does that mean we need a funeral for Bailey?"

"Something like that," Brenda replied thoughtfully. "Even though people know you're the principal, it's harder for them to accept it until the torch has been symbolically passed. What did they do to mark Phil's retirement?"

"Nothing, actually. They wanted to hold a retirement dinner, but Phil said he wouldn't come."

"That's too bad. People need a chance to celebrate both his accomplishments and his screwups, to savor the memories, and to tell stories. They need to say 'Thank you,' 'We care about you,' and 'We wish you well.'"

"But Bailey didn't die," said Rodriguez. "He retired. He doesn't need a casket. He's having too much fun on the golf course."

"But, for many people, his retirement still feels like a death in the family. To them, he's gone. They've never had a chance to mourn his loss or celebrate his life at the school, so it's harder for them to let go. If people haven't let go of Phil, it's hard for them to form attachments with you."

"So maybe I need to plan a funeral and see if we can get rid of the ghost for good."

"Remember, you're still a newcomer to the school's culture. You haven't paid your dues yet. You need to check in with the key people in Pico's cultural network. They need to plan and bless something this important."

"Who do you have in mind?"

"Didn't you say that Bill Hill is the eyes and ears of Pico?"

"Yes. He's the unofficial message center. I get the point. I need to talk to him. I also need to talk to Phyllis, because she's the school historian."

"She may be even more than that. She might be the unofficial priestess."

Rodriguez looked surprised.

"From what I've heard," Brenda explained, "Phyllis takes confessions and gives blessings. She keeps confidences. But she weaves what she hears into her portrait of the school. She celebrates things that succeed. She gives comfort when things go wrong. She's like the priests and priestesses in traditional cultures. They were storytellers, and they presided over rites and ceremonies. She may be a key custodian of Pico's culture."

"You make it sound like I'm more like a tribal chief than a school principal," protested Rodriguez.

"You've got it, and a good chief, particularly a new one, knows the tribe's spiritual leaders have to be in charge of important ceremonies. Talk to Phyllis. Ask her who should preside over your end-of-the-year ceremony. She'll know. Otherwise, you might shoot yourself in the foot."

The next morning, as Rodriguez lingered over his second cup of coffee, he felt apprehensive and even a little foolish about his meeting with Phyllis. The more he thought about it, the more he worried that Brenda might be leading him into a morass. If she had not been right so many times in the past, he might have ignored her advice.

When he and Phyllis Gleason met, he opened by saying that he needed her help again. Then he asked, "Is Phil Bailey still the presiding principal?"

"Mr. Rodriguez, I wondered when you'd ask me that. Mr. Bailey was around for a long time. He wasn't perfect, and he had his quirks, but people were used to him. He was like an old T-shirt. It's comfortable and familiar. It reminds you of memories that get better and better as time passes."

"Is it true that he said no to the idea of a retirement party?"

"Absolutely. Mr. Bailey was not the kind of person who stood on ceremony. He literally walked out on the last day, gave me the keys, and told me to send the stuff in his office to his home. He didn't even show up for our end-of-the-year party. I think that hurt a lot of people. People have leftover feelings, including Mr. Bailey. I've talked to his wife a few times. Retirement is tougher than he expected. He sometimes calls friends on the faculty to ask how things are going. They're not sure what to say. It's really past time for Mr. Bailey's official retirement party."

"Maybe for both him and me. I feel I've been in his shadow all year long."

"Do you want me to be frank, Mr. Rodriguez?"

"Of course."

"Well, you've done some things to make it worse."

"Like what?"

"Like the time you came in during Christmas vacation, cleaned out the old storeroom, and redecorated it as a faculty lounge," said Gleason.

"But teachers told me how happy they were to have the lounge," said Rodriguez.

"People don't always tell you everything. A lot of people liked the idea of the lounge. You did a nice job of decorating it. But in creating it, you threw out some things that people really cared about."

"You're telling me people thought that junk was important?"

"How would you feel if someone went up to your grandmother's attic and tossed everything out?"

"I think I'm starting to get it. It just never occurred to me that anyone would miss any of that stuff. I meant it as a gesture of how much I support the teachers," said Rodriguez.

"I wish you had asked me before cleaning out the storeroom," said Gleason. "I could have told you what might happen. It wasn't the stuff itself that was important, it was what it represented. You tossed out memories. The act itself was not so important as what it meant."

"I've learned a lot this year, Phyllis. But I know I still have a lot more to learn. I hope you'll keep on giving me a hand."

"Since you're asking, let me mention one other thing," said Gleason. "Remember parents' night, when you sent the teachers a memo telling them that everyone would be in the gym, instead of meeting parents in the classrooms?"

"Sure. The idea actually came from a couple of parents. They thought it would be a lot more convenient that way. Otherwise, they have to wander all over the school, particularly if they have more than one child at Pico."

"Maybe, but it's always been a tradition here for teachers to meet parents in their classrooms. That way, parents can see the children's work displayed, and the teachers can show off their domain. A lot of them work very hard on their classrooms, and they're proud of them. At Pico's open house, maybe convenience is not the most important thing for parents or teachers. Maybe they're more concerned about getting a sense of what it's really like in their child's classroom."

"Phyllis, have you ever seen *M*A*S*H*?"

"Sure, why?"

"Our relationship is a lot like the one between Colonel Potter and Radar. You're always way ahead of me," said Rodriguez ruefully.

"I just try to do my job. But you can't learn the ropes alone. Don't worry about Mr. Bailey. I'll take care of it, and I'll let you know what you need to do."

Rodriguez felt a twinge of annoyance at the idea of taking orders from his secretary. Remembering Connors's counsel, he resisted the urge to remind Gleason who was in charge. Instead, he simply said, "Thanks, Phyllis. Let me know what I should do."

Three weeks later, Jaime arrived at his office to find a flyer on his desk announcing the "Fiesta de Pico," to be held on a Friday evening near the end of the school year. The program highlights were to include "Give My Regards to Bailey," "The New Principal's Report Card," and "What a Guy!" Rodriguez felt his stomach tighten, particularly when he thought about getting a performance evaluation in public. Would this be a celebration or a lynching? Was the priestess going to preside over a human sacrifice? He hoped that Brenda Connors knew what she was talking about and that Phyllis Gleason would come through.

On a warm and beautiful evening in June, Rodriguez walked into the school's multipurpose room. He was bowled over. He had never seen the room look so festive. He tried to guess where all the flowers, balloons, and streamers had come from, particularly because he hadn't signed any budget requests. His attention was drawn to the large banner hanging from the wall that read simply, "Fiesta de Pico: The Beat Goes On!" He noted with relief that the room looked too festive for a lynching. But he was still nervous, because Gleason had not yet told him what he was supposed to do.

Just then, a familiar voice said, "Mr. Rodriguez, glad you came early. How do you like the decorations?" Gleason took Rodriguez aside and briefed him on his role in the event. "When Mr. Bailey arrives, shake his hand, smile, and then go find a seat in the back row. The first part of the party is for him. Whatever happens next, keep smiling, and act as if you're having a good time."

Rodriguez did not feel very reassured, but he had little time to regroup. A large crowd was pouring into the room: teachers, staff, parents on the school council, even the superintendent and all the members of the school board. Just then, he was chagrined to see Sam Shepherd and his wife walk into the room. In his ear, he heard Phyllis whisper, "Go welcome Mr. Shepherd and ask him about the hunting lodge. He's not doing so well financially. Maybe you could schedule a faculty retreat up there to give him a boost." He gritted his teeth and tried to follow Gleason's instructions. He was more than pleased at Sam Shepherd's warm response and stunned when Mrs. Shepherd took him aside and said, "I can't thank you enough for all you did for Sam and our family."

Before he could regain his emotional equilibrium, Rodriguez saw Phil Bailey and his wife walk in to enthusiastic greetings from everyone. It was the kind of entrance that movie stars make at the Academy Awards ceremony. Remembering Gleason's advice, Rodriguez went over to welcome Phil Bailey as warmly as possible before taking his seat in the back row.

What followed caught him off guard. The superintendent, Mildred Hofsteder, walked to the podium. She asked Phil Bailey to come forward. She briefly recounted Bailey's years at Pico and then asked the board chairman to unveil the draped object at the back of the room: a large oil portrait of Bailey. The room erupted in a standing ovation, and Jaime watched as tears streaked down Phil Bailey's cheeks. Though he felt jealous, he kept smiling and joined the crowd in the applause.

Bailey's speech was brief and emotional. It felt a little too emotional to Rodriguez, but he could see that many in the audience were deeply moved, He felt an unexpected sense of relief. He began to ask himself what it would take to push a raise for Phyllis through the district office.

Next at the rostrum was Margaret Juhl. Her job, she announced, was to give the new principal his first annual report card. "Heaven help me!" thought Jaime, though he forced himself to keep smiling. What followed was a delightfully humorous roast. Rodriguez received an E for effort and an N (Needs to Improve) for citizenship. He tried not to wince at his grade of Needs to Improve for "Opening Sermons to the Faculty," or his citation for "Excessive Zeal in Cleaning Out Old Storerooms." His C (average) for the discipline policy felt low to him. But all that passed when he heard the summary recommendation: "Deserves Promotion to Second-Year Principal."

Juhl then called Jaime forward. Four people shook his hand: Margaret Juhl, Phil Bailey, the superintendent, and the board chairperson. Rodriguez felt a warm flush of joy, but what followed touched him deeply. The entire faculty came to the front of the room. Some of them were off beat and off tune, but their song said it all: "If you knew Jaime, like we know Jaime, oh, oh, what a guy!"

The "fiesta" was not quite over. Joan Hilliard came to the podium to announce that the Pico School Faculty–Parent Council had a certificate to award its principal, Jaime Rodriguez. She read it: "To Jaime Rodriguez, Our Principal. In his leadership of Pico School, may he ever be right. But, right or wrong, our principal!"

After the certificate, the hug from Phyllis gave Jaime the feeling that he was finally the principal of Pico.

A few days after Fiesta de Pico, an exuberant Rodriguez was having lunch with Connors. He had taken special care to let her know that this one was his treat. Connors could sense the excitement and pride as Jaime reviewed the fiesta in loving detail. She congratulated him on his success, and he tried to express how much he appreciated her help. "It's getting late, and I have another meeting," said Brenda, "but I really want you to know how much I've valued our talks over this year. And I have a little something for you."

As Connors reached down to pick up the shopping bag she had brought with her, Jaime pulled out a gift-wrapped package from his briefcase. He placed it on the table in front of her as she brought out her own gift. "Jaime," she asked with a smile, "What's that?"

"Sort of like an apple for the teacher. Open it."

Connors unwrapped the package to find a book by Richard Rodriguez, titled *Hunger of Memory.*

"It's a very important book for me," said Jaime. "The author and I are both named Rodriguez, though we're not related. We're both Mexican Americans. He tells the story of what he went through in learning to live in this culture. He helped me find my own story. You've helped me take that story farther." On the inside cover, the inscription read, "To Brenda, an extraordinary mentor, with thanks and love, Jaime."

Brenda beamed and wiped away a tear. "You shouldn't have, but thanks. You don't know how much this means to me. Well, don't just sit there, open yours."

Jaime admired the package, then opened it slowly. His face broke into a broad smile, even as his eyes welled with tears. There were two items in the package. One was a copy of John Dewey's *Education and Experience*. The inscription read, "To Jaime: You have learned so much this year! I'm proud of you." The second was a small statue of Pico's mascot, the mountain lion, with a plaque that read, "To Jaime Rodriguez, a great friend and a great school leader, from Brenda Connors."

"You could call it recognition for the rookie," said Brenda, "but it's a lot more than that. It's a symbol of what you mean to me and what I know you'll become."

CHAPTER TEN

"I'm Just a Great Teacher!"

W hen they hung that portrait of Phil Bailey on the wall, I was almost in tears. That may have been the single best event in all my years at Pico," said Phil Leckney. There were nods around the table at Andy's among a group of teachers who had gathered for refreshments and conversation after Fiesta de Pico.

"It was fantastic!" Joan Hilliard agreed. "Before tonight, I'd never even seen Mr. Bailey, but I'd heard so many stories about him. It was almost like he was a ghost roaming the halls."

"He was," replied Margaret emphatically. "That's why we needed the fiesta."

"Was this your idea, Margaret?" asked Carlos Cortez.

"No, I wish it had been. I'm not sure who thought it up, but I know Phyllis Gleason masterminded a lot of it, with a good bit of help from Bill Hill."

"When the secretary and custodian put together the best party in years," replied Carlos, "it almost puts us professionals to shame."

"Maybe," said Margaret, "but the principal also helped in his own way. He gave it his blessing and stayed out of the way. That was pretty daring for a rookie."

"Aren't you being modest, Margaret?" Joan chimed in. "You had a big role, too. I couldn't believe how funny you were in delivering the new principal's report card to Jaime. I can't remember when I laughed so much. Even Jaime seemed to think it was funny."

For nearly an hour, people shared their favorite stories about the evening. The mood swung fluidly from laughter to tears and back to laughter again. It was Carlos Cortez who broke the magic spell with a more serious observation. "You know, this is the first time we've all had this much fun together in a very long time. We don't do this often enough."

"Yeah," added Phil Leckney. "And the sad part is that the celebration was for Bailey and Rodriguez, not for us. Why should administrators get all the glory?"

His question struck a nerve, and a long silence spread over the group. Margaret Juhl, looking even more serious than usual, finally said in a very serious voice, "Phil, you just asked the right question. Maybe something's happened to all of us. Teaching used to be magic. It still is, sometimes, but it doesn't always feel that way. Every one of us has probably been at a party and met someone who asks us what we do. We get a little embarrassed and say, 'I'm just a teacher.' That's absurd! We ought to be the proudest people on earth. Yet we're taken for granted."

"Just look what you read in the papers. Schools are failing. Teachers can't teach," Leckney chimed in. There was bitterness in his voice.

"Maybe it's partly our fault," replied Margaret thoughtfully. "We ought to see teaching as a sacred profession. *We* don't take enough time to recognize what makes our job so special."

Joan agreed. "Margaret's absolutely right! This is my first year, and I've already lost some of the spirit I had in September. I love my students. I feel good about how my class went, despite some rough spots. It's just that we don't take time as a group to laugh, share our stories, and have fun together. We did that in my last job. I kind of miss it. If something's missing for *me*, how does it feel after you've been teaching 20 years?"

The emotion in Phil Leckney's voice surprised everyone at the table. "You really want to know? You get more burned out every year. A lot of times you struggle just to get up in the morning and make it through the day. You all know I wasn't crazy about our new principal or about some of the ideas he was pushing. I'm not a fossil. I don't resent new blood. God knows, I need a transfusion once in a while. But I need something so that I don't just coast my way to retirement."

"How about you, Margaret?" asked Joan.

"Maybe I pretend a lot," said Margaret. "My union responsibilities keep me busy, and I'm pretty good at mediating battles among different factions in the faculty. But when I close the classroom door,

I sometimes wonder if I'm really making a difference. I used to be absolutely sure of that, deep down in my heart. Now, I sometimes wonder. Come to think about it, I could use a lift myself."

"Well," said Joan, "if we can have a huge celebration for our principals, why can't we have something like that for teachers? Are principals more important than we are?"

"Of course not!" Carlos responded forcefully. "What matters most at Pico is what happens in the classroom between us and our students. Joan, you've got a great idea! I love Jaime, and tonight's fiesta was wonderful. But we should do something for ourselves as well."

Then, to everyone's delight, Phil Leckney ordered a bottle of imported champagne. "In the Navy," he said, "there was always champagne whenever we launched a new ship. We're launching something just as important. It deserves a toast!"

Throughout the summer, the group continued to meet, gradually transforming themselves into an informal planning team. Initially, they had wondered how Jaime Rodriguez would respond to their plans, but the strength of his enthusiasm made him one of their strongest backers. His only suggestion was that they add Phyllis Gleason to the group. "Phyllis knows how to do celebrations," he said confidently.

It was Phyllis who was the first to suggest that some students from Pico's past be included in the ceremony that the group was planning for opening day in the fall. "You know," she said, "we've had so many students that we might have written off who have gone on to do fabulous things. Take Carla Correa, for example. She's the anchorwoman on Channel 5. Or, how about Benny Bernstein? Who'd have thought he'd become a successful neurosurgeon?"

"You must be putting us on," said Phil Leckney. "Not Benny! Anyone but Benny! He was the shyest, most off-the-wall nerd who ever graced Pico's hallways. We all thought he'd end up part of life's invisible woodwork. Benny does brain surgery?"

"Yes, Benny does—and very well," responded Phyllis. "Try another one. I'll bet none of you know which graduate of Pico is now teaching at Harvard University."

Several tried to guess, but no one hit the mark. "Charley Packer," said Phyllis finally.

That seemed even harder to believe than the idea of Benny Bernstein doing brain surgery. Everyone seemed so stunned that they could only roll their eyes in disbelief. Phil's almost inaudible whisper broke the silence. "Well, I'll be. I thought he'd be in the state pen, and instead he cracked the Ivy League. But suppose," he continued in a stronger voice, "those folks don't want to come back to Pico?"

"Nonsense," said Phyllis. "You'd be surprised!"

When September rolled around, the planning group was feeling nervous. They had invested an entire summer designing an opening day unlike anything in recent memory. Would it work? Would it flop? Would their colleagues think that they were crazy? Only Phyllis never seemed to lose her serene confidence.

Joan Hilliard heard some of the usual cynical murmurs as Pico's teachers assembled in the front corridor waiting for the opening day's activities to begin. What she overheard was not comforting. Few teachers sounded excited to be back, nor excited about what lay ahead. But when the doors to Pico's auditorium were opened and the teachers entered to take their places, the mood changed quickly. There were balloons everywhere, each carrying the name of a Pico student. Crystal apples were on display at the front of the auditorium, each inscribed with the name of a Pico teacher. The auditorium walls were plastered with words and phrases that described the profession of teaching at its best. Huge placards carried terms like *coach, mentor, guide, guru,* and *leader.* There were pictures of previous students everywhere. The room was suddenly abuzz. Even the dyed-in-the-wool naysayers seemed overwhelmed by the banner across center stage. It said simply, "I'm just a great teacher!"

The room was still astir as people took their seats. In prior years, teachers had often settled into a deadening funk in the face of a drone of announcements about procedures and policies. This time, a different spirit was in the air. But what was it, and what was to come next?

As the room quieted down, Jaime Rodriguez walked on stage. "Normally," he said, "I would give a speech, hopefully better than last year's effort. But this year, something really different is in store. And now, let the show begin."

A group of strange faces walked on stage. Wilma Worthingham, a beloved teacher who had retired a few years earlier from Pico, was followed by a group of almost-familiar faces. As Wilma began to introduce each of the strangers, cries of recognition echoed across the room. "My God! Don't tell me that's Bernie," someone said. It turned out that the strange faces had names that were very familiar—at least to their former teachers. Each of the Pico alumni said a few words thanking the teachers for everything that they had done, but it was Sid Holstrom that brought the crowd to its feet. "I was probably one of your worst, almost as bad as Charley Packer," he said. "And look at where I am now. And look at all the others here who wouldn't be where they are if you had not helped them when they were here. When you look at us, you see reflections of yourselves. We are your legacy. And we are only the tip of the iceberg. There are thousands more like us who owe you a debt of gratitude."

The ovation that followed seemed to last forever. It was not for anyone in particular, it was for everyone. As the din subsided, Phil Leckney came on. His opening words startled almost everyone present, especially those who knew him as Pico's resident cynic. "I am a phoenix. I have arisen from the ashes of a burned-out teacher. This year the magic is there for me. If it can be there for me, it can be there for anyone here."

Many in the audience were stunned. Someone murmured, "What happened to Phil?" One of Leckney's longtime friends wondered aloud what he had been drinking that morning. Seeming to anticipate the surprise and skepticism, Leckney continued, "There may be some in the room who wonder if I've gone crazy. I have not. But I'm once again crazy about teaching. I have three years left before I retire. I want to make them the best three years I ever had. I invite all of you to join me."

As Leckney left the stage to sustained applause, a young woman entered the stage. Few in the audience knew who she was. With her short, neatly coifed brown hair and tasteful, light blue summer suit, she looked as if she might be on her way to a job interview. She seemed too old to be a Pico student, yet too young to be a teacher. The newcomer walked slowly and hesitantly, almost as if she wished that she were somewhere else. But once at the microphone, she spoke in a steady voice. "My name is Rosemary Pulcini. This is my first year teaching, and I'm proud to start my career at Pico. When I interviewed for this job, someone asked me who I admired most. At that time, I wasn't really sure. But I've had the chance to talk to some of you in the past few weeks and to hear many stories about Pico's students and particularly its faculty. I want to tell you that my heroes and heroines are all right in this room. I'm looking forward to teaching here for a long time."

The third standing ovation tripled anything ever before seen on opening day at Pico. The meeting then adjourned to the cafeteria, normally a utilitarian spot with an ambiance of aluminum and Formica and a pervasive aroma of nondescript leftovers. Some teachers wondered if they had made the wrong turn when they found the cafeteria tables decorated with lace tablecloths and crystal candleholders. At every teacher's place was a name card and a large red apple. The event was hosted with gusto by an enthusiastic group of Pico parents. Luncheon was an international buffet featuring dishes from each of the ethnic groups represented at Pico. No detail was overlooked. Margaret Juhl heard one veteran say, "This lunch is better than anything I've ever imagined, even at 10 times the cost."

After the lunch, Margaret Juhl came to the microphone and said, "I came here 22 years ago because of the spirit I saw here. Over the years, that spirit has seen its highs and lows. But I think deep down it's always been here. This year, the Pico spirit is back stronger than ever. I would now like to introduce Pico's principal, Jaime Rodriguez. We are permitting him to say a few words because, frankly, we thought he deserved another chance after last year's opening-day performance."

Laughter filled the room, and Rodriguez was smiling broadly as he came to the lectern. All had been forgiven on both sides.

"What I have to say is very simple," Jaime began. "No school is much better or much worse than its faculty, and that's why I'm so proud of you and of this school. We have a great faculty here—some like Rosemary Pulcini who are just starting, others like Phil Leckney or Margaret Juhl who have served Pico for a quarter century. It's what you all do in the classroom that produces the results that we were all so proud of this morning when some of our graduates came back to say thank you. Pico has a history that we can all celebrate with pride. There have been ups and downs in recent times at Pico, and I spent much of last year just getting to know this place and its people. What I've learned convinces me that there are no limits to our future.

"As principal, my job is not to lead the charge, but to support and serve you so that you can use your talent and energy to provide the best possible educational experience for our students. Together we can bring new meaning to our watchword, Pico Pride. I want to introduce someone who can say this much better than I, because she is one of you."

Joan Hilliard walked to the microphone. Those who were close could tell she was nervous. Her voice was soft as she began. "When I came here a year ago, I thought my four years in the business world would serve me well—and they did. But there were still times this past year when I wondered whether I could, or should, stick it out. Without a lot of help and support from many of my friends in this room, I would never have made it. But I did, and there's one thing I'm sure of now—I'm just a great teacher, and so are all of you!"

With that, she brought into full view a small bronze oil lamp. With a flourish, she lit the wick of the lamp. "Now, it's time to light the lamp of learning to illuminate our spirit for another year."

From the wings, the student chorus marched confidently on stage. The school song had never sounded better. The cafeteria had never seen so many tears of joy.

Leadership Lessons

Celebrate Values and Culture

Pico's "fiesta" to honor current and past principals brought home the importance of celebration in helping people build spirit and keep the faith. Its success inspired the "I'm Just a Great Teacher" celebration, which became a transforming event in Pico's culture. Celebration and ceremony are antidotes to boredom, cynicism, and burnout. They bring members of a group together, strengthen bonds, and build spirit and faith. The following guideposts can help you apply those lessons to your own school.

Learn and celebrate the history. Cultures are created over time as people face challenges, solve problems, and try to make sense out of their experience. The present is always sculpted by powerful echoes from the past. Frequent glances in a school's rearview mirror are as necessary as having a vision of the future. Every school's history includes a mix of ups and downs, triumphs and tragedies. The triumphs deserve celebration. The tragedies, laced with ample doses of humor, can be turned into stories that are as instructive as they are entertaining.

Diagnose the strength of the existing culture. Some schools have very strong cultures: Beliefs, values, and practices are clear and widely shared; people are proud of the school and its traditions. Others have weak cultures: There is little agreement about or pride in the school's identity. In schools with strong cultures, as soon as you walk through the front door you're likely to see banners, slogans, photos, trophies, and displays of student work. The message is "We're proud of who we are and we want to share it with you." In schools with weak cultures, the only sign you see may be one instructing visitors to report immediately to the principal's office. Weak cultures often call out for change; they are an invitation to strong leadership. Strong cultures are the reverse: They resist change and reject newcomers who are seen as enemies of tradition. The good news is that strong cultures are usually built on a history of success and progress. But unfortunately, the educational landscape is littered with too many toxic schools that have developed an entrenched culture of blaming, defeatism, and circle the wagons. If you sign on with one of those, you'll need patience, persistence, and a lot of support from somewhere to have much hope of making a positive difference.

Reinforce and celebrate the culture's strengths. Even in schools with weak or threadbare cultures, it is usually possible to find something worth celebrating. Some alumni have gone on to lead successful lives. There have been some star athletes, merit scholars, performing artists, or just some individuals whose never-say-die persistence against the odds is worth celebrating. Those stories, values, traditions, heroes, or heroines provide a vital starting point for updating, reinvigorating, and reframing the school's identity and culture.

Mark transitions with ceremony. Beginnings and endings, like triumphs and tragedies, require some form of symbolic recognition. The beginning of school, the end of a school year, the attainment of tenure, or the death of a student all cry out for cultural events. The military learned long ago that a change of command has to be marked with pomp and circumstance. Otherwise, the unit suffers, and the new person in charge has a hard time. In most schools, principals come and go without any special event. This leads to cultural sterility. The ups and downs, comings and goings of life in schools need cultural attention and support.

PART VI

Values, Ethics, and Spirit

CHAPTER ELEVEN

Teaching and Leading

Finding a Balance

The spirit of Pico's opening day extravaganza endured well into fall. Teachers said this was the best start they remembered. The school felt alive and energized. People *wanted* to spend time there. Teachers who had never gone beyond their contractual obligation were arriving early to chat with colleagues and prepare for the day. Many parents commented that their children were enjoying school more than ever before. Residents who passed by on their way home from work on fall evenings were often impressed to notice so many lights still on and cars still in the parking lot.

The planning team for the opening celebration had grown in numbers with the addition of new volunteers and continued to meet regularly under its new name, The Pico Pride Pack. Everyone agreed that the approaching holiday season was the perfect time for another event—an ecumenical holiday party for the Pico community. Careful planning and a lot of sweat brought their idea to fruition. Phil Leckney, buoyed by his best fall in years, was a jovial and spirited master of ceremonies. Jaime Rodriguez donated what many thought must be the world's largest piñata. Margaret Juhl brought her still lovely voice to a medley of Hanukkah songs. Heidi Hernandez wowed everyone with her ballet solo from the *Nutcracker*. The students went wild when Roscoe, dressed as Santa Claus and accompanied by his elf, Armando, missed the piñata

12 times in a row. His final effort spread candy and small gifts across the entire cafeteria. Never had the first semester ended on such a high note.

Two weeks later, on a Saturday evening between Christmas and New Year's, Margaret Juhl received a tearful middle-of-the-night telephone call from Joan. "Margaret, the bottom just dropped out. Larry and I just had our biggest fight ever. It was the same thing he's been harping on for the last year. He said he was sick of playing second fiddle to my students. He gave me an ultimatum: either I cut back on my work, or he's cutting out. I got furious, but I tried to stay calm. I just said, 'I don't tell you how to do your job. What gives you the right to tell me how to do mine?' He yelled back at me, 'That's it! I've had it!' He walked out and slammed the door behind him. I was devastated. I thought we were starting to get past all this and that he understood how important teaching is to me, just as his work is important to him. It's as if in his mind, work is important if it's all about numbers and bottom lines, but not if it's about children! I don't know, maybe I'll never understand men. Maybe we'd be better off without them. But I've been crying since he left."

The conversation continued for more than an hour. Margaret mostly listened and tried to give Joan as much support as she could. Just before saying good-bye, they agreed to have lunch the next day.

When they met, Joan looked tired; her eyes were red and puffy. She acknowledged that she had sobbed much of the night, but she seemed more composed than she had the previous night. As the two sat together over pasta at La Trattoria, the conversation gradually moved from Joan's breakup to a bigger issue.

It was Margaret who signaled the transition. "You know, Joan, as we were talking last night, some real painful stuff came up for me. The early days at Pico felt a lot like they do today. We all did things together, we enjoyed each other, and we did great things for kids. But it also took a big chunk out of our personal lives. You probably wonder why I've stayed single for so long. Partly it's because someone special walked out of my life, too, for pretty much the same reasons Larry did. I still wish I'd found a better way to balance teaching and the rest of my life. It's great for everyone to say teachers should take a more active leadership role, but not if it keeps them from having a life outside of school."

Joan was frowning. "Margaret, you sound just like Larry. Why do women have to do all the compromising and balancing, while men just go on doing their thing? If you're a man, you can be committed to your work *and* have a family. Women can do one or the other, but not both. Men get to work as much as they want, and we get the mommy track!"

"When you put it that way, it doesn't seem fair, does it?"

"It sure doesn't."

"Have you said all this to Larry?"

"I've tried, but whenever we try to talk about it, it pushes too many buttons for both of us. We just get angry and fight. We never seem to get past that to have a real conversation."

"I wish I had the answers," replied Margaret. "It seems to me there's more than one problem here. One involves relationships between men and women. It's about sex roles and about what men and women need from each other. It's also about power and about what it means to be male or female. There's a second issue of overload—we all feel rushed and too busy these days. That can affect any teacher, male or female. Right now, we're stuck—we don't know how to move on either issue."

"Maybe that's just how things are." Joan looked and sounded discouraged.

"Do you really believe that?" asked Margaret skeptically.

The question seemed to mobilize Joan's more optimistic side. "No, not really. I'm just down after last night. In fact, an idea just came to me. What if we talk about this stuff at the next Pico Pride meeting?"

"That's a terrific idea. Because maybe what we're talking about here is not problems, but dilemmas."

"What's the difference?" asked Joan.

"Problems have solutions. Dilemmas don't exactly *have* solutions, because you're caught between different values—like between commitment to teaching and commitment to family. It's not a tension that ever really goes away. You just have to look for better ways to manage it. That's why it makes sense to talk about this with the Pico Pride bunch. Right now we're all dealing with symptoms. We need to get a better handle on what's going on and what we can do about it. I don't know of any better way to do that than to talk with some colleagues who have the same concerns."

At the next Pico Pride meeting, Margaret and Joan presented the issues they had discussed. The nodding heads confirmed that others shared their concerns. On the surface, everything was going extremely well at the school, but something more troubling was bubbling underneath.

Phil Leckney led off the discussion. "I'll tell you one thing. You don't have to be female to worry about all this. I'm feeling caught in the middle myself. On the one hand, I've never felt better about my teaching. My classroom is running better than it has in years. The kids are learning, and I look forward to coming to school every day. But on the other hand, I miss all the spare time that I used to have. When I came to school at 7:30 and left at 2:30, I had time to do other things. I could work on my boat, spend time in the yard, and make a few bucks as a referee. I haven't been near my boat all year. The yard's a mess so it's a good thing it's covered with snow. My wife nags me about needing the extra money."

"Wait a minute, Phil. I understand what you're saying," responded Rosemary Pulcini, "but I'm not sure you really got Joan's message—because you've got a wife. You have someone who takes care of the home front while you focus on your career. Joan and I don't. I know what she's trying to say. For me, being a first-year teacher is simply *overwhelming*! There's never enough time to do it all. Lesson plans, correcting student work, talking to parents, going to meetings—it never ends. And I'm not sure how long it's going to take before my husband tells me he's fed up. Your wife doesn't work, does she, Phil?"

"Not now, but she used to before the kids." Phil paused and smiled as if to say that Rosemary's message hit home. Then he looked directly at Joan. "Maybe I'll always be a fossil in your eyes, Joan. You're right, my marriage is pretty traditional. But I wouldn't give up on Larry yet. Thinking back, I remember a time when I thought you were always on the attack, and I felt my best bet was to dive for cover. But all that changed when we started to listen to one another. If this old dinosaur can learn from you, I'll bet he can, too."

Joan rose from her chair, walked over to Phil, planted a kiss on his forehead, and calmly returned to her seat. Phil turned beet red. Everyone in the room was silent for a few moments before a wave of laughter spread over the group.

"You know," said Phyllis Gleason, "this conversation is a blessing. I've been worried for the last couple of months. I hear things. In one way or another, you all share what Margaret and Joan are talking about. What's happening now is a lot like what happened in Pico's heyday. That was more than 20 years ago. It almost broke my heart. We had drinking, divorces. This is a *déjà vu* that I never want to go through again. It's not just you teachers. I was talking to

Jaime's wife last week. She was telling me she's worried because she never sees him anymore."

"That's a good point," agreed Carlos. "We're not the only ones who worry. As we get deeper into this stuff, it's important to include Jaime as well as other teachers and staff. What do you think? Should we invite Jaime to our next meeting?"

The group quickly accepted Carlos's suggestion. At the next meeting, Rodriguez agreed that the issues deserved attention but seemed as perplexed as everyone else. "It's a dilemma. I've never been more proud of our school and what we're doing for our students. But the whole thing could crash if everyone burns out."

"If we all have the same concerns," said Carlos, "why not plan a retreat to see if we can get to the bottom of it?"

"I think it's a great idea," said Jaime. "I'll talk to the superintendent about some funds."

Joan responded angrily, "Now, wait a minute. Here we go again! If we do it over a weekend, it's another big chunk out of our personal lives."

"You're right, Joan," said Margaret. "It's a real catch-22. But I think we're going to have to spend some time in order to get more. Another possibility would be to ask the district to cover a day's worth of substitutes. That way, we could spend an evening on Thursday, a whole day on Friday, and a half-day on Saturday. Is that a compromise that people would buy? I think the union could go along with that, as long as it's voluntary for teachers."

"Well, Jaime, it's up to you. You have to sell it to Dr. Hofsteder. Would she buy it?" asked Joan.

"I think so, if the faculty is really behind it," Jaime replied.

As it turned out, getting faculty support was relatively easy. Many shared the same concerns and worried about how long the school could continue at the same pace. The superintendent threw her full weight behind the idea. She and the school board were so pleased with what was happening at Pico that they did not want to see their lighthouse project run out of steam.

An expanded Pico Pride Pack planned the retreat and developed a theme—"Thriving and Surviving." As they wrestled with how to organize the event, Margaret Juhl offered an idea. "A few years back," she said, "I took a course on school leadership."

"You wanted to be a principal, Margaret?" asked Phil Leckney skeptically.

"No. I just wanted learn more about how they think. And I remember this one framework that's really been very helpful for me. It talks about four main issues that every organization, schools included, needs to address. The first is to create a structure that works. The second is to respond to people's needs and provide the skills that they need. The third is to manage conflict effectively, and the last is to develop a shared sense of meaning and commitment. I think each of these may be important to the issues of balance and burnout that we're trying to get at. What if we had groups working on each of them?"

"Margaret," said Joan. "This all sounds *awfully* familiar. Haven't I heard this before somewhere?"

Margaret smiled. "You sure have. Many times. They're ideas that worked for me. I hoped they would for you, too."

"Well, I think they've been seeping in, even if I didn't always realize it," replied Joan.

"I don't know whether this conversation is a commercial or not, but it sounds like it's worth a try," Carlos commented.

Using Margaret's suggestion, the planning group broke the faculty and staff into groups, each charged with exploring one of four issues: (1) How can we use our time more efficiently? (2) How can we deal with conflict more productively? (3) What in-service training would help? Or is needed? (4) How can we balance schoolwide cohesion and commitment with family and other outside obligations?

Despite some tense moments, the retreat was a huge success. A range of issues and feelings came to the surface, but they were almost always framed in a way that allowed the group to get below what people were thinking and feeling to the real reasons and move forward. The group produced a number of new initiatives. It also identified areas where more information was needed. The efficiency team identified several structural avenues to make better use of time. One was to use team teaching to reduce duplication of effort. Another involved reducing the number of meetings that teachers attended. The overall impact was to free up time for individual teachers to do preparation and grading at school rather than taking it home.

The conflict group and the in-service groups collaborated to develop workshops on both alternative strategies for managing conflict and on techniques for time management. The cultural cohesion group concluded that the school needed to sponsor schoolwide events that included spouses, partners, and families to reduce the separation between work and personal life. The group also remembered what the original Pico Pride Pack had demonstrated about the importance of symbolic beginnings and endings. They ensured that the retreat ended on a high note with a series of skits that left everyone rolling in the aisles.

CHAPTER TWELVE

A Talk About Values

His Wednesday breakfast meeting with Brenda Connors was the most sacred item on Jaime Rodriguez's calendar. As their relationship deepened, both had come to value their own two-person support group that served as vital nourishment for mind and spirit. Over time, they delved ever more deeply into issues that principals often recognized but rarely voiced.

On a particular Wednesday in February, only a few weeks after the weekend retreat, Rodriguez wanted to talk about values. He had grown up in a family that put a strong emphasis on doing the right thing. His parents always had clear answers to every question of right and wrong. Now that he was a school principal, things often seemed fuzzier. "Somewhere I heard that the difference between management and leadership is that managers do things right and leaders do the right thing," he mused. "That sounds good, but how do you *know* what the right thing is?"

"Doesn't it come down to what you believe in and what your values are?"

"Sure, but that's what I'm trying to sort out," replied Rodriguez. "It's easy to say that I'm committed to education for all children. I really believe that. But I've been thinking about some of the tough situations I was up against last year. What made them so hard was trying to sort out conflicting values."

Brenda smiled. "You figured that out a lot quicker than I did when I was a young principal. Value conflicts are the real struggles. That's when it's real hard to tell the difference between a ball and a strike. It's like shifting from being an umpire to being a philosopher."

"I've been thinking about an article I read that talked about four important values in education," said Jaime. "Excellence, caring, justice, and faith. I like all of them, but they're often in conflict.

"The first value, excellence, is one that we always hear about. Our job is to help kids achieve as much as possible. In terms of that, the role of the leader is like an engineer or an architect—diagnosing how things are working and figuring out how to do it better."

"I'm all for excellence, but how can you champion mediocrity?" Brenda replied. "But I worry when that's the only thing people focus on. A school is not a factory. We're dealing with people, not widgets."

"That's why the second value is caring. It's the whole idea of schools as families, that people have an obligation to care about one another and to look out for each other's welfare. At its deepest, it's the whole issue of love," said Jaime.

"I like that," Brenda said. "It fits with the idea of the leader as servant—that my job is to understand people's needs and concerns, and to serve them as well as possible by building a caring community."

"But then sometimes you run into a conflict between caring and excellence. Maybe that's what I was wrestling with in dealing with Sam Shepherd. I didn't like what he did with kids, but I still wanted to treat him with respect. If I'd hurt him, it would have set a bad example for everyone else. I was caught between caring and excellence, and I had to find some way to balance them," said Rodriguez.

"That's exactly what you did," Brenda responded. "But where does justice fit in?"

"Well, as I understand the article, the basic idea of justice is fairness. It's like the statue of the blindfolded goddess with the scales. People have a right to fair and equal treatment. In dealing with Shepherd, it was important to be fair to him and to the students."

"That makes sense. Maybe the newsletter is another example. You felt that people didn't care about you, and they felt that you didn't care about them. Maybe the deeper issue was justice: They felt you weren't being fair. Like when Leckney said you were favoring the Chicano teachers."

"These things are really complicated," said Jaime. "Everything is layered on top of something else, and a lot of times different layers are pitted against each other."

"Was that true for the discipline issue, too?"

"Probably. On the one hand, we were trying to do what's best for children, so it was an issue of excellence. But we were also trying to balance the interests of teachers, parents, kids, and others. It wasn't going to work unless people felt that the process and the product were fair."

"But I think there's even another layer. Maybe this is where that fourth value comes in. You could say that the whole process was a ceremony in search of a cultural anchor for your school community. You wanted something that everyone could believe in. The search for justice was also a search for faith."

"In a way, that's what my whole first year was about. That's what I think I was trying to do with my vision speech last fall. Teachers need to believe they make a difference. We both know a lot of teachers who burned out somewhere along the line. Education is so tough, and the rewards are so intangible. It's a challenge to keep the faith, particularly when so many people are bashing schools and teachers."

"Jaime, that's the most important thing a principal does. Keep the faith, so everyone else doesn't lose theirs."

"Sounds right, but I sure had some moments of doubt this past year."

"We all do. Every year. But the longer I've been a principal, the more I'm convinced that a principal has to be a spiritual leader. We have to help people recapture the meaning of their work, and we have to talk about the things that touch their hearts. Remember the Fiesta de Pico? When the Pico faculty anointed you as their new principal, I got goose bumps. When you're dealing with a generation of children in a school, every day should give people goose bumps."

CHAPTER THIRTEEN

The Essence of Teaching

Leaving a Legacy

No one expected it. Margaret Juhl was close to retirement, but everyone assumed that she would go on forever. The news that she had cancer knocked the wind out of everyone in the Pico community. Each day, people waited for an update on her condition. Had the surgery been successful? Was the chemotherapy working? When would she be back to work? What if she never returned?

Phyllis Gleason became a human hot line for news about Margaret's progress. Bill Hill served as the primary link to parents and the community. Grapevines sometimes distort the news in the direction of worst-case scenarios, but Pico's gossip network was remarkably accurate and positive. Everyone hoped that positive thinking would help Margaret's recovery and speed her return to the school she loved so much.

On a warm and sunny spring morning in late April, Joan Hilliard, Carlos Cortez, and Phil Leckney were the first to visit Margaret at St. Joseph's Hospital. Phyllis Gleason had declined an invitation to come along. "The best medicine for someone who loves teaching as much as Margaret is a visit from a few of her closest buddies. I know Mr. Rodriguez feels the same way. He and I will be over at St. Joseph's another time. Just be sure to call me as soon as you finish your visit."

As the three teachers walked down the shiny floor of a hallway that felt sterile and smelled of antiseptic, they wondered how Margaret would look and what her condition would be. As they entered Room

203, they were pleasantly surprised. Margaret was propped up in bed with a book, her wire-rimmed, half-circle reading glasses sitting crooked on her nose. The color in her face looked normal, although they suspected that makeup made it so. But the twinkle in her eye and the smile on her face were genuine—the good old Margaret look that they would recognize anywhere.

"Joan! Carlos! Phil! So good of you to come. I told the doctors if they didn't let me have some visitors, I was going to walk out of here against medical advice. Come on in! Sit down! Tell me the latest scoop. How's my class? Who's subbing for me? Are the kids behaving? Has Jaime been called in a rescue mission yet?"

Margaret's visitors wondered if they had wandered into an interrogation chamber rather than a friend's hospital room. As the hail of questions continued, they looked in vain for somewhere to sit. With the overflow of flowers, plants, balloons, and gifts, there were no empty spots. They were hard pressed even to find a place for the philodendron that they had brought as a gift from the faculty. Carlos started to move a huge bouquet of multicolored spring flowers from the chair by Margaret's bed in the hopes of clearing a place to sit.

"No, Carlos, don't move that one. That's from my kids. Every one of them signed the card, can you believe it? Where did they ever get the money to pay for something that gorgeous? Come on, two of you can sit on the foot of the bed. Phil, lean against the sink. I want to be able to see you while you bring me up to date. So what's new at Pico? I'm dying to know."

Everyone winced at Margaret's choice of expressions, but Carlos started the briefing, only to be interrupted by Joan with a story about Phil's failed attempt to play a classic "trick-the-rookie" prank on Rosemary Pulcini. Pulcini had caught on so quickly that the prank backfired and Phil himself became the butt of the joke. Phil blushed while everyone else in the room laughed uproariously. Margaret laughed so hard that tears rolled down her cheeks, streaking her rose-colored makeup. For the next half-hour, her visitors talked nonstop, sometimes with all three talking at once.

Margaret took it all in as if she were reconnecting to a vital source of energy from which she had been shut off for too long. As Phil was filling Margaret in on some of the latest community gossip via Bill Hill, Joan saw a hint of pain cross Margaret's face. She gently nudged her colleagues. "We could go on for hours and that might be just what Margaret wants, but I know the doctors will have our heads if we overstay our welcome." Margaret seemed both disappointed and relieved when her guests agreed that it really was time for them to go.

"Before you go, I want you to take all these envelopes with you. One is for my substitute, to give her some details of where to find things and some sage warnings about the students who are most notorious for driving off subs. The other envelope is for my students. I want Horace to read the first part to the class and then give it to Sally for the finale. Horace will be great in getting the funny stuff across, but he'd flub the last part. There's also a note for Phyllis and for Bill, so that they can help get the word around. And this one is for Jaime. He sent me a note a couple of weeks ago asking about some personnel decisions. Tell him I'm sorry I wasn't able to get back to him sooner. I know these things have been bothering him."

As Joan was wondering to herself whether there was any message that Margaret wanted to send to her colleagues, Margaret picked up the book that she had put down as they came in. "The last thing I want you to do is go by Barry's bookstore and pick up some copies of this book, *The Courage to Teach*, by Parker Palmer. I know some people have already read it, but all of us should. It's a challenging book, but if you stay with it, it really gets to heart of what it means to be a teacher. I find that every chapter really gets me thinking about myself and my teaching and reminds me how much I really want to get back to my classroom. It would make me feel good to know that others are reading it too. In fact, the assignment for all of you is to read it before the next time you visit."

Joan, Carlos, and Phil all promised to do their homework. Each gave Margaret a hug and left carrying the envelopes that Margaret had entrusted to them.

"She looks great," observed Phil as they walked down the hall.

"She does," Joan replied, "but even though she seemed like her old self when we got there, she wore out fast. Did you notice the pain in her face just before we left? I'm not sure she's as good as she looks. I just hope she's going to make it."

"Don't even say that, Joan," replied Carlos. "She will. She's got to."

"Why do you think she wants us to read that book?" asked Phil.

"I guess we'll find out when we read it," Joan replied. "Let's stop by Barry's on the way home. It's only about four blocks from where I live. We can get the books before you drop me off. That way we can take them to school tomorrow."

When Margaret's three visitors arrived at Pico the next morning, they were in such demand that they felt almost like visiting rock stars in the presence of admiring fans. But the fans were not looking for autographs. They wanted to know how things were going with Margaret. Joan distributed the envelopes as Margaret had requested. Phyllis and Bill greeted theirs with such enthusiasm that Joan knew they could not wait to begin making their rounds to spread the news.

Two weeks later, Joan was sitting in her apartment on a rainy May evening when the phone rang. When she answered, it was Margaret at the other end.

"Margaret, how are you? You know, you're still the only thing we talk about at Pico anymore. Everyone keeps asking why we were all supposed to read the book."

"Well, that's part of why I'm calling. Joan, I'd really like to talk to you. I know how busy you are these days, but could you find time for another hospital visit in the next few days?"

"Is tomorrow afternoon too soon? Four o'clock?"

"That would be perfect. Just you, O.K.?" said Margaret.

Joan went to bed still pondering the meaning of Margaret's phone call. Nothing was said directly, but they had known each other so long that they often needed no words to understand what the other was thinking. Joan hated even to think it, yet she was almost sure that Margaret's call had not been prompted by good news.

When Joan arrived at Margaret's hospital room the next day, she was again greeted by the same cheerful Margaret, this time perched in the chair next to her hospital bed. Cards and writing materials were spread in a series of neat piles across her bed. "Joan, thanks for coming. I'm still writing thank-you notes. It's just amazing all the cards I've received. I was just reading one from a girl I taught more than 20 years ago, and I hadn't heard from her since. Let me clear some of this stuff away so you have someplace to sit."

"How about if I just move the stuff on this chair over to the window ledge?" At Margaret's nod, Joan sat down. "You're looking better every time I see you," said Joan, trying to sound as cheerful and convincing as she could.

"Well, the truth is I look a little more tired every time you see me. At least that's how I feel. Look, we've never tried to kid each other. The news from my doctor isn't as good as I'd hoped. I probably won't make it back to school this spring. This might have been my last year teaching." Margaret's voice was soft and there were tears forming on her cheeks, though hardly visible through Joan's own tears.

Fighting the impulse to break down and sob, Joan came over and hugged Margaret awkwardly. "Please go sit down!" said Margaret. "There are some things I need to say."

Joan returned to her seat, fumbled through her purse for tissues, and struggled to compose herself.

"I've had a lot of time to think while I've been here—about my life, and even more about my career and how teaching has touched every corner of my life in some way. I've been asking myself whether I would do anything differently if I had it all to do over. You tried another career before becoming a teacher. I never even considered other options. And there are a few times when I did something pretty silly or said something that hurt someone else. On these things I wish I had a second chance. But the thing I feel surer about than anything else is that I made the right choice when I decided to be a teacher. I've started to think about what I'm giving back to a profession that's done so much for me."

Joan knew she should not interrupt, but the import of Margaret's talk about her legacy was too upsetting. Did it mean that she was giving up? Joan blurted out, "Let's talk about the future, not the past."

Margaret smiled and responded calmly, "The future is exactly what I'm talking about. That's why I wanted to speak to you alone. You're very special to me, Joan. Have you read the book I assigned?"

"Every word. It was wonderful."

"I knew you'd like it. As I was reading it, it got me thinking again about the spiritual side of what we do. In earlier times, schooling was basically religious instruction. Somewhere along the line, we got confused and started to think of schools as factories instead of temples. As teachers, we have to hold on to the essence of what we're about. Otherwise, we stand to lose everything. Tracy Kidder has a beautiful way of talking about it in his book, *Among Schoolchildren.* Wait a second, I have his book here somewhere. O.K., here it is. 'Good teachers put snags in the river of children passing by, and over time, they redirect hundreds of lives . . . There is an innocence that conspires to hold humanity together, and it is made up of people who can never fully know the good they have done'" (Kidder, 1989, p. 313).

"I love it! Isn't that what we were trying to get at with our celebration of teaching last year?"

"Yes, that was a great beginning, probably one of the best things we ever did at Pico," said Margaret. "But there's a deeper level of what we're about that we didn't quite get to. It's a level we're almost embarrassed to talk about—the spiritual dimension that makes teaching a calling. It's about values: the values we live by and the values we pass on to our students."

"Isn't caring the core value in teaching?" asked Joan.

"It's critical, but there are other important values that we often overlook. Take Roscoe, for example. You certainly cared about him, but it took more than caring. Being loved was not all that Roscoe needed. He also needed to master some basic skills and learn to set higher standards for himself."

"That makes a lot of sense. One of the toughest challenges I had with Roscoe was deciding when to tell him how much I liked him and when to really push him to do better work and set higher standards for himself. So there are really two values in teaching?"

"We're only halfway there. In deciding when to support or push Roscoe, you also had to consider fairness for everyone in the class. Roscoe's like a lot of children these days. When they look around them, they feel the world is unjust. You agree. In trying to make it fairer for them, you can create injustice for others—particularly the kids in the middle. You know how much your students insist on fairness. They want a just classroom."

"That's what happened to me when we finally got Roscoe straightened out. Some of the other parents complained that their children were getting shortchanged," replied Joan thoughtfully.

"Can you begin to see that when you try to take all these competing values into account, there's always going to be tension? A classroom has to be caring, it has to be just, and it has to value performance and results. But even deeper than that, it has to be a place of hope. It has to have meaning and to build faith."

"What do you mean by faith?" asked Joan.

"Faith is believing in things when everything tells you not to. It's believing in Roscoe even when his record tells you you're fooling yourself. It's convincing Roscoe to believe in himself even though almost no one else ever has. It's getting his parents to have faith in him and what school can mean for him. Even more important, teachers have to believe in themselves and in their work. That's where I think we've fallen down. Just pick up any magazine or newspaper. Listen to the conversations in restaurants. Thinking about how we teachers talk when we're together. The public has lost faith in us, and we've lost faith in ourselves."

"But what about the opening-day celebration or the holiday party? Weren't we on the right track?" asked Joan.

"Of course. They were both very important. So was the retreat, because it gave us a chance to talk about balancing conflicting values. For me, that's one of the things that makes Parker Palmer's book so poignant. He said some things I'll never forget, and I want to make sure that people remember them at Pico even if I'm not there. That's why I wanted you to distribute the books. And I want you to promise me that you'll have the same conversation with your colleagues that we're having now. It'll be even more powerful coming from you, because you've tasted life on the other side. You chose to be a teacher after trying a career in business. I don't know why I feel so strongly about this, but I do. I have my own faith, and it's really a comfort now. But I'm also drawing heavily on my faith in teaching. I want to make sure others carry on these values while they have more time than I do to do good things for kids. Do you promise?"

CHAPTER FOURTEEN

Passing the Torch

J oan's promise reverberated on the drive from the hospital to her apartment. When she arrived to an empty apartment, she had an impulse to call Larry, just to have someone to talk to. But she resisted, remembering how rarely Larry had understood her dedication to teaching. Instead, she picked up Tracy Kidder's book and started to read the final chapter again. As she drifted off, the last few sentences kept replaying in her mind. "She belonged among schoolchildren. They made her confront sorrow and injustice. They made her feel useful. Again this year, some had needed more help than she could provide. There were many problems that she hadn't solved. But it wasn't for the lack of trying. She hadn't given up. She had run out of time" (Kidder, 1989, p. 342).

It was still dark when the sound of her telephone woke Joan the next morning. Startled, she looked at her clock to see that it was only 5 A.M. She was almost afraid to answer. Her worst fears were confirmed when Jaime Rodriguez said, "Joan, she's gone."

"Margaret? Oh, God, no! What happened?"

"They aren't sure yet. The operation and the chemotherapy took a lot out of her, but even the doctors were surprised."

"I can't believe it," said Joan, crying softly as she spoke. "I saw her yesterday. She looked tired, but I never expected this."

"I'm planning to have a brief schoolwide assembly this morning. I think we should tell everyone at once. I'd like to say a few words and then have a couple of teachers talk about her. I'm hoping to get someone like Phil Leckney or Vivian Chu—someone at Pico who's known Margaret for a long time. Bill Hill will be great because so many of the kids know and trust him. I also wanted you to say something, because I know how close you and Margaret have become."

"I don't know, Jaime. I'm not sure I can do it. I might just stand up there and cry."

"I'm not sure I can do it either, but I figure as the principal, I have to give it my best. I'm pretty sure that if there's anyone Margaret would want up there, it's you. You're the last person who saw her alive."

"That's why this is so hard to believe." She was crying softly as she spoke. "But you're trying to do too much too soon. Have the assembly today, but make it brief. We need more time to plan the right way to remember Margaret."

After a moment's hesitation, Rodriguez agreed. He went to work to plan for a brief assembly. Joan began to think about how Pico could celebrate Margaret's life.

The news of her death had spread quickly. There was hardly a sound as students and staff filed into the auditorium later that morning. The mood was somber. Only a few muffled sobs punctuated the heavy silence. Rodriguez was calm and controlled as he made the brief announcement of Margaret Juhl's death. He informed them when the funeral would be, and when visitors could pay their last respects. He also announced that Pico would hold its own memorial assembly the day after the funeral. "And now," he said, his voice beginning to crack, "let's make the rest of the day just what Ms. Juhl would have wanted it to be—a day when everyone learns. That's the highest tribute we can pay to a teacher we all loved and admired."

Many staff and students sat in silence for a few moments before slowly moving to the aisles. The only noise was the shuffling of feet. The usual din of conversation gradually picked up as people moved back to their classrooms. At the end of the day, several teachers remarked that even though students were subdued, they seemed focused and eager to do their best.

On the day following the funeral service at Largren's Mortuary, Pico held its own celebration of Margaret's life. Jaime Rodriguez and members of the Pico Pride Pack had spent hours planning an event that would mirror Margaret's importance to the school. But without her steady hand and unflappable spirit, the planning process had little of the joy and humor always there in the past. Everyone felt her absence, but it spurred them on to work with more intensity and focus than ever before.

Pico's memorial service was comforting, moving, and uplifting for everyone. Before it started, Joan Hilliard felt almost like an emotional wreck. Yet as she began to speak, the words flowed. Steadily, smoothly, and straight from her heart. Only after sitting down did she see the visible signs of her impact. Staff and students were in tears all over the auditorium. It was then that Joan herself began to feel the full force of what she had said.

As the service drew to a close, Joan's mind wandered back to her first days at Pico and especially to the day that Margaret first came into her classroom, just after Roscoe and Armando had destroyed her day. She beamed through her sadness as she reviewed how far she and the school had come since then. She thought about Roscoe and how well he had been doing in Margaret's class before she died. Just as she began to wonder how well Roscoe would cope with Margaret's loss, she saw him enter the room with Heidi, Armando, and several other students pushing a wagon toward the podium. Perched unsteadily on the wagon was a large tree, its burlap-wrapped root ball hanging over the sides. As the entourage approached with its swaying cargo, Joan's eyes met Roscoe's, and she noticed the tears rolling down one of the largest grins she had ever seen on his face. It was different from the mischievous grin that she had seen so many times in the past. This was the earnest, self-satisfied look of someone who was confident he had done something really *right*.

The tree was not in the script, but a smiling nod from Phyllis to Rodriguez was the only signal he needed to welcome the group and invite them to the stage. To Joan's astonishment, it was Roscoe, not Heidi, who came to the microphone. His words came out in a confident tone. "Ms. Juhl is going to heaven, but we don't really want to give her up. So we students took up a collection and bought this tree. We want you all to come outside with us and watch as we plant it in front of the school and water it. That way, we can keep Ms. Juhl's spirit with us and remember what she done for us."

Heidi Hernandez followed Roscoe to the microphone and read a poem that she had written. It was about a teacher who planted seeds of learning every day. All the seeds began to grow into beautiful plants, each different from the other. Over the years, so many plants grew that no one could even count them, but everyone could

had become. Joan tried

tears, but gave up as she

approached by a man wear-

sociated with lawyers and

former student of Margaret

d, and she made a big differ-

u for the eulogy—it meant a

oo," Joan replied. There was

very comforting to her, and she

'I'm Steve Riley. I'm a lawyer in

the school board."

argaret told me about you. She was

have been proud of. I was a pretty

her class. Anyway, thanks again for

get together some time, and share

d he meant it when he promised to call.

***

"Where did the years go," Jaime Rodriguez asked himself, as he was about to begin his sixth year as Pico's principal. His mind had begun to wander as he sat in the first principals' meeting of the new school year, half listening to the associate superintendent's announcements of new district policies. His thoughts floated over Pico's past five years. Being recognized as a school of excellence had been an enormous satisfaction to everyone at the school. But he felt even more gratified at how far he, the staff, and the community had come. Just then, his thoughts were interrupted when the associate superintendent asked, "Why are you smiling? Is there something funny about this policy?"

"I guess I was admiring all the work you put into it," Jaime responded. The associate superintendent droned on, and Rodriguez returned to his memories. This time he thought about Brenda Connors and what an important force she had been in his career. She had retired and moved to Florida, and Rodriguez often thought about how much he missed her. If she had been there, he would have expected a note under the table complimenting him on his quick recovery. He thought about how much of her wisdom had been incorporated into his own philosophy. Just then, his eyes wandered down the table to Sandy Dole, the new principal at Hillview Elementary School, only a few miles from Pico. She definitely was not smiling. She seemed to be losing a difficult struggle to follow every word in the associate superintendent's presentation. More than anything, she looked plain scared. Was she feeling the same way he had five years ago?

At the end of the meeting, he made a special point of pulling her aside. He introduced himself and asked her, "How's it going?"

She paused, gulped, and stammered, "You want the truth?"

"Nothing but."

"Well," she hesitated, then plunged ahead. "I'm buried in paper. The school secretary quit two weeks before I started, and we still don't have a replacement. Classes start next week, and I'm short two teachers. I'm not sure I'll make it through the week."

Jaime felt a wave of nostalgia. Smiling warmly, he said, "That sounds pretty much on target for your first week. I felt the same way my first year at Pico. How about a cup of coffee?"

Two weeks later, Joan Hilliard found herself sitting with a new teacher, Francesca King, on the carved wooden bench by the oak tree in Pico's Margaret Juhl Patio. It was a beautiful September day, and Francesca had asked if they could meet somewhere away from her classroom. Joan automatically suggested the patio—whenever she went there, she felt Margaret's presence.

As Francesca started to talk, it was clear that she had wanted a setting well away from the chaos that had been her classroom that day. When Joan asked, "How's it going?" Francesca's words tumbled out in an almost frantic stream.

"It's going downhill fast. My class is out of control, and I don't know what to do about it. I'm afraid I'm in over my head. Maybe I should quit now before it gets any worse. I've always wanted to be a teacher, but I never thought it could be this tough. I'm working day and night, but I'm still losing my class, and my love life is going to hell. I feel like I'm drowning!"

Joan smiled as memories of her first encounter with Margaret flooded back. "This tree is beautiful, isn't it? It was planted here six years ago in honor of a wonderful teacher, Margaret Juhl. She was my best friend." Joan noticed the puzzled look on Francesca's face and went on. "You're probably wondering what that has to do with you. At about this point in my first year as a teacher, I was ready to quit, too."

"That's hard to believe," Francesca protested. "People say you're one of the best teachers here."

"That's where the tree comes in," said Joan with a smile. "I wouldn't have made it through the first term if Margaret Juhl hadn't taken me under her wing. Tell me about your day. If we put our heads together, we might be able to figure out some ways to make it a little easier."

Epilogue

Before her arrival at Pico School, much of what Joan Hilliard knew about teaching and Jaime Rodriguez knew about leading was based on course work, reading, and a few gleanings from earlier experience in teaching or in the business world. It was all helpful—anything was better than nothing. But it was only the beginning of their education. Working in the trenches day to day helped each of them gradually develop the know-how and wisdom that can only be gained from experience and practice. While their appreciation for books, and for new ideas and concepts, actually grew over time, they also came to understand that ideas were useful only when you know how to use them. This book tries to illustrate the process of converting knowing-about into know-how. In the dialogues between Juhl and Hilliard, Rodriguez and Connors, you witness a continuing process of reflection and dialogue about practice. Reflection is something that readers can and should do by themselves, but its value is enhanced immeasurably with help from others—friends, colleagues, and mentors.

A book is only a partial substitute for the kind of sustained, intense, and personal relationship that a young professional can develop with an experienced and wise senior colleague. But we hope that our effort can help you reap some of the same benefits by raising provocative questions, offering new perspectives, challenging your thinking, and encouraging your heart.

We hope that it will also encourage you to ensure that dialogue and mentoring are a rich and continuing part of your professional life. Both teachers and principals often feel isolated and trapped in their classrooms and offices. Though rarely alone, they are often lonely. They are starved for opportunities to talk freely and openly with other adults who can really understand what their life is like. Fellow teachers and administrators can become allies and guides for each other. Like Juhl and Hilliard, Brenda and Jaime, they can help one another create an inspiring and elegant conversation.

Annotated Bibliography

A. GENERAL

Bolman, L. G., & Deal, T. E. (1997). *Reframing organizations: Artistry, choice, and leadership* (2d ed.). San Francisco: Jossey-Bass.
This book presents a systematic overview of our ideas about leadership and organizations, with many illustrations and examples from schools, colleges, government, and the private sector.

Bolman, L., & Deal, T. E. (2001). *Leading with soul: An uncommon journey of spirit.* San Francisco: Jossey-Bass.
In *Leading with Soul*, we explore the spiritual underpinnings of leadership. We argue that effective leadership ultimately resides in soul and faith and that spirited leaders develop their own gifts so that they may share them with others.

Gardner, J. W. (1989). *On leadership.* New York: Free Press.
If you could read only one book on leadership, this would be a very good choice. Gardner packs a lot of wisdom and experience into a highly readable and valuable book.

Johnson, S. M. (1990). *Teachers at work.* New York: Basic Books.
Johnson's book provides a very insightful view of how schools function as workplaces for teachers. She documents many of the barriers and frustrations that teachers encounter in bureaucratic organizations and offers many helpful ideas about how to make schools better places for teaching and learning.

Kidder, T. *Among Schoolchildren.* (1989). New York: Houghton Mifflin.

Palmer, P. (1997). *The courage to teach: Exploring the inner landscape of a teacher's life.* San Francisco: Jossey-Bass.
This book was Margaret Juhl's gift to her colleagues because it expressed so well her belief that teaching has to come from the heart and be rooted in each teacher's identity.

B. POWER AND POLITICS

Kotter, J. P. (1985). *Power and influence: Beyond formal authority.* New York: Free Press.
This book is written for corporate managers, but school leaders will still find it very useful. It provides very clear and comprehensive discussions of power and politics in organizations. Kotter's discussion of the "power gap" in administrative jobs and his chapters on managing your boss are invaluable.

C. RESPONDING TO HUMAN NEEDS

Barth, R. (1990). *Improving schools from within.* San Francisco: Jossey-Bass.
This is Roland Barth at his best, offering a clear and compelling vision of how principals, teachers, parents, and children can work together to build learning communities.
Kouzes, J. M., & Posner, B. Z. (1988). *The leadership challenge: How to get extraordinary things done in organizations.* San Francisco: Jossey-Bass.
A stimulating and inspiring discussion of the practices of managers operating at their personal best.

D. UNDERSTANDING STRUCTURE IN SCHOOLS

Weiss, C., Cambone, J., & Wyeth, A. (1992, August). Trouble in paradise: Teacher conflicts in shared decision making. *Education Administration Quarterly, 28*(3), 350–367.
This provocative paper documents many of the promises and pitfalls of shared leadership and teacher empowerment. In a

national sample of high schools, Weiss found that there is a price to be paid for participative approaches to decision making, a price about which teachers are often ambivalent. The article suggests that even in progressive schools, teacher leadership is conspicuous mostly for its absence, but we think it also shows how important it is for teachers to become more active leaders.

E. SYMBOLS AND CULTURE IN SCHOOLS

Bolman, L. G., & Deal, T. E. (1992, Autumn). What makes a team work? Inside the soul of a new machine. *Organizational Dynamics*, 34–44.
This article uses a famous case of an unusually effective design team to illustrate the symbolic and cultural elements that are critical to peak performance in teams.

Deal, T. E., & Kennedy, A. (1982). *Corporate cultures.* Reading, MA: Addison-Wesley.
A groundbreaking best-seller that first popularized the idea of organizational culture. This is the original and still one of the better overviews of what culture is, how it works, and how it can be shaped.

Deal, T. E., & Peterson, K. (1990). *The principal's role in shaping school culture.* Washington, DC: U.S. Government Printing Office.
A down-to-earth, practical guide to analyzing and changing school culture.

F. ETHICS IN TEACHING AND LEADING

Bolman, L. G., & Deal, T. E. (1992). Images of leadership. *The American School Board Journal, 179*(4), 36–39.
This article spells out the four values that Joan and Margaret discuss in Chapter 7 and relates them to four different images of what a school is: family, factory, jungle, and cathedral.